Ethical, Legal, and Social Issues in Medical Informatics

Penny Duquenoy, Middlesex University, UK

Carlisle George, Middlesex University, UK

Kai Kimppa, University of Turku, Finland

WITHDRAWN

TOURO COLLEGE LIBRARY
Kings Highway

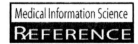

MEDICAL INFORMATION SCIENCE REFERENCE

Hershey · New York

Acquisition Editor:	Kristin Klinger
Development Editor:	Kristin Roth
Senior Managing Editor:	Jennifer Neidig
Managing Editor:	Jamie Snavely
Assistant Managing Editor:	Carole Coulson
Copy Editor:	Larissa Vinci
Typesetter:	Chris Hrobak
Cover Design:	Lisa Tosheff
Printed at:	Integrated Book Technology

Published in the United States of America by
    Medical Information Science Reference (an imprint of IGI Global)
    701 E. Chocolate Avenue
    Hershey PA 17033
    Tel: 717-533-8845
    Fax: 717-533-8661
    E-mail: cust@igi-global.com
    Web site: http://www.igi-global.com

and in the United Kingdom by
    Medical Information Science Reference (an imprint of IGI Global)
    3 Henrietta Street
    Covent Garden
    London WC2E 8LU
    Tel: 44 20 7240 0856
    Fax: 44 20 7379 3313
    Web site: http://www.eurospanbookstore.com

Library of Congress Cataloging-in-Publication Data

Ethical, legal, and social issues in medical informatics / Penny Duquenoy, Carlisle George, and Kai Kimppa, editors.
    p. ; cm.
  Includes bibliographical references.
  ISBN 978-1-59904-780-5 (hardcover)
  1. Medical informatics—Moral and ethical aspects. 2. Medical informatics—Law and legislation. 3. Medical informatics—Social aspects. I. Duquenoy, Penny. II. George, Carlisle. III. Kimppa, Kai.
  [DNLM: 1. Medical Informatics—ethics. 2. Access to Information—ethics. 3. Confidentiality. 4. Medical Informatics—legislation & jurisprudence. 5. Medical Records Systems, Computerized—organization & administration. 6. Social Responsibility. W 26.5 E837 2008]
  R858.E82 2008
  174.2—dc22
                      2007049519

British Cataloguing in Publication Data
A Cataloguing in Publication record for this book is available from the British Library.

Ethical, Legal, and Social Issues in Medical Informatics

Table of Contents

Foreword... vi

Preface... x

Section I:
The Internet and Healthcare

Chapter I
Online Medical Consultations: Legal, Ethical,
and Social Perspectives... 1
Carlisle George, Middlesex University, UK
Penny Duquenoy, Middlesex University, UK

Chapter II
Applied Ethics and ICT-Systems in Healthcare.. 29
Göran Collste, Linköping University, Sweden

Section II:
Trust, Values, and Healthcare Information Systems

Chapter III
Trust and Clinical Information Systems... **48**
    Rania Shibl, University of the Sunshine Coast, Australia
    Kay Fielden, UNITEC New Zealand, New Zealand
    Andy Bissett, Sheffield Hallam University, UK
    Den Pain, Massey University, New Zealand

Chapter IV
Values of an Electronic Social Record.. **65**
    Karin Hedström, Örebro University, Sweden

Section III:
Responsibility and Healthcare Information Systems

Chapter V
Are Agency and Responsibility Still Solely Ascribable to Humans?
The Case of Medical Decision Support Systems **84**
    Hannah H. Gröndahl, Formerly of CTE Centre for Applied Ethics,
        Linköpings Universitet, Sweden

Chapter VI
Responsibility in Electronic Health: What Muddles the Picture?............**113**
    Janne Lahtiranta, University of Turku, Finland
    Kai. K. Kimppa, University of Turku, Finland

Section IV:
Quality Management in Healthcare Information Systems

Chapter VII
Compliance and Creativity in Grid Computing **140**
    Anthony E. Solomonide, University of the West of England, Bristol, UK

Chapter VIII
Clinical Safety and Quality Management in Health IT............................ **156**
    Benedict Stanberry, Medical Imaging Group Limited, UK

Section V:
Privacy and Data Protection Issues Regarding
Electronic Healthcare Information

Chapter IX
The Impact of Information Technology in Healthcare Privacy 186
  Maria Yin Ling Fung, University of Auckland, New Zealand
  John Paynter, University of Auckland, New Zealand

Chapter X
Compiling Medical Data into National Medical Databases:
Legitimate Practice or Data Protection Concern? 228
  Boštjan Berčič, Institute for Economics, Law and Informatics,
    Ljubljana, Slovenia
  Carlisle George, Middlesex University, UK

Section VI:
Emerging Technologies

Chapter XI
Biometrics, Human Body, and Medicine: A Controversial History 249
  Emilio Mordini, Centre for Science, Society and Citizenship, Rome, Italy

Chapter XII
Prospects for Thought Communication:
Brain to Machine and Brain to Brain 273
  Kevin Warwick, University of Reading, UK
  Daniela Cerqui, Université de Lausanne, Switzerland

About the Contributors 291

Index 297

Foreword

Over a century ago, with the work of Alexander Graham Bell, the motivation under-lying the first use of the telephone in communication had a health-related origin: a doctor attempted to be in contact with his deaf mother and sister. Early developments in electronic patient records took place over 40 years ago through the pioneering work of Ed Hammond and his interest in community and family medicine. Very soon, the European Union will be celebrating a 20-year history of co-financing eHealth research and development initiatives. Multiple eHealth programmes and projects around Europe have been the result.

Since the publication of the European eHealth action plan in 2004[1], many more concrete steps have been made in European countries towards deploying and imple-menting medical informatics whether in primary, secondary, or tertiary healthcare. Today, all the European Member States have a strategy or vision for the achievement of eHealth in their country and many are well on their way towards the practical implementation of these roadmaps.

A vast amount of other work on eHealth is also being undertaken in a very concrete and practical way around the whole globe. While the countries of the European Union and the Organisation for Economic Cooperation and Development are among the pioneers in the application of physical eHealth systems and services, the World Health Organisation also endeavours to ensure that the health systems and services of its worldwide members are also well-served by information and communication technologies.

eHealth is a topic that lies at the crossroads of multiple disciplines, both hard and soft: including, on the one hand, engineering and computer science and, on the other, psychology and the social sciences. It can therefore be seen as an academic discipline, or rather, being at the crux of several academic disciplines, that under-pin these activities and interests. These key specialisms are often reflected in the discourse outlined in the papers in this volume.

The first advances in eHealth were often based around the computer science or engineering tools and techniques used to progress the field of medical informatics. eHealth may be related to either medical or health informatics. It is however always concerned with an understanding of the skills and tools required to use and share the information appropriate to the provision of healthcare services and the promotion of good health. Given the essential grounding of health and medicine in the human condition, ethical, legal, and social issues did not remain long outside the field of endeavour, discussion, and debate.

United Kingdom and Finnish-based academics, Penny Duquenoy, Carlisle George, and Kai Kimppa, have brought together a set of contributors from largely Scandinavian, United Kingdom, and eastern and southern European countries to explore a number of key non-technical issues surrounding eHealth. All are deeply concerned with the ethical, legal, and social issues surrounding eHealth, whatever the relative range of complexity of the technologies involved: some of these applications are very simple, others complex and futuristic. The authors' themes are principally three: the Internet; today's ethical, legal, and social issues; and the challenges of future developments in eHealth.

A 15-year journey has taken place since a canine in a *New Yorker* magazine cartoon warned early online users, "On the Internet, no one knows that you're a dog"[i,ii,] While this observation is pertinent to many areas of public service information, it is especially important in the health sector where health information needs to be valid, appropriate, vetted, and often confidential. The focus on Internet and Web-based technologies is self-evident throughout this volume. Its collection of papers has special relevance for the concerns of citizens, patients, health consumers, and healthcare professionals, given recent announcements made by some of the most internationally well-known software and health service-related companies, institutions and not-for-profit associations on keeping health data safe and sound[iii].

Contemporarily, trust, responsibility, and the quality of information are all major concerns that lie at the foundation of eHealth. As the technologies that support healthcare increasingly mix, merge, and converge, giving us "connected" or "connecting" health, these matters grow progressively, sometimes even disruptively, in importance. Patient safety and reduction of medical risk is a perceived basic benefit of eHealth[iv]. Work undertaken in developing tentative recommendations on the interoperability of eHealth systems and services, at least in Europe, due for publication in spring 2008 by the European Commission[v], goes further to cover the provision, connectivity, equity, quality, cost, and safety offered by the various technology applications involved. As some of the most obvious and yet profound ethical, legal, and social issues in healthcare information, these matters are all given due attention in this volume.

Educationalists and policy-makers do not care to look only at contemporary developments, they also examine their crystal balls to see what future developments are emerging. The latter chapters of the book therefore focus on issues relating to bio-medical developments, new genetic and proteonomic data, sensors, engineering initiatives, implantations and close-to-body devices, and the way in which these advances are considered today and could be perceived tomorrow.

Currently, these research and application topics are to the forefront in Europe's laboratories and research centres. Data information, which originates as our own, may lead to profound insights into health—and, particularly, public health—trends, threats, and challenges.

Contemporary studies, such as Scenarios4Health[vi] on ICT-enabled healthcare developments, will surely lead to interesting and provocative visions as they publish their final reports this year or next. It is perhaps not surprising, therefore, that a 13 September 2007 foresight workshop held at the home of the Institute for Prospective Technology Studies in Spain, rather than focus on the developing applications and technologies that underpin eHealth, deliberately concentrated on the ethical, legal/regulatory, and social challenges that need to be faced in electronic support of the health domain.

As we look towards the future, and particularly that peak in the West of baby-boom ageing around 2030, all citizens in our societies need to ask themselves certain basic questions[2]. How in a flat world[3], will societies find a balance between those populations which are ageing and those which are relatively young and healthy; between those of whatever age who are experiencing more and more chronic diseases; between those who need care and support and those few(er) who are economically active; between those regions and states which are blessed with abundant healthcare professionals and those which have insufficient; between those countries and institutions which extract the benefits of advanced telemedicine and teleconsultation and those which remain as yet unconnected? How too can we move towards a more innovative and evolutionary view of thinking about and organising our healthcare systems and services?[4]

Let us look forward eagerly to a continuation in this kind of debate and dialogue. The preliminary questions outlined in this volume are preliminary, concrete, but fundamental, steps on a journey, which will permit the asking of many more challenging and provocative questions. We will all need to face a health-permeated future that, while it is full of aspirations about technological and scientific possibilities, at the same time is replete with ethical, legal, and social challenges. A structured debate and dialogue on these questions is now of pending, and indeed of major, concern.

Diane Whitehouse
October 27, 2007
Paris, France

Endnotes

[1]   COM(2004)356 final. *e-Health - making healthcare better for European citizens: An action plan for a European e-Health Area.* I am indebted for many of these insights to Dr Petra Wilson of Cisco Systems Internet Business Group and her observations made during and industry leaders session at the World of Health IT conference held in Vienna, Austria, 22-25 October 2007. For more information on the conference itself, see http://www.worldofhealthit.org/

[2]   I am indebted for many of these insights to Dr Petra Wilson of Cisco Systems Internet Business Group and her observations made during and industry leaders session at the World of Health IT conference held in Vienna, Austria, 22-25 October 2007. For more information on the conference itself, see http://www.worldofhealthit.org

[3]   Thomas L. Friedman (2005) *The world is flat: A brief history of the twenty-first century.* Farrar, Strauss, and Giroux

[4]   Although not on the topic of healthcare *per se*, some of the ideas contained in a recent book contain innovative and thoughtful reflections on collaborative ways of working in new fields. See Don Tapscott and Anthony D. Williams (2006) *Wikinomics: How mass collaboration changes everything*, Atlantic Books: London, UK

[i]   Cartoon designed by Peter Steiner. *The New Yorker*. 5 July, 1993. Vol 69 (LXIX), no. 20, p61

[ii]   Although this observation was first made a decade and a half ago, Ms Celia Boyer of the Health on the Net (HON) Foundation, Geneva, Switzerland, very pertinently reminded her audience of it at an ePractice high impact services workshop held in Brussels, Belgium on 10 September, 2007. For more information about HON's work, see http://www.hon.ch/

[iii]   See The *Economist*, 4 October, 2007 'The vault is open' on the notion of a 'health vault'.

[iv]   V.N. Stroetmann, J-P. Thierry, K.A. Stroetmann, A. Dobrev (October 2007) *eHealth for safety. Impact of ICT on patient safety and risk management.* European Commission: Brussels

[v]   Based on earlier work published by the Commission Services: European Commission (2006) *Connected Health. Quality and safety for European citizens.* Luxembourg: European Communities

[vi]   http://www.scenarios4health.org/

Preface

Over the last 50 years, the integration of computer technologies within all sectors of society has increased exponentially year on year, providing fast and easy access to information in a timely and cost-effective way. The capabilities of such technologies to manage large amounts of data and provide access regardless of physical distance have been exploited both by commercial enterprise and public sector organizations, giving rise to terms such as e-commerce, e-learning, e-government, and e-health. The drive to fully exploit the potential of this technology together with a keen interest by individuals to use it has resulted in a rapidly changing social landscape—encompassed in the concept of the "e-society" or "information society."

In the last 10 years, particularly since the introduction of the World Wide Web (WWW), we have seen radical changes within society as more and more individuals and organisations adopt this "digital" world—founded on what are commonly known as information and communication technologies (ICTs). The delivery of information is no longer just within the domain of the traditional computer and keyboard interface, it incorporates the convergence of computer technology with any digitally capable means of transmission, including mobile wireless devices such as mobile phones. What is significantly different in this digital context is the inclusion of the general public in a two-way information exchange, taking a role whereby they are not only the recipients but also the creators of information and who moreover, have a potentially global audience.

The impact of global information exchange on traditional organizational processes and social expectations poses several challenges. When we consider that this exchange spans cultural as well as national boundaries, and that the creators and providers of information include experts and non-experts (in a particular domain, as well as in technology use and understanding) we can see that the challenges to accessing, understanding, regulating, and distinguishing the valid from the invalid are not trivial. However, whilst some of the issues are challenging they are not insurmountable and great strides have been made in meeting and addressing the issues by those working in the relevant disciplines that include both computer science and the social sciences, and particularly cognitive science, psychology, philosophy, and law.

In all of the different sectors that have incorporated computer technologies the ethical, legal and social issues that arise have an impact that affect all stakeholders—from individuals within the society through to the professionals working in a particular domain. These issues have not often been clearly seen or anticipated—largely because many of the applications present new ways of doing things in unfamiliar contexts. In familiar contexts, we have in place processes and rules that inform and accommodate work and social practices. Where situations are presented that are unfamiliar it is not clear how the rules we are used to map into the new situation. (Consider, for example, a visit to a culturally different country—the ways of doing things may be quite different and take some time to rationalize.)

These differences are important to understand when technology is introduced to the medical sector. Whilst computers and medicine have for a long time been linked together[1], for example in monitoring systems, their use has broadened and touches on almost all spheres of patient care that have an effect on practice within the traditional care setting, as well as in radically new areas such as patient "self-help" and embedded chips (see Chapters I and XII respectively).

It is for these reasons that this book has come together. The ethical, legal, and social issues that arise from the introduction of ICT's in the medical sector need to be considered not only in the specific context of their use, but also in a wider context that highlights the transforming effect of such technologies. The terms that have emerged to cover the convergence of computer technology and medicine are various: health informatics, healthcare informatics, biomedical engineering, e-health, and medical informatics. The areas all overlap and share a common theme, but for us the term medical informatics emphasizes the "technical" information application area that is bound together with the medical profession—a domain to which the ethical, legal, and social aspects are at the moment most relevant.

The Scope of Medical Informatics

Medical informatics touches most people in the world today in the developed and not so developed countries. Its scope is vast, covering the full range of information support to medical practice provide by computer technology—from computerized records in doctor's surgery's at one end to decision-support systems in hospitals at the other. In terms of academic research, the scope of medical informatics includes the management of information from a range of healthcare sources: "hospital management information, patient records, clinical examinations, laboratory results, physiological measurements, medical images of all kinds, primary care information, and epidemiology."[2] Although this list does describe the different types of information gathered, and considered to be part of the medical information domain, it does not fully capture the complexity or breadth of inter-organisational, cross-organizational, and indeed global, exchange.

With the advent of global communications, in the form of information communication technologies (ICTs), developments in mobile wireless devices and most recently the grid[3], medical care has been revolutionized bringing new opportunities for improving practice, improving healthcare, and reducing costs. At the same time, these radical changes accentuated by the fast pace of development and innovation, raise significant challenges to traditional health care models. The opportunities offered by the Internet for the sharing of information across the globe on a "many to many" basis has for the first time opened the door to a "do it yourself" type of approach to personal healthcare. Individuals can find their own health information, and act on it without consultation with a healthcare professional (e.g., their local doctor).

The standards and regulations that have hitherto served to protect individuals in such a vitally important area of life can no longer be guaranteed when healthcare moves into the public arena. Agreeing common standards and regulatory procedures across the globe is hard—enforcing them is another matter. At a more local level, the introduction of computer—mediated healthcare changes the processes and practices of the care professionals—not least in learning to operate and manage ICTs, individually and as part of a team.

In all of these different situations and contexts, the ethical, social, and legal environment can be substantially changed but, as mentioned earlier, presented in such an unfamiliar setting that initially the differences may not be clearly seen. In this interim stage difficulties are experienced by the users of the technologies, as well as by those individuals and communities who are impacted by the changes that have been brought about. It is at such a transitional time (i.e., where stakeholders are making adjustments to accommodate new technologies), that discussion, debate, and the exploration of new ways of doing things are common.

With this extension to the availability of healthcare information both within the profession and to the general public, the scope of medical informatics as suggested in the first paragraph above is not enough for current purposes. It excludes the participation of the general public—as current or potential patients—from the information domain. Some might argue that including this aspect is going too far, and that public access to information (that may or may not be scientifically proven or accurate) goes outside the boundaries of the professional field. However, we would argue that the source of the information accessed is not the point—the fact that it is available and widely used by the general public has an impact both on patient health and welfare, and on the profession. Therefore, the definition of medical informatics given by Shortliffe and Blois for example, as "the scientific field that deals with biomedical information, data, and knowledge—their storage, retrieval, and optimal use for problem-solving and decision-making" (2001, p. 21) more appropriately covers the scope, and although it may not intentionally be including the broader 'self help' aspects of the Internet or other patient devices and aids, the definition does not constrain the scope to a purely organizational one.

The Issues Raised

We have previously said that the increasing integration of ICT within healthcare systems changes traditional processes that have come into use in an evolutionary way to accommodate key healthcare ethical principles and social policies. The issues arising from this changed environment concern the transference of the embedded principles of best practice standards and regulation to the new technologically informed processes and models. For example, the process of delivering prescription medicines have traditionally been mediated by pharmacists who are trusted experts—it is their responsibility to ensure patients receive the correct medication. How does this model transfer to the situation we now see where prescription drugs can be bought from online (Internet) pharmacies? Other issues arise where the trust that has previously been placed in medical personnel is mediated by technology—where is that trust now placed in this situation? How can previous models of trust be transferred to information mediated by technology?

The role played by ICT as mediators of information and as "aides" in working practice is a difficult one to distinguish, where levels of responsibility are blurred. In a process that involves extremely complex negotiations and data retrieval how can practitioners distinguish between the boundaries of responsibility? Understanding these boundaries is important, not simply for staff accepting responsibility but also so that they are aware of displaced responsibilities—and errors that could occur. In including mediating technologies it should be recognized that the cognitive load on users, and difficulties in compartmentalizing "human habit" and "computer characteristics" have an impact on the perceptions of those using the technology. This behaviour is often seen where users attribute human characteristics to machines, resulting in confusion over roles and responsibilities.

Further confusions over boundaries between the human and technical occur when the two become more closely connected. There are differences that need to be thought about when proving personal identity is a choice between using some form of paper card, a computer chip, or parts of the body that have been converted into a digital record (such as fingerprints) as is the case with the security technologies known as "biometrics." Where computer chips are implanted into the human body what then are the boundaries? Is it important to know and recognize the boundaries?

Physical boundaries inform our thinking, allowing a separation between behaviour and expectations attributed to humans (and animals) and other physical objects. Boundaries have also traditionally distinguished cultural differences and preferences. Laws and other forms of regulation are culturally informed, admittedly with some sharing of principles across cultures. These boundaries disappear when using ICT—either in using the Internet to buy drugs from another country, or exchanging information with other countries that have different views on privacy and confidentiality. How does this impact on our traditional information processes? What are the areas at risk when regulation may not apply across territorial boundaries?

All of the previous are some of the serious questions that need to be explored, and which the chapters in this book attempt to address.

Structure of the Book and Outline of Chapters

The book is divided into six sections offering different perspectives, or themes. If we take a technology perspective, the book begins with a look at the impact of the Internet on healthcare and doctor-patient relationships and takes us through a technological domain that includes information systems in use in health institutions, new technologies in research, and emerging technologies that connect to the patient. Taking a "human focused" perspective the chapters follow a structure that highlights issues of ethics, trust, quality of care, responsibility, patient confidentiality and regulation, both from an individual perspective and a wider social and legal perspective.

It begins with two chapters that investigate the phenomenon of the Internet in respect of new forms of patient autonomy—that is the increased access to health information and medicines. In the first chapter the focus is on the sale of prescription drugs by online pharmacies and the ethical and social impact of this practice, what it means to traditional models of healthcare practice when patients become "shoppers" and how the regulatory controls manage to control not only the remote delivery of prescription drugs (i.e., without the local physical presence of a dispenser), but also how the law copes with this transnational environment (George & Duquenoy). In the second chapter, Collste takes an ethical perspective and puts the remote and internationalization aspects of Internet healthcare within the context an ethical framework in order to see more clearly how this type of healthcare delivery conforms to the ethical principles that have always been at the core of medical practice.

Section II moves into the domain of medical practice and takes the core aspects of trust and values for investigation. Both chapters in this section use empirical research to further explore these aspects, and understand the perceptions on those immediately involved in using technology in practice. Bisset et al. are interested in how clinical decision support systems (i.e., systems that rely on an existing knowledge base to provide information) are regarded in terms of trust, and whether these perceptions are supported by the chains of responsibility in the system provision. Their study incorporates views from the suppliers of the knowledge base, the software developers, and end users in the context of a New Zealand primary care environment.

The second chapter in this section is also set in the context of primary care, this time in Sweden, where Hedström aims to assess the changes in practice that may arise from the use of electronic journals. In this study, which takes the aspect of elderly care and the social journal—a device that is used to share information about an individual with those involved in their care. Taking the view that information technology systems are naturally embedded with the values of the development process, Hedström uses a value framework (that incorporates the values relevant to this aspect of the health work) as a tool to compare and assess impact on practice arising from the change in recording medium (i.e., paperbased to digital).

Questions of responsibility are the focus of Section III. Taking the issue of decision support systems (as previously summarised) a step further, Gröndahl (Chapter V) asks where the responsibility for action rests. When computer systems are used to inform and support decision-making and those systems become ever more complex, is it reasonable that practitioners using them should be assigned responsibility for the results of their decisions? Using a series of arguments as leverage for discussion, Gröndahl explores the issue of moral agency in respect of systems using what is known as artificial intelligence techniques, as well as the associated question of legal responsibility. As such systems are infiltrating medical practice more and more answers to these questions become imperative. A similar theme is followed by Lahtiranta and Kimppa where the concept of "agentization" (whereby the technology becomes the agent) is employed to illustrate how easily we are moved to attribute responsibility to mechanical artifacts. They particularly look at how the patient-doctor relationship may be affected when machines are integrated within the healthcare process, to the extent that they may become naturally accepted inclusions in the relationship, and how issues such as informed consent are dealt with in this mediated environment. One recommendation is to make it quite clear to those involved the distinction between human agent and artifact.

The two chapters that make up Section IV emphasise the technical systems in their role as supporting technologies to healthcare practice. In the opening chapter of this section Solomonides introduces a relatively new concept, for example, the grid, which utilizes shared and distributed computer processing power in order to provide the capacity needed for large scale data management (such as medical images). The storing and exchange of medical images is crucial to providing a knowledge base for practitioners, and clearly it is also crucial that the images from which judgments are made are reliable. Quality of information is vital. The grid also raises some challenging ethical, legal, and social issues due to the characteristics of its operation—the same characteristics that inspired its creation.

As such large-scale utilization of ICT becomes more prevalent, and IT projects become more ambitious, the quality of the system becomes more difficult to control and keep track of. This is particularly the case where national programmes are rolled out, as with the NHS (National Health Service) *Connecting for Health* programme in the United Kingdom. This programme is just one of many government projects that have received enormous criticism and bad press in the UK. Suppliers of systems are increasingly under pressure to address issues of quality and reliability, for their own professional sakes as well as in the interests of patient safety. Stanberry (Chapter VIII) gives a comprehensive account of the trials and tribulations of informatics deployment in the health sector so far, the legal and professional imperatives for improving performance, and the emerging standards and best practice that are being developed in response to these problems.

Section V addresses one of the key issues at the forefront of current debates on medical information. Patient confidentiality has always been at the heart of medical practice, and this is severely challenged by information transfer to digital media, and the global operation of the Internet that allows the exchange of medical information not just nationally, but globally.

Fung and Paynter (Chapter IX) discuss the issue of privacy in relation to patients' medical information and the risks to privacy that the more open electronic exchange facilitated by Internet technology has promulgated. They show that despite legislation and assertions as to the value of privacy (of medical data) there are major vulnerabilities in following this through to strong privacy policies and the upholding of privacy standards using technological means, such as in system set-ups and security technologies. In their analysis of the health information situations in New Zealand and the United States, they categorise the different sources of risk and solutions used to tackle the problems. Their conclusion is that as new technologies appear bringing new risks so strategies must be developed that include a comprehensive approach and utilization of available technologies in order to maintain the benefits that ICTs offer.

Similar concerns regarding personal medical data are raised by Berčič and George in Chapter X. In this case, they focus on Europe (EU) and the collection of medical records in national databases, which are compiled from local databases and file systems. Given the special level of legal protection pertaining to medical data in the EU issues of access, legitimacy of data held and subject access rights, amongst others, need to be considered and addressed.

Having critically assessed, analysed, and discussed the various applications of medical informatics in current use, we end our investigative journey with two chapters that discuss emerging technologies and their prospective uses. In Section VI, the final section in this book, the focus is on the convergence of technology with the human body. The first chapter (Chapter XI) brings together the issues of personal information and privacy together in a discussion on identity and the technical means of identity verification—biometrics. The use of this technology responds to the growing problem of medical identity theft (using unlawfully gained medical information) that provides fraudulent access to health care. Biometric technology is based on using unique personal attributes such as fingerprints, retina patterns, and others to verify identity. Although more effective than many other methods of authentication, biometric information is also medical information and as such provides more than just a positive affirmation of a valid identity. Mordini takes us through the technical characteristics of biometrics, issues of privacy, and the benefits and risks of adopting this technology.

The book concludes with a chapter that describes the integration of computer technology with, and into, the body. Although the title "Prospects for thought communication: Brain to machine and Brain to Brain" has a futuristic implication the chapter describes past research with neural interfaces, which has provided the groundwork for the claims in the title. The focus of the discussion is between the use of this technology for therapy or enhancement —and whether there is a difference as far as ethical use is concerned. As the authors, Warwick and Cerqui, hold different positions on this research (Warwick as the motivator and subject of much of the research and Cerqui as interested anthropologist), the benefits together with the moral issues make for an interesting dynamic.

Conclusion

This book brings together the perspectives of authors from a variety of disciplines: computer science, information science, medicine, law, philosophy, and the social sciences, to offer an international overview of the ethical, legal, and social issues inherent in the application of information communication technologies in the healthcare sector.

As we move into an era that relies more and more on technology to assist work practices, enhance knowledge, improve healthcare, and facilitate patient autonomy and independence it becomes crucial to understand and assess the impact of current and future technologies. In seeking more efficient, faster, and large-scale implementation of our technological creations, we should not lose sight of the human factors—the ethical and social dimensions. We must also pay due regard to the regulatory controls that exist and the challenges that these technologies pose.

Each of the chapters in this book raise key questions that deserve attention and reflection, and through this process can offer recommendations for improving the implementation of new technology in this domain.

The aim of the book, in addition to providing the basis for reflection in its case studies, arguments, and analyses, is to provoke thought, stimulate debate, and provide a foundation for further work in the field—in education, research, and practice.

Penny Duquenoy
Middlesex University, UK

References

Shortliffe, E. H., & Blois, M. S., (2001). The computer meets medicine and biology: Emergence of a discipline. In E. H. Shortliffe & L. E. Perreault (Eds.), *Medical informatics: Computer applications in health care and biomedicine* (2nd ed.) (pp. 3-40). New York: Springer Verlag.

Endnotes

[1] Shortliffe and Blois note the use of "electromechanical punched-card data-processing technology" which was widely used for epidemiologic and public health surveys during the 1920's and 30's (2001, p.23).

[2] The scope outlined as relevant to the journal *Medical Informatics and The Internet in Medicine*, Informa Healthcare, Taylor and Francis Group.

[3] The grid is a term used to describe the utilisation of distributed computing power to increase computing capacity (explained further in Chapter VII of this book).

Acknowledgment

The editors would like to acknowledge the help of all involved in the collation and review process of the book, without whose support the project could not have been satisfactorily completed. Most of the authors of chapters included in this book also served as referees for chapters written by other authors, and thanks are due to them for their constructive remarks and suggestions. Thanks also to our colleagues and experts from the health sector, Diane Whitehouse and Chris Zielinksi, who were kind enough to review chapters.

More thanks are due to Diane Whitehouse for agreeing to write the foreword for this book, and finding the time to do it amongst all the other demands on her time.

Special thanks also go to the publishing team at IGI Global, particularly Meg Stocking and Deborah Yanke who provided support throughout the process. Whether it was emails to remind us of deadlines, or in offering help and advice, our communications have not only been at a consistently professional level but have also been conducted in an open and friendly manner.

Finally, to the authors—a thank you for your staying power, insightful contributions, and continued support throughout.

Penny Duquenoy
Carlisle George
Kai Kimppa

Section I

The Internet and Healthcare

Chapter I

Online Medical Consultations:
Legal, Ethical, and Social Perspectives

Carlisle George, Middlesex University, UK

Penny Duquenoy, Middlesex University, UK

Abstract

The growth of the Internet over the last 10 years as a medium of information and as a communication technology has provided the opportunity for selling medical products and services online directly to the public. This chapter investigates on-line medical consultations used for the purpose of prescribing and hence selling prescription drugs via the Internet. With consumers in mind, this chapter takes a critical look at this growing phenomenon from three perspectives—legal, ethical, and social—as a basis for discussion and to illustrate the problems raised by using the Internet in this way. The chapter concludes that online medical consultations pose greater dangers to patients compared to traditional off-line consultations. The chapter also concludes that while new technologies may aid doctors in making better diagnoses at a distance, they often bring new concerns. Finally, the chapter gives suggestions on safeguarding online consumers.

Introduction

The growth of the Internet over the last 10 years as a medium of information and as a communication technology has, not unsurprisingly, provided a foundation for the growth of direct-to-the-public online sales. Amongst the many commercial activities that are now flourishing in this environment are Internet pharmacies (e-pharmacies, cyber pharmacies), providing a variety of products (e.g., health and beauty products) as well as prescription drugs. Some pharmacies only dispense drugs with a valid prescription, some provide online consultations for prescribing and dispensing medicines, and some dispense medications without a prescription (Radatz, 2004).

Internet pharmacies provide various benefits to consumers but also bring many problems for regulators and consumers (George, 2005). Benefits include the ease and convenience of 24-hour shopping, increased consumer choice of products, increased consumer information, and information exchange between patient and pharmacist, generally lower costs, privacy, and availability of alternative treatments. Problems include uncertainty about the purity and quality of drugs sold, risks of buying drugs online, for example, related to foreign labels and use of different drug names in different countries, dispensing prescription drugs without a prescription, and the issuing of prescriptions through online consultations but without prior physical examination by a licensed physician. This latter aspect provides the focus of this chapter.

The chapter will first discuss online consultations, identifying various concerns. It will then discuss the various legal, social, and ethical issues related to this growing practice. The role of information technology both in terms of creating such problems but also possibly facilitating solutions will be examined. Finally, the chapter provides some suggestions on how consumers can be safeguarded in the future.

Online Medical Consultations

Many Internet pharmacies provide online consultations as a first step towards selling prescription medicines online. These consultations usually require that a potential customer fill out an online questionnaire. A 2007 study by the U.S. National Centre of Addiction and Substance Abuse (CASA, 2007) concluded that:

- Between 2004 and 2006 there was an increase in the number of Internet pharmacies (not requiring prescriptions) offering an online consultation: 2004—53% (76), 2005—57% (84), and 2006—58% (90);

- In 2007, of the 187 sites that offered to sell controlled prescription drugs over the Internet, 85% (157) did not require a prescription. Also, 53% (83) of the sites not requiring a prescription offered clients an online consultation.

A typical online consultation questionnaire may consist of three parts. The first part asks for personal details such as name, address, contact telephone numbers, date of birth, height, body weight, and gender. The second part of the questionnaire asks about medical history including whether a particular drug requested has been used before, what drugs are currently being taken, a history of allergies and side-effects to certain medicines, what complaint is the drug requested for, and whether the customer has suffered from a range of conditions such as heart disease, kidney disease, liver disease, diabetes, epilepsy, hypertension, asthma, and chronic bowel disorders. The third part asks for payment details and shipping information.

After the questionnaire is completed, it is then reportedly evaluated by a licensed physician/doctor affiliated to the pharmacy in order to either approve or decline a prescription request. If a request is approved, a prescription is written by the physician then sent to the pharmacy for dispensing and shipping of the medication. In addition to the medication, a customer will receive contact information for the pharmacy and information on usage, dosage, and precautions relating to the medication.

Consultations made online, by their very nature, do not involve a physical examination in person by a licensed physician. Therefore, they may be dangerous both in terms of making a correct diagnosis and determining drug interactions (Henney, 2000), amongst other problems discussed throughout the chapter.

In some cases, physicians/doctors who issue online prescriptions ("cyberdoctors") are either not licensed to practice medicine in the consumer's state/country or are not credible. A 2003 U.S. study reported that many cyberdoctors recruited by Internet pharmacies were previously unemployed, semi-retired, or had declining practice incomes (Crawford, 2003). Also, investigations into the backgrounds of some online prescribing physicians have found that some had previous convictions for either forgery, fraud, or sexual assault, revoked or suspended licences, and addiction to drugs or alcohol (BDA, 2004).

Legal, Ethical, and Social Perspectives

In the following pages, the practice of online medical consultations is looked at from the three different perspectives: legal, ethical, and social. In a context of use, it can often be difficult to distinguish between these three. Although legal aspects should be more easily identifiable (through citizens' familiarity with law), there are particular laws that are applicable to specific situations and domains—as in this case. Similarly, non-experts in ethics can often recognise some ethical difficulties but may confuse ethical with social issues. The different aspects are discussed in this chapter under the relevant headings, but some explanation of the differences may be helpful at this point.

Activities within public life necessarily have an impact on other people that may be beneficial or harmful. Benefits and harms are determined according to the values of the people within a society, and come under the domain of ethics. The rules governing social activities, and which promote benefits and prevent harm, are formally expressed in legislation, and less formally in, for example, professional codes of conduct, or practice. Thus legislation formally upholds social values (within democratic societies at least) and in this way supports the ethical position of that society. However, not all "bad" actions are regulated by law, and not all laws are necessarily ethical. Ethics is a complex subject, but one could say that the "laws" of ethics are expressed as ethical principles, which are used in this chapter to give a reference point for discussion. Finally, the social perspective is a broader perspective that looks at society as a whole (rather than individuals within society). This perspective is needed to see the "bigger picture"—that is the application of a technology within society and the impact that it is likely to have.

Thus an assessment of the benefits and harms of a new technology on individuals and the general public can be done by using a framework that refers to the law (formal social rules guiding behaviour), ethical principles (personal and social views of behaviour), and social aspects.

The Legal Perspective

Regulation in the UK and U.S.

Online consultations are an important first step in aiding patients to legally purchase prescription drugs online. In both the UK and U.S., drugs classified as "prescription drugs" require a prescription issued by an appropriate licensed healthcare professional before such drugs can be dispensed by a pharmacist. In the UK, the Medicines Act 1968 (as amended), classifies medicines into three classes namely: (1) Prescription only (Section 58), which can only be sold with a valid prescription; (2) Pharmacy only (Section 60), which must be sold in consultation with a pharmacist; and (3) General Sales List (Section 5), which do not require any prescription or consultation before sale. Under Section 58, it is illegal to supply prescription only drugs except through a registered pharmacist with a prescription issued by an appropriate practitioner. In the U.S., under the Federal Food, Drug, and Cosmetic Act (i.e., Title 21 of the United States Code – 21.U.S.C.), drugs are classified into two categories namely: prescription drugs and over-the-counter drugs. Under 21.U.S.C.353(b)(1), pharmacists are prohibited from dispensing prescription drugs without a valid prescription issued by a licensed practitioner (physician). Over-the-counter drugs do not require a prescription for sale.

As noted earlier, online consultations are an important aspect of the online selling of prescription drugs since these consultations are used to issue prescriptions to enable the sale of drugs. All medical consultations, however, are subject to certain professional standards, and in many instances consultations done online fall below the accepted professional standards (of a medical consultation) as set out in the regulation of medical practice.

In the UK, medical practice is regulated by the General Medical Council (GMC) and to some extent the British Medical Association (BMA). The GMC was established by the UK Medical Act 1983 (as amended) and its primary functions are "to protect, promote, and maintain the health and safety of the public" (Section 1). All doctors practising medicine in the UK must be registered with the GMC. Registration involves the granting of various privileges (e.g., the right to prescribe drugs, access to medical records, authority to sign medical certificates) and obligations (e.g., confidentiality, adherence to code of practice). Under Section 36, the GMC has the authority to suspend or remove from the register any fully registered person found guilty of professional misconduct or convicted of a criminal offence (even if not committed in the UK). In 2004 the General Medical Council (GMC) issued new practice guidelines (further revised in 2006) which detail conditions to be met for remote prescribing (via telephone, e-mail, fax, video, or Web site) in situations where a doctor: (a) has responsibility for the care for a patient, (b) is deputising for another doctor responsible for the care of a patient, or (c) has prior knowledge and understanding of the patient's condition and medical history and has authorised access to the patient's medical records (GMC, 2006, paragraph 38). If these situations are present, the doctor is advised that he or she must have an appropriate dialogue with the patient to:

- "Establish the patient's current medical conditions and history and concurrent or recent use of other medications including non-prescription medicines;
- Carry out an adequate assessment of the patient's condition;
- Identify the likely cause of the patient's condition;
- Ensure that there is sufficient justification to prescribe the medicines/treatment proposed. Where appropriate you should discuss other treatment options with the patient;
- Ensure that the treatment and/or medicine/s are not contra-indicated for the patient;

- Make a clear, accurate, and legible record of all medicines prescribed." (GMC, 2006, paragraph 39)

In the absence of situations (a) to (c) discussed above the GMC does not expressly forbid remote prescribing but gives additional conditions, which a doctor must satisfy if remote prescribing is to be used. The prescribing doctor is advised of the additional conditions as follows:

- "Give an explanation to the patient of the processes involved in remote consultations and give your name and GMC number to the patient;
- Establish a dialogue with the patient using a questionnaire to ensure that you have sufficient information about the patient to ensure you are prescribing safely;
- Make appropriate arrangements to follow the progress of the patient;
- Monitor the effectiveness of the treatment and/or review the diagnosis;
- Inform the patient's general practitioner or follow the advice in paragraph 9 if the patient objects to the general practitioner being informed." (GMC, 2006, paragraph 40)

Paragraph 9 states that:

If the patient does not want their general practitioner to be informed, or has no general practitioner, then you must: (a) Take steps to ensure that the patient is not suffering from any medical condition or receiving any other treatment that would make the prescription of any medicines unsuitable or dangerous or (b) Take responsibility for providing all necessary aftercare for the patient until another doctor agrees to take over. (GMC, 2006)

The GMC guidelines give further advice to doctors if they prescribe for patients who are overseas. These include the need to be aware of differences in the licence names, indications and recommended dosage of medical products, the need to ensure adequate indemnity cover for such practice, and the need to be registered with the appropriate regulatory body in the jurisdiction where the prescribed medicines are to be dispensed.

In the U.S., all physicians/doctors practising within a state are required to be licensed by that state. Each state has a state medical board that is responsible for regulating physicians according to state medical practice laws, investigating complaints, and upholding professional standards among others. All U.S. state medical boards belong to a representative organisation called the Federation of State Medical

Boards (FGSMB) that is committed to developing and promoting high standards of medical practice by physicians. In 2002, the U.S. Federation of State Medical Boards published, "*Model Guidelines for the appropriate use of the Internet in Medical Practice*" (FSMB, 2002). Some of the guidelines specifically addressed the issue of remote prescription practices stating the need for "documented patient evaluation" (including a patient history and physical evaluation), and that "Issuing a prescription based solely on an online questionnaire or consultation does not constitute an acceptable standard of care" (FSMB, 2002). The FSMB Guidelines further state that "e-mail and other electronic communications and interactions between the physician and patient should supplement and enhance, but not replace, crucial interpersonal interactions that create the very basis of the physician-patient relationship." (FSMB, 2002),

Guidelines issued by the American Medical Association in 2003 (regarding the prescribing of medicines to patients via the Internet) state that a physician who prescribes medications via the Internet must establish or have an established a valid patient-physician relationship (AMA, 2003). This includes among other things: obtaining a reliable medical history and performing a physical examination of the patient; having sufficient dialogue with the patient regarding treatment options, and risks and benefits of the treatment; and having follow-ups with the patient where appropriate. In the U.S., therefore, the use of an online questionnaire without a physical examination of a patient, will not amount to the existence of a legitimate patient-physician relationship. Indeed many U.S. States have passed laws which add prescribing without first conducting a physical examination to the definition of unprofessional conduct (e.g., Arizona Revise Statutes Title 32, Chapter 13 Article 1; California Business and Professions Code Section 2242 and 4067; Kentucky Revised Statutes 311.597(1)(e); Missouri Statute 334.100.2(4)(h); Nevada Revised Statutes 453.3611). A listing of the policies of state medical boards and state legislation regarding Internet prescribing can be found at FSMB (2007a).

In both the U.S. and UK, doctors have been prosecuted for using online consultations to prescribe drugs. For example, in the UK, Dr. Richard Franklin was found guilty of serious professional misconduct by the GMC after prescribing drugs online (BBC, 2002). Patients were required to fill out an online questionnaire, which was then reviewed by Dr. Franklin and used to prescribe drugs. The GMC stated that the questionnaire was closed and did not allow for a dialogue between doctor and patient. Also, that Dr. Franklin did not carry out an adequate assessment of his patients' conditions, and therefore did not act in the best interests of his patients (BBC, 2004). Regarding the U.S., details of the convictions (e.g., fines, suspensions) and other disciplinary actions (from 1998-2007) of numerous U.S. physicians for online prescribing are given at FSMB (2007b). A typical example is Dr. Shreelal Shindore of Florida (U.S.) who was forced to relinquish his medical license after "prescribing a Schedule IV controlled substance to a patient who completed an Internet questionnaire without conducting a physical examination, obtaining a complete history, making a diagnosis, or establishing a treatment plan" (NYSBPM, 2004).

One of the purposes of a professional medical body (or other professional body) is to provide protection for those seeking expertise, that is, those who are less expert and therefore vulnerable in their lack of knowledge (e.g., RPS, 2006; Duquenoy, 2003). The case of Dr. Franklin illustrates this aspect where the GMC stated that Dr. Franklin did not act in the best interests of his patients. Whilst the law has taken action in this particular case, it may become increasingly difficult to monitor the activities of doctors practicing in this way—and in particular in areas where either no medical body exists, or where a medical body does not have the weight of established professional bodies such as the GMC in the UK, and FSMB in the U.S..

Liability for Patient Care

A person becomes liable if he or she fails to perform a legal obligation or duty. Such legal obligations or duties may arise from fiduciary relationships between parties, existing laws (statute, common law), or contractual agreements among others. Liability can be civil or criminal and can arise under various areas of the law such as professional malpractice, negligence, negligent misstatement, and breach of contract.

In the traditional doctor-patient relationship, if a patient suffers loss or damage caused by negligent or intentional acts committed by the doctor (in the course of performing his or her duties) then professional malpractice claims may arise. It may be the case however, that for online consultations, only civil liability issues may arise since liability for professional malpractice may not be clearly established where an online prescription is issued (Kahan, Seftel, & Resnick, 2000). This is because whereas in a traditional doctor-patient relationship a clear duty of care exists, it is debatable whether a doctor who prescribes medication online (without any direct verbal or physical contact with a patient), forms a traditional doctor-patient relationship and therefore attracts the same duty of care.

Although the same level of "duty of care" as in a traditional doctor-patient relationship may not exist in an online consultation, a prescribing doctor will still be required to exercise a duty of care to prevent loss or injury to a patient. A breach of that duty (e.g., through careless acts or omissions) leading to loss which is a direct and natural result of the breach (i.e., consequential loss) will result in liability for negligence. Where a prescribing doctor gives incorrect medical advice, which leads to loss, then liability for "negligent misstatement" may be established. For a breach in negligence, an injured patient can be awarded damages or compensation, and the prescribing doctor can incur financial and/or criminal penalties, depending on the seriousness of the breach.

Finally, a contractual relationship will exist between an online prescribing doctor and a patient, due to the fact that the patient is making payment for a service. Therefore, a prescribing doctor will be bound by his or her contractual obligations, which include express contractual terms as well as terms implied by law (e.g., regarding the quality of service). Failure to perform his/her contractual obligations will result in the prescribing doctor facing an action of breach of contract and possibly incurring a financial penalty.

Confidentiality and Data Protection

The writing of prescriptions via online consultations raises important legal issues of confidentiality and data protection. Confidentiality focuses on maintaining the secrecy of information and data protection focuses on the legal framework governing the processing (collection, storage, security, and use) of personal data.

During an online consultation, a patient places his or her trust in a prescribing doctor and in turn, the doctor has a duty to faithfully discharge his responsibility. It is therefore widely accepted in law that there exists a fiduciary (trust) relationship between doctor and patient because of the vulnerable position of the patient. By virtue of the fiduciary (trust) relationship that exists between an online prescribing doctor and a patient, the prescribing doctor will be under an obligation of confidence not to disclose any medical information divulged to him/her unless authorised to do so. Confidentiality issues may arise because information given for online consultations may be prone to be seen by people other than the consulting doctor, unless strict security and protocols are in place (Kahan et al., 2000). Staff assisting a prescribing doctor in the provision of medical care will most likely be authorised to have access to patients' medical data and therefore will also have an obligation of confidence. However, the transmission of data between doctor and patients over the Internet poses an inherent risk that such data may be accessed in transit by an unauthorised person. This has important implications within the European Union/ United Kingdom (EU/UK) with regard to obligations under data protection law. In the EU/UK medical data is classified as "sensitive personal data" (Data Protection Act, 1998, Section 2(e)) and acknowledged as a special category (amongst others such as ethnic origin, religious belief) which requires a higher level of protection compared to ordinary personal data. Amongst eight data principles in the 1998 Act, the seventh principle states that "data must be kept secure from unauthorised access, unlawful processing, destruction, or damage" (Schedule I). This implies that online transactions must have adequate security to prevent the unauthorised access to medical data.

Jurisdiction

The Internet crosses geographic and state boundaries and hence creates a global market for commerce. It is thus relatively easy for a medical practitioner to be located within one jurisdiction and to administer an online consultation to a patient located in a different jurisdiction, without being licensed to practice medicine in either of the jurisdictions. The practice of medicine within any jurisdiction without an appropriate licence is a criminal offence, since it places citizens at a serious risk. It may, however, be difficult to successfully prosecute a medical practitioner located in a jurisdiction different to that of the patient. This is especially true where it is prohibitively expensive to do so or where the appropriate legal agreements between jurisdictions (especially countries) are not present.

In the European Union, all member states are signatories to the Brussels Regulation (i.e., Council Regulation (EC) No 44/2001 of 22 December 2000 on jurisdiction) and the recognition and enforcement of judgments in civil and commercial matters. This legal instrument details the rules for determining jurisdiction (i.e., which courts are entitled to adjudicate on an action) in EU states in matters of tort (civil wrongs) and contract law. As mentioned earlier, an online medical consultation may give rise to a legal action (e.g., a tort committed over the Internet), where a doctor makes a negligent misstatement such as giving incorrect medical advice. Under the Brussels Regulation, a patient can bring an action in tort against an Internet doctor (defendant) in the courts of the state where the doctor (defendant) is domiciled, or in the courts of the state where the harmful event occurred (i.e., the place where the wrongful action was carried out or the place where the damage occurred).Where the regulation does not apply (e.g., the defendant is not in an EU state or a criminal charge is contemplated), then various other rules (e.g., common law rules) may be used to determine jurisdiction.

The Ethical Perspective

The ethical issues are closely related to the legal concerns expressed above. In the cases reported in the previous section, national legislation serves to protect patients and uphold the established ethical practices of the medical profession. The foundation for the ethical principles of the medical profession (in the western world) is the Hippocratic Oath (Nova, 2001a). The principles referred to in the Hippocratic Oath recognise the responsibilities of the expert to those who seek their professional help, amongst which are prevention of harm, justice, respect for the person, and maintaining confidentiality (interpreted to privacy in a modern version (Nova, 2001b)). Setting out, and abiding by these principles gives grounds for a relationship whereby the patient can feel secure and trust that their interests are taken into account, and that they are not going to suffer harm. Establishing and maintaining this relationship is vital in the medical context where the patient seeks to improve their health and is absolutely reliant on the doctor to achieve their goal. Doctors, for their part, are equally reliant in purely pragmatic terms (if not for humanitarian reasons) on helping them to achieve that goal. What is the impact, then, of online consultations on this relationship?

We begin the discussion by looking at the impact on trust (as a precondition for health care) of an online relationship, and follow with an assessment on the prevention of harm and injustice and confidentiality. Finally, we consider the aspect of acting in the patient's best interests, and whether online consultations can provide the reassurance that the patient needs.

Trust

The question of "duty of care" raised in the previous section, whilst expressed in legal terms, captures some sense of the secure and trusting relationship we are arguing is the foundation of a healthcare relationship. The lack of physical presence and its impact on trust has been taken up by Bauer (2004) who argues that the empathy and sense of connected-ness built through trust and understanding, encourages healing. A key point of his argument is that trust is built in the doctor-patient relationship through a certain amount of risk-taking, particularly on behalf of the patient. In the case of online health care he claims that "cybermedicine makes risk-free interactions easier and more commonplace" thus reducing the opportunity for building trust. His conclusion, founded on arguments from moral philosophy, is that as the pursuit of healing is the fundamental ethical principle of medicine, the diminishing of the healing practice is immoral and that "cybermedicine encourages morally inappropriate physician-patient relationships."

If we accept this argument, we should ask: What risks are there in the healthcare relationship, and are they reduced in the "diagnosis at a distance" setting? The patient is putting their health and intimate information in another person's hands and thus implicitly accepts some risk, whether in terms of correct advice and treatment, or confidentiality. The doctor's risk is in the reliability of the information received, knowledge of the patient's history and circumstances, and reliability of the prescribed course of action. These issues of validity, reliability of information, confidentiality and the impact on them of remote consultations are discussed in the following paragraphs.

Prevention of Harm and Injustice

The questionnaire approach used in online consultations as a means of ascertaining medical needs, typified in our early example, illustrates the degree to which the "empathetic" doctor-patient relationship has been stretched. Even if we were to discount Bauer's argument regarding interconnectedness, and return to the more generally accepted principles of the Hippocratic Oath—which by its existence attests to the recognition of the power imbalance between professional (expert) and layperson—it is hard to see how the questionnaire approach to medical consultations can adequately address the prevention of harm, and the imbalance between expert and non-expert, which could result in injustice. The dialogue between doctor and patient that is traditionally conducted face-to-face is an important aspect of a doctor's practice especially with regard to his duty to prevent harm (as far as is reasonably possible). In practical terms, it is within the face-to-face context that doctor makes an assessment of the condition presented at that time, based on a number of factors that give an overall picture of the health of the patient—such things as skin tone and texture, condition of eyes, tongue, reaction to touch, emotional state, and many others. Thus, a rich picture of the patient is built based on the doctor's experience (and tacit knowledge). In respect of the risk factor, which Bauer argues contributes to the trusting relationship, the validity of information received from the patient is more easily assessed, and for the patient it is more likely that their doctor's credentials are professionally accepted. So under these circumstances it seems that risks are reduced.

Doctors in this familiar setting are also in a position to share information with the patient, and are in a much better position to establish that the patient understands what they are saying—whether it be information about the condition, or, vitally, information concerning drug use. Thus some measure of informed consent (an underlying principle of an ethical action) can be achieved. Whether informed consent is usual when patients are receiving prescriptions for drugs may be debated (as opposed to surgery where signed consent is explicitly required) but consent is certainly implicit in accepting the prescription. However, when completing an online questionnaire, the level of language competence and understanding within the medical context (discussed later) has serious implications for this generally held principle of informed consent—how informed is the consumer under such circumstances? This aspect is pursued later under the heading of "social perspective."

Confidentiality

We questioned earlier the legal status of patient confidentiality, and raise it again as an ethical issue. Doctors who prescribe drugs online could argue that the precautions they take to ensure confidentiality are at least as good as the measures used in more traditional settings. We cannot say that patient files are secure from unauthorised access in either the off-line or online environment (and some could argue that as patient records are transferred to electronic storage there is little difference). However, it would be safe to say that there is an increased opportunity to gain access to confidential material online, with much less risk of being caught, even where the best security measures are in place. If security measures are not in place, then patient confidentiality is not provided for. What is more, if access to this information is inadequately protected online, the extent of the spread of this information is potentially on a "massive" scale. Once leaked it would be impossible to contain, or conduct any damage limitation. Whilst the vulnerability of personal data is a general concern in online activities, and not exclusive to online medical practices, personal medical information is highly sensitive and warrants special care (under EU data protection legislation). We would argue that because this information is valuable to third parties (pharmaceutical and insurance companies, for instance) it is especially at risk online.

In some cases doctors and others are required to pass information to health authorities for the purposes of building data banks of public health information providing sets of statistics, which can be used to inform government policies regarding public health initiatives. Cooper and Collman (2005) note that "to operate effectively physicians need complete and accurate information about the patient" and are therefore in a position to provide detailed information for such statistic-gathering. Although this information in its statistical form is anonymous (that is, having no identifier to any patient) the amount of information collected, and the use of data-mining techniques can isolate and identify to a surprising extent. The authors point to studies by Sweeney (1997) who demonstrated that birth date alone can uniquely identify names and addresses of individuals from a voting list (12% success rate), when combined with birth date and gender the results increased to 29%. Additional information increases the chance of identification, with a full postal code and birth date bringing the identification rate up to 97%. We can see that just because the data has been anonymised confidentiality and protection of medical information is not assured for the individuals concerned.

Aside from the (legitimate) passing on of medical information by doctors, health data can be gleaned from the Internet activities of the patient/customer (Cooper et al., 2005). The authors refer to instances where IP addresses (the unique address of the computer accessing the Internet) "have been linked with publicly available hospital data that correlates to DNA sequences for disease." Of course, anyone using the Internet can be routinely tracked to find out the sites they have visited in order to build profiles of Web users, but the linking to medical data is taking this a step further and into more serious waters.

Patients' Best Interests

We began this section with reference to the Hippocratic Oath. In a modern version the following has been added:

I will remember that there is art to medicine as well as science, and that warmth, sympathy, and understanding may outweigh the surgeon's knife or the chemist's drug. (Nova, 2001b)

In part the sentence quoted underpins the notions of empathy expressed earlier, and its importance in the healing process. In doing so it is recognised that surgery or drugs may not be the best way forward. It could be argued that the practice of prescribing drugs online favours the assumption that drugs are the best solution to the problem. There is already a questionable cultural trend in the U.S. and the UK to use drugs as the first line of attack for many conditions. Patients visit their doctor and expect a solution to their condition in the form of pill, and it is often easier for doctors under pressure to prescribe drugs than investigate other possible causes (such as living conditions or life style for example). McCoy (2005) refers to this trend as the "over-biomedicalisation of healthcare" that is, the lack of attention to life context, and the reduction of illness to something that can be solved by prescription. This trend, according to McCoy, is as a result of pressure exerted by pharmaceutical companies, directly and indirectly through advertising (McCoy, 2005). The question that arises is whether, in the case of online medical consultations, the advising doctor would recommend against the use of prescribed drugs and offer instead "warmth, sympathy, and understanding?" Reducing the relationship to the completion of a questionnaire and the provision of a prescription drug supports Bauer's argument that "cybermedicine makes risk-free interactions easier and more commonplace" thus diminishing the healing relationship. This type of approach resembles more of a commercial transaction than a mutual effort to promote wellbeing, and if this is all that is needed why not have questionnaires at Pharmacy counters in towns, and bypass the doctor? The issue of questionnaires and the wider implications of conducting online transactions in the healthcare sector are further explored below.

The Social Perspective

The two cases reported at the beginning of this chapter (i.e., concerning Drs Franklin and Shindore) raise a number of social issues. In general terms, buying prescription drugs remotely encourages a culture of independence from recognised institutional practices and undermines the ethos of risk associated with such drugs. Drugs that are designated prescription-only are considered to carry risk under certain conditions—if they were not they would be available for anyone to buy. The issuing of a prescription implies that an expert has taken the medical, and possibly emotional, characteristics of the patient into account, the risks, and benefits of prescribing the drug, and has recommended a course of treatment based on those factors. This assessment has taken place traditionally face-to-face, and incorporates the visual clues and existing personal knowledge of the patient referred to in the section "prevention of harm and injustice" above. By offering an "easy" route to buying drugs, it could be argued that the practitioner prescribing online is complicit in undermining the best practice advice of recognised professional bodies.

There is also a wider social implication to bypassing the traditional route and using an e-commerce model, and this is the issue of patient protection. Both the issuer of the drug and the receiver are taking a risk that has hitherto been mitigated by the levels of protection provided by regulation, whether it be legislation or professional codes of conduct. For example, The Royal Pharmaceutical Society of Great Britain (RPSGB)—the professional body for pharmacists in the UK—in their draft version of a revised Code of Ethics (RPS, 2006) offers substantial guidance on the professional role when dispensing drugs. Some of the principles they list are: making the care of patients your first concern, act in the best interests of individual patients and the public, obtain consent for … treatment, care, patient information, encourage patients to participate in decisions about their care. Some of these principles have been discussed in the previous section (patients' best interest, confidentiality) others such as consent and participation in decisions are discussed below.

In the previous section we introduced the notion of informed consent, and suggested that doctors in a face-to-face diagnosis were in a better position to gain feedback on the patient's understanding of the diagnosis and treatment, and could to some extent be reassured that the treatment was consensual. In this section we discuss the impact of the remote approach to diagnosis and treatment via online methods on the notion of "informed." At the level of individual applications for online prescriptions, the online questionnaire takes no account of the level of literacy of the patient—either in terms of understanding the terminology used in the context of health, competence in the language used in the questionnaire, or specific cultural interpretations. Under Section 4 of the RPSGB Code of Ethics "Encourage patients to participate in decisions about their care" (RPS, 2006) it is stated "Listen to patients and their carers and endeavour to communicate effectively with them. Ensure that, whenever possible, reasonable steps are taken to meet the particular language and communication needs of the patient" (Item 4.2 RPS 2006). Clear communication is considered to be important in the delivery of medicines. They also instruct the pharmacist to "make sure that patients know how to use their medicines" (Item 1.5 RPS, 2006).

It is hard to see how an online questionnaire can fulfil these communication needs. When completing an online medical questionnaire, a respondent may not completely understand a question and may "guess" an answer, or may misinterpret a question and give an invalid answer. These issues are extremely relevant where drugs are bought and sold in a global market place, where language competence and understanding of medical terminology can vary. A lack of understanding of the medical context, and particularly familiar medical culture, could have drastic effects.

To illustrate our point, the following questions (below) are taken from an actual online consultation questionnaire at https://meds4yourhealth.com. Notice that some of the questions are expressed in medical terms, which are not immediately obvious to a non-medical person.

- Do you suffer from or currently have Cardiac or (ischemic) heart disease?
- Do you suffer from or currently have Transient ischemic attack(s) (TIA's)?
- Do you suffer from or currently have Diabetes?
- Do you suffer from or currently have Epilepsy?
- Do you suffer from or currently have Hypertension (exceeds either value of 80/120 mm Hg)?
- Do you use MAO-inhibitors like phenelzine or moclobemide?
- Do you use NSAID's (nonsteroidal anti-inflammatory drug - f.i. salicylates, diclofenac, naproxen)?

While terms such as "diabetes" and "epilepsy" may be familiar to many, we suggest that it is doubtful that someone would know whether they had a "transient ischemic attack" or whether they suffered from hypertension that "exceeds either value of 80/120 mm Hg." Also medical terms such as "MAO-inhibitors" and "NSAID" are not commonly used amongst the general population. These terms may be familiar to the local, or national, community from which the Web site is generated—but it cannot be assumed that they would be understood by people outside of that community.

So what of informed consent? According to the Council for International Organizations of Medical Science (CIOMS) International Ethical Guidelines, informed consent is defined as: "Consent given by a competent individual who: Has received the necessary information, has adequately understood the information, after considering the information, has arrived at a decision without having been subjected to coercion, undue influence or inducement, or intimidation" (CIOMS, 2002). These guidelines refer to the research environment, as do the following noted by Tavani (2006) in a discussion concerning genomics research and quoting Alpert (1998): (1) individuals must "know and understand the nature of the information being released," and (2) consenting individuals must be made aware of the party or parties to whom the information about them can be released. These requirements, he notes, are similar in ethos to conditions laid out in the Office of Technology Assessment (OTA) Report "Protecting Privacy in Computerized Medical Information" (OTA, 1993) whereby patients must (1) have adequate disclosure of information about the data dissemination process, and (2) be able to fully comprehend what they are being told about the procedure or treatment. In a footnote he points out that the OTA also say the patient must be "competent" to consent.

Thus, important questions are Who is considered competent, and what competencies are required? Do competencies vary according to context? Does online communication require different competencies? And finally, how would anyone operating in an online context offering consultations and selling prescription drugs know whether their client was competent or not?

The patient/client/customer (depending on which relationship model one uses) places themselves at risk in this context from the point of view of fully understanding the situation and thereby not being fully informed. Patients also run the risk that a legitimate consulting physician may not be present to evaluate the online questionnaire. Further, use of general questionnaires may not provide the necessary information for the determination of a number of important issues such as whether a particular drug (FTC, 2001): (1) will work for an individual, (2) is safe to use, (3) is more appropriate than another treatment, (4) may cause adverse reactions if an individual is taking another medication, or (5) may be harmful due to an underlying medical condition such as an allergy.

The risk, however, is not just on the part of the patient. Even with the best of intentions, a doctor entering into an online consultation, and pharmacist conducting an online transaction, may not be in a position to fulfil their professional responsibilities. The procedures used for assessment are less able to offer reassurances than face-to-face transactions. For example, if online questionnaires are not completed truthfully then medications will be prescribed on false information. Another important aspect is the authenticity of the patient request —does this person really have the symptoms the drug will alleviate, are they buying for someone else, or buying to sell on to others? We should bear in mind that it is possible for a minor (under 18 years old) to buy drugs. In a 2003 briefing to the U.S. Congress, an investigator reported that his 9-year-old daughter successfully ordered a prescription weight-loss drug on the U.S. Drug Enforcement Administration (DEA) controlled substance list (Lueck, 2003). In addition, his 13-year-old son ordered and received Prozac, a drug on the United States Food and Drug Administration's (FDA) Import Alert list (Lueck, 2003).

The responsibility of the medical practitioner does not end in the prescribing of a drug. Follow-up treatment may be required. In the case of Dr. Shindore, one of the reasons given for withdrawing his licence to practise was that no treatment plan was established. One wonders whether some purchasers are choosing to get the drugs online because they prefer a one-off interaction, and whether they appreciate the potentially harmful implications of such a one-off deal. Even if advice is given as to the period of time the drug should be taken, when a reassessment is due or what contra-indications may appear, the purchaser may not (a) take any notice, or (b) not fully understand. Furthermore, the purchaser of online drugs may find it difficult to effectively communicate concerns, developments, or changes in symptoms either through the lack of established online procedures or even where a facility is available difficulties may be experienced since he/she cannot be physically assessed by a medical practitioner.

Concerning the extent of responsibility in the online environment, it is interesting that the following disclaimer is included in the questionnaire.

I declare without any restriction:

(a) that I have read the terms and conditions and the disclaimer on this Website and agree with their content and applicability

It should be noted that this is only the first of a total of four clauses. This approach is surely very different from the type of doctor/patient interaction that takes place in a surgery—patients in the traditional role are not asked to agree to any "disclaimer."

Future Trends

As technological developments advance and are incorporated into commercial practices some of the issues noted in the previous sections may be alleviated. We have not so far discussed the use of Web cams for example in overcoming the issue of face-to-face consultations, direct measuring techniques for aiding diagnosis, or legitimate access to a shared database of patient records (overcoming the problem of patient history). These technologies are in existence, and are currently used in the medical domain between trusted parties.

In the sub-sections that follow, we look at the previous three examples of available technologies and assess how they may help in the online consultation context. In each case we show how the legal, ethical, and social difficulties previously highlighted might be addressed.

Web Cam (Problem Addressed: Face to Face Consultations)

Legal

The U.S. Federation of State Medical Boards guidelines clearly state that "e-mail and other electronic communications and interactions between the physician and patient should supplement and enhance, but not replace, crucial interpersonal interactions that create the very basis of the physician-patient relationship." (FSMB, 2002), It is rather doubtful therefore whether in the U.S. a Web cam can be used as a substitute for a face-to-face physical interaction between a physician and patient (who has not previously been physically examined). In the UK however, the GMC's guidelines for online consultations (as outlined in detail earlier) appear to indicate that it is possible to use a Web cam (video) subject to certain conditions (see GMC, 2006, paragraphs 39 and 40).

Some criteria relevant to utilising a Web cam are:

- Establish a dialogue with the patient, using a questionnaire;
- Adequately assess the patient's condition (which may include performing a physical examination of the patient as far as is practicable via video);
- Discuss alternative treatments;
- Assess any contra-indication effects;
- Have sufficient dialogue with the patient regarding treatment options;
- Inform the patient's general practitioner.

Ethical

The ways by which some of the ethical issues might be addressed are listed following the headings used within the ethical perspective section.

- **Trust:** The visual clues could encourage a trusting relationship, and help the patient feel more engaged in the consultation process.
- **Prevention of harm and injustice:** The lack of visual clues for the doctor discussed under this heading would be addressed with this technology, for example assuring the doctor that the patient understands the treatment (e.g., dosage), and the language competence of the patient.

- **Confidentiality:** The issue of vulnerability of data over a public network (the security issue) is not addressed by using this technology. An additional ethical issue may in fact be raised here with regard to the storage of visual data. This may be appropriate and helpful as a record of care, but visual data adds to the issue of confidentiality and security of data. It also reduces anonymity (which could be seen as a beneficial outcome or a disadvantage).

- **Patients' best interests:** Using this technology may have a benefit in diminishing the sense of engaging in a purely commercial transaction (as described earlier), thus fostering a better relationship between the patient and consulting clinician.

Social

Under this heading, we noted how online consultations could give the impression that the patient is engaged in something akin to a commercial transaction, thus reducing the import of prescription drugs. Using a Web cam could have the effect of elevating the apparently "casual" transaction of buying drugs to a more formal setting and thus reinstating a sense of medical "best practice." In addition this type of visual interaction allows for a more meaningful interpretation of "informed" both on the part of the practitioner, and the patient (each receiving feedback from the visual clues). It should be noted of course that this only applies to non-visually impaired participants. However, it should also be noted that when using a Web cam the voice is normally transmitted at the same time and therefore for the visually impaired the traditional consulting room setting is fairly represented. An interaction using a Web-cam would address some of the communication concerns of the Royal Pharmaceutical Society of Great Britain (discussed under this section).

Diagnostic Measuring Techniques (Problem Addressed: Lack of Physical Contact and Capability to Make a Full Patient Assessment)

Technologies are being utilised to aid diagnosis and to transmit data to a central database, or General Practitioner. For example, trials are being conducted in the UK that use devices to monitor blood sugar levels as an aid in the management of diabetes and transmitting the patient data to a central location, such as a local general practitioner (Farmer et al., 2005).

Legal

Returning to the GMC guidelines the following are addressed by using diagnostic measuring techniques.

- Adequately assess the patient's condition;
- Assess any contra-indication effects;
- Perform a physical examination of the patient.

Ethical

- **Trust:** In some ways using a technology such as this may encourage trust in that the patient and the consultant have a clearer indication of the patient's condition. However, this depends to a large extent on the trust placed in the technology itself, which is playing a mediating role. While it could be said that any technology used in a consultation (i.e., in traditional face-to-face settings) also needs to be trusted, the presence of the doctor who can oversee the technology at first hand would arguably give some confidence to the patient, and the doctor, that all is working correctly.
- **Prevention of harm and injustice:** Using this type of technology helps to build a "rich picture" of the patient's condition and thus contributes to the prevention of harm.
- **Confidentiality:** As previously described, the vulnerability of transmitted and stored digital data constitutes a risk to confidentiality.
- **Patient's best interests:** As above, using a diagnostic device may alleviate the sense of a purely commercial transaction, fostering more of a relationship between the patient and consulting clinician.

Social

Making use of technology that is specific to the medical profession could have the effect of elevating the "casual" transaction of buying drugs into a more formal setting, thus reinstating a sense of the medical aspect and confirming social norms that are described as "best practice." It may also encourage the patient to participate in decisions about their care (in the case of the research with sugar levels and diabetes, which serves as the example for this section, the ethos is about encouraging patient "self-management" of their condition). As further information is provided this technology serves to further "inform" the patient, and also helps to address the issue of the "authenticity" of the patient.

Shared Patient Record Database (Problem Addressed: Adequate Medical History and Feedback)

Legal

The GMC (2006) suggest that practitioners should:

- Justify medicines/treatment proposed;
- Assess any contra-indication effects of medicines/treatments proposed;
- Keep a record of all medicines prescribed.

The U.S. FSMB (2002) asks for:

- Documented patient evaluation (including a patient history and physical evaluation).

A patient record would satisfy these requirements.

Ethical

- **Trust:** Where consultants have access to the patient's records—as on a shared database—it would be argued that the reliability of the information received and the knowledge of the patient's history and circumstances are improved. Such a situation is likely to improve the reliability of the prescribed course of action. However, the reliability of the information on a shared database cannot be assured—in which case there is a risk that the consultant assumes the correctness of the information (which may be an error) and the prescribed treatment is therefore not fitting. The outcome of this could have extremely serious consequences (perhaps fatal).

- **Prevention of harm and injustice:** Although using a database to access a patient's records contributes to the rich picture (providing increased relevant information about the patient) harm may not be prevented, as noted in the previous paragraph.

- **Confidentiality:** Issues of the security of the information are still an issue, particularly as the patient data is stored (i.e., available over a prolonged period of time), and accessible by many authorised personnel who also may alter and update the record (which can be a source of error).

- **Patients' best interests:** Providing a patient history and maintaining up-to-date accurate records would further the patient's best interests. This information also enables follow-up treatment, and a feedback mechanism.

Social

Access to the patient's records would eliminate the reliance on a questionnaire such as the one described earlier, where questions using medical terminology could cause confusion and misunderstanding. The consultant would be able to see at a glance the relevant and most recent medical situation of the patient. Thus in this respect there is a benefit. The records could also serve to provide an additional means of authenticating the patient (i.e., that this is the patient claimed, that they do have the condition they are claiming to have, and when they last had a prescription issued).

We can see from the previous examples, and reference to the earlier discussions and drawbacks of the remote consultation, that introducing new technologies (as described in the examples above) could alleviate some of the problems. As with the introduction of most technologies, other problems may be generated—such as the reliability of electronic patient records—but a trade-off is an inevitable part of the decision-making process.

Summary and Conclusion

In this chapter, we have provided an overview of the practice of online healthcare, highlighting some of the benefits and problems associated with this phenomenon. We focused on the use of online consultations to facilitate the sale of prescription drugs, and outlined the related regulatory frameworks, which exist in the United States and United Kingdom. Further, we discussed some legal, ethical, and social issues of concern, which may arise with regard to the use of online consultations.

Some legal issues of concern discussed were liability for patient care—medical malpractice (in light of the extent to which a duty of care in an online consultation is comparable to that which exists in the traditional doctor-patient relationship), negligence and contractual obligations, confidentiality of patent information, EU/UK data protection law regarding the security of medical data, and jurisdiction issues (related to the relative locations of an online doctor and a patient, and bringing a claim against an online doctor).

In our discussion of ethical issues, we questioned the reasons for buying online. One reason may be that someone may want large quantities of a particular drug—much easier to get online by visiting different sites. The purchaser may be contemplating suicide, or may be planning to sell the drugs on at a profit and bypassing any regulations that protect the user. Other issues were patient confidentiality; informed consent, and finally, the implicit assumption that prescribing drugs is the most appropriate form of treatment for the patient.

With regard to social issues, the subtle but clear move from a face-to-face interaction towards a simple "form-filling" exercise is likely to encourage a casual and less informed approach to drugs that carry some risk, and has an added impact in undermining the status of the medical profession. We are also concerned about the level of understanding on the part of the purchaser, the verification of authenticity of the patient request and the potential for a lack of continuous monitoring and advice concerning the patient's medical condition. Finally we suggest that with online consultations, the risks to the consumer are greater and the level of protection less, compared to the traditional off-line medical consultation.

All of the present concerns previously discussed are relevant to future developments. Technology is moving on, and the Internet has brought with it an irrevocable cultural change. Opportunities have arisen that allow consumers more choice in how they purchase goods, and from whom. With developments in mobile technologies and increased access to the Internet, the preponderance and use of online pharmacies is likely to grow.

Many of the concerns we have raised will continue to be relevant. These include:

- **At the medical level:** Issues related to disassociation of remedy from cause, disassociation from personal expert advice and the consequent clinician/patient relationship that is formed over time (which includes knowledge of the patient's personality, medical history, and social context).

- **At the purchaser level:** Language competence and understanding in multicultural states, and cross-national transactions.

- **At the technological level:** Issues of confidentiality and security of personal data.

- **At the legal level:** Liability for malpractice, negligence or contractual obligations, issues of confidentiality, data protection, and enforcement of interjurisdictional offences.

Advances in technology can impact on the provision of online healthcare, both in terms of providing solutions to present difficulties and in creating further legal, ethical, and social concerns. Technology can provide solutions by aiding doctors in making better diagnoses at a distance, for example: use of Web cameras for examining patients and use of medical instruments that can be used to carry out various medical tests on a patient (as we have previously discussed). Technology can also provide better security for information, aid regulatory bodies, and enforcement authorities in their duties and help promote public awareness of important issues. Unfortunately technologies are also likely to be abused or subject to malfunction or failure. This further raises legal concerns such as where legal liability for failure of a technology lies, ethical concerns such as the potential for misuse of a new technology, and social concerns such as how a technology impacts on current norms and practices.

The previous discussions imply a need for continuing regulatory and ethical scrutiny of the evolving social phenomenon of online medical practice. Present regulatory frameworks and ethical codes of conduct may not adequately address the future scenarios that could develop. Although legitimate Internet pharmacies appear to adhere to the provisions of the existing regulatory frameworks, as discussed earlier, the problem really lies with rogue pharmacies that are driven by commercial profits and operate without regard to either regulatory or ethical guidance.

Having seen the rather futile efforts to dissuade Internet users from utilising its resources (for example, by the music industry to prevent the sharing of music files), we argue that the medical profession will need to consider how they can best adapt to Internet practices using technology, policy and legislation, and consumer education, to adequately protect the patient. Any adaptation, however, should not lower the established medical standards and hence put patients at potential risk. The global risk to the health and well-being of everyone dictate that ethical codes of conduct and regulatory frameworks need to be constantly reviewed and updated not only to address online medical practitioners, but also other players that facilitate this commercial activity. Thus appropriate ethical guidance and regulation should be aimed at technologists, delivery specialists, and credit card companies among others in the stream of online medical commerce. The need to protect consumers from the potential harmful consequences of online consultations should be a core principle, guiding the conduct of all commercial entities. We argue, finally, that perhaps the only way forward into the future is for more international consensus, cooperation, and agreement to establish global ethical and regulatory standards for online medical practice, to safeguard medical practitioners and recipients of medical advice and treatment.

References

Alpert, S. A. (1998). Health care information: Access, confidentiality, and good practice. In K. W. Goodman (Ed.), *Ethics, computing, and medicine: Informatics and the transformation of healthcare* (pp.75-101). New York: Cambridge University Press.

AMA. (2003). *H-120.949 guidance for physicians on Internet prescribing.* Retrieved June 21, 2007, from http://www.ama-assn.org/apps/pf_new/pf_online?f_ n=browse&doc=policyfiles/HnE/H-120.949.HTM

Bauer, K. (2004). Cybermedicine and the moral integrity of the physician-patient relationship. *Ethics and Information Technology, 6,* 83-91, 2004. Kluwer Academic Publishers.

BBC. (2002). *Viagra Web doctor suspended.* BBC News, 10th January 2002. Retrieved June 21, 2007, from http://news.bbc.co.uk/1/hi/england/1752670.stm

BDA. (2004). *Importing foreign medicines: Good or bad idea for Americans?* Retrieved June 21, 2007, from http://investigations.com/files/onlinepharma- cies.pdf

CASA. (2007). "You've got drugs!" IV: Prescription drug pushers on the Internet. *A CASA White Paper*, May 2007. Retrieved June 21, 2007, from http://www. casacolumbia.org/absolutenm/articlefiles/380-YGD4%20Report.pdf

CIOMS. (2002). *International ethical guidelines for biomedical research involving human subjects.* Prepared by the Council for International Organizations of Medical Sciences (CIOMS) in collaboration with the World Health Organiza- tion (WHO), Geneva 2002. Retrieved June 21, 2007, from http://www.cioms. ch/frame_guidelines_nov_2002.htm

Cooper, T., & Collman, J., (2005). managing information security and privacy in healthcare data mining: State of the art. In H. Chen, S. S. Fuller, C. Fried- man, & W. Hersh (Eds.), *Medical informatics knowledge management and data mining in biomedicine* (pp. 95-137). Springer Science+Business Media, Inc. 2005.

Crawford, S. (2003). Internet pharmacy: Issues of access, quality, costs, and regula- tion. *Journal of Medical Systems, 27*(1), Feb 2003.

Duquenoy, P. (2003). Models for Internet ethics. Risks and challenges of the net- work society. In P. Duquenoy, S. F. Hübner, J. Holvast, & A. Zuccato (Eds.), *Proceedings of the 2nd IFIP 9.2., 9.6/11.7* (pp.51-60). Summer School, Karl- stad, Sweden.

Farmer, A. J., Gibson, O. J., Dudley, C., Bryden, K., Hayton, P. M., Tarassenko, L., & Neil, A. (2005). A randomized controlled trial of the effect of real-time telemedicine support on glycemic control in young adults with type 1 diabetes (ISRCTN 46889446). *Diabetes Care, 28,* 2697-2702. © 2005 by the American Diabetes Association, Inc. Retrieved June 21, 2007, from http://care.diabetes- journals.org/cgi/content/full/28/11/2697

FSMB. (2007a). *Internet prescribing—State medical board policies/state legisla- tion.* Retrieved June 21, 2007, from http://www.fsmb.org/pdf/smb_policies- state_laws_internet.pdf

FSMB (2007b). *Internet prescribing overview by state.* Retrieved June 21, 2007, from http://www.fsmb.org/pdf/internet_prescribing_table.pdf

FSMB. (2002). *Model guidelines for the appropriate use of the Internet in medical practice.* Retrieved June 21, 2007, from http://www.fsmb.org/pdf/2002_grpol_Use_of_Internet.pdf

FTC. (2001). *Offers to treat biological threats: What you need to know.* Federal Trade Commission, Consumer Alert. October, 2001. Retrieved June 21, 2007, from http://www.ftc.gov/bcp/conline/pubs/alerts/bioalrt.htm

George, C. (2005). Internet pharmacies may not be good for your health. In C. Zielinski, P. Duquenoy, & K. Kimppa (Eds.), *The information society: Emerging landscapes, IFIP International Conference on Landscapes of ICT and Social Accountability.* Turku, Finland, June 27-29, 2005, USA: Springer

GMC. (2006). *Good practice in prescribing medicines.* Retrieved June 21, 2007, from http://www.gmc-uk.org/guidance/current/library/prescriptions_faqs.asp#p38

Henney, J. (2000). Online pharmacies—Maintaining the safety net. *Medscape Pharmacists, 1*(1), 2000.

Kahan, S., Seftel, A., & Resnick, M. (2000). Sildenafil and the Internet. *The Journal of Urology, 163,* 919-923, March 2000.

Lueck, S. (2003). Drug industry enlists an ex-cop lobbyist. *The Wall Street Journal.* October 22, 2003.

McCoy, D. (2005). Strong medicine. *RSA Journal,* June 2005. pp 48-53.

NYSBPM. (2004). *Report on professional medical misconduct.* New York State Board for Professional Misconduct. Retrieved June 21, 2007, from http://w3.health.state.ny.us/opmc/factions.nsf/0/7d54e09e72517b5485256f50006d5f06/$FILE/lc112252.pdf

Nova. (2001a). *Hippocratic Oath—Classical Version.* Retrieved June 21, 2007, from http://pbs.org/wgbh/nova/doctors/oath_classical.html

Nova. (2001b). *Hippocratic Oath—Modern Version.* Retrieved June 21, 2007, from http://www.pbs.org/wgbh/nova/doctors/oath_modern.html

OTA. (1993). Protecting privacy in computerized medical information. Office of Technology Assessment. *Washington, DC: U.S. Government Printing Office.*

Radatz, C. (2004). Internet pharmacies. Wisconsin Briefs, Brief 04-5, March 2004. Retrieved June 21, 2007, from http://www.legis.state.wi.us/lrb/pubs/wb/04wb5.pdf

RPS. (2006). *Consultation on the revised Code of Ethics for Pharmacists and Pharmacy Technicians.* Royal Pharmaceutical Society of Great Britain. Retrieved June 21, 2007, from http://www.rpsgb.org.uk/pdfs/coecons0611.pdf

Sweeney, L. (1997). *Guaranteeing anonymity when sharing medical data*. The Datafly System. *Proceedings of AMIA Symp* (pp. 51-55).

Tavani, H. (2006). Environmental genomics, data mining, and informed consent. In H. T. Tavani (Ed.), *Ethics, computing, and genomics*, Jones and Bartlett Publishers, Inc. 2006.

Chapter II

Applied Ethics and ICT-Systems in Healthcare[*]

Göran Collste, Linköping University, Sweden

Abstract

What are the ethical implications of information and communication technology in healthcare and how can new ICT-systems fit in an ethically based healthcare system? In this chapter, new ICT-applications in healthcare are assessed from an ethical perspective. The first application assessed is a system making patient information accessible for all healthcare units at a district, county or even national level. The second application, the so-called patient portal, is a system for patient Internet access to his or her medical record. The third application is the use of the Internet as a source of medical information, a means for medical consultation and for marketing of drugs. The systems are primarily assessed by the following ethical principles; the principle of doctor-patient relationship, the principle of responsibility and the principle of autonomy.

Introduction

Healthcare is going through a transformation caused by the use of ICT. While healthcare basically is a moral enterprise, aiming at the health and well-being of patients, the transformation should be assessed in regard to how the new organisation and the new technology affect the possibilities to realise the values of healthcare. In this chapter, I will ethically assess three different kinds of ICT applications in healthcare: a system for patient information, a system for patient access to his or her medical record, and e-medicine.

What does it mean to make an ethical assessment of technology? This is a kind of technology assessment (TA) using ethical criteria. It is also the kind of activity that one finds in applied ethics.

What should I do? What is right? These questions are the point of departure for ethics. In ethics, the moral content of our actions is analysed. How should we act in order to achieve human well-being and avoid harm, respect human dignity, human rights, and privacy? Human beings are social animals and, hence, we act in different spheres of society—as individuals, as professionals, and as citizens. In applied ethics, the questions of what we should do and what is right are related to social action. Applied ethics is an expanding field. One reason is the increasing complexity of human action. With the help of new technology we can do more complex things, but we also face new and difficult moral problems. This is not least true in medicine.

Much of the discussion in medical ethics concerns new medical possibilities provided through new scientific discoveries and new technological inventions. Ethical problems related to pre-natal genetic diagnosis and embryonic stem cells research are just two examples of current hot topics for discussions in medical ethics. However, it seems as medical ethicists generally have overlooked the thoroughly technical transformation of healthcare the last decade or so caused by the implementation of information and communication technology (ICT) in healthcare.

All kinds of actions in healthcare (i.e., patient registration, medical consultations, medical diagnosis, therapy, drug prescriptions, etc.) are nowadays supported by ICT. While, as medical philosophers Pellegrino and Thomasma state, "Medicine is at all levels a moral enterprise where 'moral enterprise' means action involving values" (Pellegrino & Thomasma, 1981, p. 112), the changes of medicine due to the application of new ICT have implications for the "moral enterprise" of medicine and should be assessed from an ethical point of view.

In this chapter, I will discuss some different ICT applications in healthcare. The first application is a system making patient information accessible for all healthcare units at a district, county, or even national level. The second application, the so-called patient portal, is a system for patient Internet access to his or her medical record. The third application is the use of Internet as a source of medical information, a means for medical consultation and for marketing of drugs. The three cases are different examples of recent ICT applications in healthcare that highlights partly different ethical problems.

ICT In Healthcare

A System for Patient Surveys

Patient information is usually stored in many different registers. There are, for example, systems for patient administration, patient's medical casebooks, patient records at clinics for intensive care, laboratory records, admission notes etc. A system collecting all kinds of patient information has recently been introduced in Swedish healthcare. It makes it possible for healthcare providers to have access to patient information in a given region, for example a county's regional healthcare. A requirement for access is that a person stands in a relation of care to the patient as doctor or nurse. The care providers must also log into the system with a personal code.

The patient information system provides information about the patient's previous consultations structured according to the time for a medical consultation, the kind of consultation, the care provider, and the place of the consultation. When the user clicks on one of the consultations, he or she gets information about that particular consultation, for instance information about a laboratory result or a diagnosis. A few healthcare units have been excluded from the system for reasons of confidentiality. One is psychiatry and another is women disease. The reasons for exclusion are that the information from psychiatry and women disease is considered to be too sensitive to be included. Why, it is asked, should a doctor have access to information about a patient's psychological status or about facts about previous abortions etc when wanting information about for example blood pressure.

Healthcare is becoming more and more divided and specialised. This development is sometimes described as the "care chain." In order to get the best treatment patients must consult various clinics and other healthcare centres. This development towards specialisation is not consistent with a patient information system that is decentralised to local healthcare centres. Hence, the new system fits the specialisation of healthcare. In this way, the system is "mediating" the value of specialisation.

The system will make patient information more accessible for doctors and other healthcare professionals irrespective of localisation, it will speed up treatment and it will decrease the number of medical tests and examinations. Thus, there is a potential for a less time consuming and more efficient healthcare.

Another reason for developing the system is that it will fasten up treatment of patients who meet with an accident away from home. When the patient is taken to a casualty department, doctors and nurses can immediately have access to the medical information they need.

Patient Portal

Patients are more and more involved in their own treatment. According to Swedish law, a patient has a right to access to his or her medical record. However, in practice it is rare for patients to request to read their records spontaneously (Ross & Lin, 2003).

The so-called patient portal gives a patient Internet access to his or her medical record. The patient can then have direct access to all medical information about him/herself that is available at the clinic. This implies for example that the patient will have access to information about diagnosis and laboratory results before meeting a doctor.

The technique that is used for the patient portal is similar to the technique used for Internet banking. The patient will get a personal certificate with a pin code that secures that no one else can get access to the information.

Even the introduction of the patient portal can be explained by tendencies in modern healthcare. There is an ongoing cut of healthcare costs and a need for prioritisation. When bank customers could do their bank affairs on the Internet, the number of customers visiting the bank offices decreased substantially, and consequently a number of bank employees were dismissed. As for banking, one can expect that the more patients have access to his or her medical casebook at the Internet, the less he or she has reasons to visit the healthcare centre. However, this assumption is not yet proven. According to a survey of patients using the patient portal, the number of visits to the health clinics was equal for a majority but had decreased for a minority (Bruzelius, 2004)

Another reason behind the patient portal is the emphasis put on patient autonomy in modern healthcare. The patient is expected to be actively involved in his or her own healthcare. However, autonomy requires information. If we expect that the patient increasingly should take responsibility for his or her own healthcare, the patient must be well informed. The patient portal can be used as a tool for achieving this goal. Furthermore, having access to his/her medical casebook gives the patient an opportunity to correct erroneous data.

E-Medicine

The Internet is used more and more for marketing and for providing medical information, medical consultation, and drug prescriptions. Medical information can be accessed from an increasing number of medical information sites, and drugs can be bought online. Hence, healthcare is going through a transformation due to different applications of e-medicine.

When a patient uses the Internet as a source of information about a disease, medicines, or ways of treatment, it is an example of, what has been called, "do-it-yourself healthcare." Consultation via the Internet is a way for those with sufficient economic resources to obtain a second opinion, yes, even a second doctor. There might be many possible reasons for this demand: the patient may have lost confidence in his or her ordinary doctor, he or she has heard of some specialist on the particular disease he or she is suffering from, he or she finds him or herself in a desperate situation, etc. E-medicine is also a potential asset for healthcare in poor countries with limited healthcare resources.

The number of health sites on the Internet is increasing. At the turn of the century, there were between 15,000 and 100,000 health-related sites in Great Britain and they had been visited by approximately 30 million people (Brann & Anderson, 2002; Parker & Gray, 2001). A Swedish survey showed that of those individuals that accessed Internet, about 20% had been looking for health-related information (Garpenby & Husberg, 2000).

The Internet has also become a market place for drugs. Here, customers can get hold of drugs without prescriptions or quality control.

The aim of this chapter is to make an ethical assessment of new ICT-applications in healthcare. But what does it mean to make an assessment from an ethical point of view? In the next section I will try to answer that question.

Framework for Ethical Analysis

Applied ethics focuses on the moral content of human practices. We act in different roles and capacities—as individuals, as professionals, and as citizens. A human practice is a social setting for human action. Through the introduction of new technologies, for example ICT, this practice might change in different ways

Ethics raises the questions of what are one's obligation, duty, and virtue and of what ideals and ends one should pursue (Williams, 1993). These are questions that any human being who takes his or her life seriously will reflect on. To make an ethical analysis or an ethical assessment is to deal with the ethical questions in a more systematic way. What obligations, duties and virtues are well-founded? How should they be ranked or prioritised? What ends are intrinsically valuable and what goals are instrumentally valuable?

To analyse an action (including a practice or a technology) from an ethical point of view is a systematic task. First, we must have information about the action. We examine how it influences the life and well-being of human beings. However, this empirical examination is only the first step of the ethical analysis. The second step is to assess the action normatively. Then the following kinds of question will be raised: Is the action beneficial or harming? Does it violate any rights? Does it show respect or disrespect for human dignity?

Clearly, an analysis of actions from an ethical point of view requires criteria. Why is a particular act right or wrong? What is the normative basis for a demand to change a practice? In order to answer these questions we must refer to ethical theory and principles. Ethical principles are generated from "ordinary morality" or "common morality". In ethical theory, the common morality is philosophically scrutinised with the aim of constructing a rational foundation for ethics. Ethical theories differ regarding what is to be considered as imperative or of basic value. For example, according to one common ethical theory, utilitarianism, only human wellbeing has intrinsic value. According to another ethical theory, Kantianism, respect for human dignity is a basic moral imperative.

The theoretical discussion in normative ethics concerns arguments for and against ethical principles and ethical theories. It is nowadays a common position that there is more than one ethical aspect that is important for an ethical assessment. This could mean, for example, that we should take both human well-being and human dignity into consideration. The most famous modern exponents of such a "mixed" ethical theory are the medical ethicists Beauchamp and Childress. They argue for a normative view that contains elements from both utilitarianism and Kantianism (Beauchamp et al., 2001)

When analysing moral problems and dilemmas in medicine, Beauchamp et al. refer to four ethical principles that, in their view, can be supported by different ethical theories and doctrines. The four principles are the principle of beneficence, the principle of non-maleficence, the principle of respect for autonomy, and the principle of justice. Two things are important to stress. First, these principles are vague and broad in scope and, hence, they must be interpreted and specified. Secondly, these principles do not provide any easy answers to moral problems. Rather, they work as a point of departure for normative reasoning and as framework for ethical reflection.

Beauchamp et al.'s four principles are general and applicable to different moral problems in healthcare. They can also be applied to moral problems in other spheres of society. When assessing ICT-systems in healthcare I will primarily refer to three principles. ICT influences how care is provided. Hence it will have implications for the shaping of the relationship between doctor (or any other healthcare provider) and patient. Responsibility for care is also of crucial importance. Two principles I will use as criteria when ethically assessing ICT in healthcare are the principle of doctor-patient relationship and the principle of responsibility. Further, access to new ICT-applications will influence the role of the patient. Hence it will affect patient autonomy. For this reason, the principle of respect for autonomy is the third principle of assessment I will use. I will now describe each of the principles.

The Principle of Doctor-Patient Relationship

The clinical encounter has for many years been an issue for discussions in medical ethics (Beauchamp et al., 2001; Pellegrino et al., 1981; Ramsey, 1970). The patient is in a vulnerable situation when his or her health or life is threatened and the clinical encounter is a means to recovery and/or of caring with the doctor as a mediator. (Pellegrino et al., 1981) With this bare description of the relationship between doctor and patient as a starting-point, I will outline the clinical interaction in different models, each focusing on specific aspects of the encounter.

According to the *engineering-model,* the patient is an object for treatment, in relevant aspects similar to a broken car taken to the garage for repair. In the engineering-model of a clinical encounter, the doctor collects information in order to make a diagnosis and a decision on therapy. The information needed is for example data on temperature, blood pressure etc. This model fits Engelhardt's description of "Medical care from passing strangers" (Engelhardt, 1986, p. 261)

Secondly, the doctor-patient relationship may also, in accordance with Pellegrino et al., be modelled as a *"healing relationship"* (Pellegrino et al., 1981, p. 64). Then, it is seen as an encounter between two persons, the doctor and the patient, which serves a specific purpose. The purpose of the encounter is to achieve a mutual understanding, or, in the words of philosopher Buber, an "I/Thou relationship" (Buber, 1923). This model pays attention to the fact, that a disease in many cases not only is a threat to the health of the patient but also to his or her existential balance.

Trust is closely related to the model of healing relationship (Pellegrino et al., 1981; Ramsey, 1970). Trust is based on two pillars, competence and sympathy. The patient can trust the doctor knowing that he or she is competent and knowing that he or she cares. The latter pillar highlights the moral aspects of the clinical encounter. According to this model, the relationship between doctor and patient is similar to one between friends, however, with the difference that the relationship between doctor and patient is asymmetrical. The patient needs the doctor for advice, care, and cure, but the doctor does not need the patient.

Thirdly, the relationship between doctor and patient can be modelled as a *contract.* Then the focus is on the rights and duties of the patient and the doctor, respectively. The professional ethical code of doctors can be seen as a framework for a formulation of the duties on the part of the doctor. However the duties of the patient remain, so far, tacit.

These models stress different aspects of the relationship between doctor and patient. They rather complete than exclude one another and a good doctor-patient relationship will balance these aspects. The engineering model with its emphasis on scientific and technical competence is essential for good treatment but the hermeneutical approach of the "healing relationship" is needed to allow the doctor to make the right decision and to involve the patient in the treatment. The relation between doctor and patient is embedded by values of commitment, trust, privacy, confidentiality, and responsibility. A principle of doctor-patient relationship stresses the moral duty of healthcare personnel to live up to these values and to establish a healing relationship. As a consequence, the organisation of healthcare, as well as the technology used in healthcare, should facilitate the realisation of this principle.

The Principle of Responsibility

Information and consultation via the Internet is associated with some problems concerning responsibility in healthcare. Hence, I will discuss the impact of these ICT-applications on responsibility in healthcare. The ethical criterion is then a principle of responsibility. But what does responsibility mean and why is it important from an ethical perspective?

We say that some person P is responsible for the outcome O of an action A, when P has intentionally done A in order to achieve O. P who is responsible must be able to answer questions like: *Why did you do A? Why did you want O? If O is a bad outcome, as a result of being responsible, this is a reason to blame or punish P and, vice versa, if the outcome is good this is a reason to praise P* (Lucas, 1995).

However, in order to hold a person responsible, there are some conditions that have to be fulfilled. If the outcome, due to some factors that P reasonably could not foresee, is different from what P intended, say O1 instead of O, P is not responsible for O1. However, if P acts without bothering to get the necessary information, P is responsible for O1, if O1 could have been foreseen, had she bothered to inform herself sufficiently. Neither is it reasonable to say that P is responsible for O, if O is caused by an action that P was forced to do.

In ethical discourse, responsibility is also seen as a character trait or a virtue. A "responsible person" is a person who takes his or her responsibility serious.

The term "responsibility" is used both in moral and legal senses. The main differences are the criteria for evaluating the outcome and the sanctions following a blameworthy action. In law, a sovereign legislator formally decides the criteria for evaluation and sanctions. In morality, on the other hand, the social ethos provides the criteria for evaluation and sanctions.

There is also a third usage of responsibility, referring to the profession. Professional responsibility is a kind of responsibility that combines traits of legal and of moral responsibility. The criteria for evaluation are basically moral, outlined in professional ethical codes. However, professional responsibility is similar to legal responsibility when the professional organisation has decided on some sanction (e.g., expulsion from the profession) for those who do not comply with the professional moral duties.

Let us now apply the concept of responsibility to medical practice. P, the doctor, recommends or prescribes A, for instance medication or surgery, in order to achieve O (i.e., the restoration of a patient's health). The doctor is responsible for medical treatment. This means that the doctor with the best intentions, and to the best of his or her knowledge, makes a decision on treatment. If something goes wrong, the doctor will be questioned "Why did you recommend or prescribe A?" Maltreatment will result in some kind of sanctions, for example a warning.

A *principle* of responsibility in healthcare implies that it is morally desirable that healthcare professionals take responsibility. They have as professionals even a moral obligation to be responsible.

The Principle of Respect for Autonomy

Healthcare is traditionally a paternalistic institution, relying on the assumption that the doctor knows what is best for the patient. However, paternalism is challenged and the principle of patient autonomy has increasingly become important in modern healthcare and it is as we have seen one of Beauchamp et al.'s four bioethical principles. The principle of respect for autonomy implies that anyone who is affected by a decision should be able to influence it and if a decision only concerns one individual, he or she should have the right to decide for him or herself. When applied to healthcare, the principle implies that the patient should be empowered to play a more active role in his or her own care. One way to do this is that the patient has the opportunity to give informed consent to the decisions that concern his or her own treatment.

The realisation of the principle of respect for autonomy, or, of the derived principle of informed consent, depends on at least three conditions. One is that there are alternatives available in the decision-making situation. Only in situations where patients have a choice is it meaningful to speak of patient autonomy. Another condition is that the patient is competent. In order to be able to make an autonomous decision the patient must be competent. Competence implies an ability to understand and process information and to form a decision on the basis of the information. A third condition is that the patient has access to reliable, non-biased and relevant information. (Beauchamp et al., 2001)

Privacy means, for example, control of sensitive information about oneself. Hence, respect for privacy means that the person her or himself should decide who has access to this kind of information. Hence, the principle of autonomy also implies respect for privacy.

To sum up: In the following I will discuss the ethical implications of new ICT-systems in healthcare. As ethical criteria, I will use the principles of doctor-patient relationship, responsibility, and respect for autonomy. Thus, the following questions (seen in Table 1) are raised.

Table 1.

Principle of doctor-patient relationship	Does ICT- application x contribute to or prevent a good doctor-patient relationship?
Principle of responsibility	Does ICT-application x strengthen or weaken responsibility in healthcare?
Principle of respect for autonomy	Does ICT-application x strengthen or weaken patient autonomy?

Ethics and New ICT Applications in Healthcare

Ethics and Patient Information Systems

There is an ethical argument for developing systems for patient information. The possibility to make patient information more accessible for doctors and other healthcare professionals and the subsequent speeding up of treatments can be justified by the principle of beneficence. The expected decrease of the number of blood tests and other painful examinations can be justified by the principle of non-maleficence.

However, there are also ethical problems connected to the system. I commented earlier that the system fits well with and even facilitates specialization of healthcare. One can have doubts about whether the development towards specialization is beneficial for the patient. This development can be justified by the effort to provide competent and appropriate medical care. However, there is an obvious risk that the personal aspects of the clinical encounter will get lost, and hence, the system will be an obstacle to the realisation of the principle of doctor-patient relationship. In that case, this is a morally relevant unintended effect of this new technology. However, another alternative scenario is also possible. The system can be used as a means for decentralization. It can provide local clinics with patient information helping the GP to provide treatment of a kind that otherwise would require specialized care. Hence, the system is malleable and whether it will contribute to centralization or decentralization of healthcare is dependent on decisions taken by those involved in its design and introduction.

Of ethical relevance is also the question whether to exclude information about psychiatry and women disease or not. The reason for exclusion is that information from these clinics is considered to be too sensitive regarding privacy. If any care provider can have access to psychiatric information or information about (venereal disease), this will imply a privacy violation. Thus, this kind of information should not be accessible to any user of the system.

There are two possible objections to this exclusion. First, it can further stigmatize these kind of diseases. For example, the view that a psychiatric disease is in some way more problematic or shameful than a physiological is a prejudice. Exclusion of this kind of information from the system will possibly strengthen these prejudices. The same can be said about the exclusion of women disease. The second objection is that the system will be less reliable if some information is excluded. One can imagine situations of emergency when this information would be needed.

On the other hand, there seems to be good reasons for a policy of exclusion. When considering possible privacy violations, the relevant question is what kind of information is considered privacy sensitive now and by most people, not what information ought to be considered sensitive. Sensitive information is according to Parent, "…facts about a person, which most individuals in a given society at a given time do not want widely known about themselves" (Parent, 1983, p. 216) And, as a matter of fact, in our society, at this given time, information about psychiatric diseases and abortions are of this kind. Furthermore, if this information was included many patients would probably refuse to give their informed consent to participate. On the other hand, this kind of information is also prevalent in primary care and can, thus, anyway be accessible in the patient information system.

This leads us to another ethical question. Through this technology, more healthcare staff will have access to confidential information. Earlier, this kind of information was normally kept between the patient and his or her doctor. Now it is available at clinics all over the region. The wider access to patient information, the greater the risk for privacy violation.

How, then, can privacy violations be avoided? First, the patient has the right to give his or her informed consent to have his or her medical data registered in the system. The patient's wish to give informed consent is dependent on the security of the system. If this cannot be guaranteed in a reasonable way, the patient will probably refuse to consent. We know from experience that no system is completely secure. There is always a possibility that some hacker will crack a code or that a healthcare professionals will misuse the system. However, these fears should not be overemphasized. There are fewer motives for hackers to crack a code to a healthcare system than to, for example, a military security system. The provision of access can be designed in such a way that any non-authorized person can be traced. Thus, if the protection of privacy is taken seriously when designing the system, we should expect very few cases of privacy violations.

The principle of informed consent implies also the right to give an informed non-consent. But what happens to those patients who refuse to consent to have their medical data registered in the system? In public healthcare, where all citizens have a right to healthcare, this should of course also be provided to those who refuse to consent, in a similar way as those who refuse to take part in medical experiment all the same should get an equal care. However, for obvious reasons non-consent will have some consequences for the patient. In situations of emergency, a refusal to give consent could imply impediment to efficient and fast treatment.

Ethics and Patient Portal

Access to information is one condition for patient autonomy in healthcare. There is so far little empirical evidence of how electronic patient access to the medical records will influence patient autonomy. However, the evidence from other forms of patient access is predominantly positive. Ross et al. refer to several studies reporting that for the majority of patients reading their own medical records educated them about their medical condition. Further, these studies do not confirm that the access generated anxiety or concern among the patients. Especially seems the access of obstetric patients to their records have had a positive effect on their sense of autonomy and self-efficacy (Ross et al., 2003). But, in contrast to the patient portal this access was mediated by a doctor or a nurse, who could explain the content and answer questions.

Through the patient portal, patients will potentially be better informed about their health status. However, more information does not necessarily contribute to patient autonomy. For a patient to be able to handle information and use it in a constructive way, information provided must be comprehended and relevant. No doubt, through access to the medical record the patient will gain access to much information but, one may ask, does he or she have the tools to handle it? If not, the information will not help in empowering the patient, but instead leave the patient confused and insecure. Some studies of non-electronic patient access to medical records confirm that patients commonly have difficulties in understanding parts of their medical records (Ross et al., 2003).

The introduction of patient portals will affect the way medical records are written. As a consequence of the direct patient access the notes in the medical record should be of a "reasonable person standard" (i.e., understandable for an "average" patient) rather than of a "professional practice standard" (i.e., understandable for doctors only) (Beauchamp et al., 2001). However, this may also imply that the doctors write their notes with this restriction in mind and that some important information that requires to be written in a professional and technical language will be left out.

Then, is it a good idea to give the patient full access to his or her medical record? The record might contain information about the patient that is— according to the principle of responsibility—necessary for the doctor to record, but that can be harmful for the patient to read. For example, a doctor may have to record that a patient is untalented and will not be expected to take his or her medicine as prescribed, or that battering may have caused some wounds on a child's body etc. The fact that the doctor has to record even unfavourable facts about patients in their best interest can be seen as a kind of weak paternalism. Thus, in this kind of cases, what is in the best interests of the patient may come into conflict with the patient's right to have full access to his or her own medical record.

Thus, there are two problems with giving the patient direct access to his/her medical record. It may lead to a less precise way of expressing relevant medical information and it may contain for the patient harmful information. A possible solution to these problems is that the information given to the patient is filtered. However, this would be very costly and also very difficult to implement. It would also lay a too heavy burden on the "filterer" who is to decide what information that could pass through and according to what standard of language.

Ethics and E-Medicine

E-medicine includes consultation, information, and marketing of drugs via the Internet. How will the relation between doctor and patient, doctor's responsibility and patient autonomy be affected by Internet consultation? Consultation is made at a distance. Personal encounter and face-to face relationship between doctor and patient is lacking. Instead, the clinical encounter fits Engelhardt's description of "Medical care from passing strangers." (Engelhardt, 1986, p. 261)

However, the lack of face-to face relationship might change when the technical possibilities for a Web-based dialogue and interactive media communication between doctor and patient are developed. In an assessment of how nurses interpreted "telecare," including videophone communication for the care of frail elderly persons, Sävenstedt writes: "The apprehension was that ICT applications could facilitate genuiness in relations through an increased possibility of having an ongoing dialogue...Superficiality was connected to a general fear that the use of ICT applications would contribute to a caring situation for frail elderly where the closeness and intimacy of face-to-face communication was reduced and replaced by a remote form of communication" (Sävenstedt, 2004, p. 34) As Sävenstedt's empirical investigation illustrates, videophone communication has a potential even for the care of frail elderly. For young people who are used to electronic communication and who have established relationships on Web-sites etc., Internet mediated medical consultation will probably pose less problems.

What implications will access to medical consultation and information via the Internet have for patient autonomy? Access to medical information via Internet gives the patient access to new sources of information, one requirement for patient autonomy. Access to Internet-consultation gives the patient a choice of a second opinion. Hence, one could argue that the patient is empowered through e-medicine. On the other hand, there are problems related to Internet-consultation. When the patient contacts a doctor via Internet, how can she judge the quality of the doctor? Is it a competent doctor or just a quack?

A similar problem is connected to medical information accessible on the Internet. One can, at present, find a lot of Web sites for any disease and treatments. Many of these Web sites are trustworthy and contain reliable information but there are exceptions. A study by American gastroenterologists found that one in ten of the health-related sites in the field offered unproven treatments (Barkham, 2000). In another study of 25 health sites, only 45% of the English health sites and 22% of the Spanish were judged to be completely accurate (Brann et al., 2002).

Pharmaceutical companies are responsible for some medical sites. Although they are presumably normally of a high standard, they may be biased for commercial reasons. Thus, the patient will have problems distinguishing between reliable and less reliable sites. As a consequence, a patient looking for information about his or her disease and possible ways of treatment runs the risk of being misinformed (Brann et al., 2002; Silberg, Lundberg, & Musacchio, 1997)

Besides, all the problems connected to the transfer of information from healthcare provider to patient in ordinary healthcare will be present in e-medicine in more aggravated forms: Is the information provided in an understandable language? Is it adjusted to the ability of the patient to process the information? Does the patient really understand the prescription?

Beauchamp et al. distinguish between three standards of disclosure of informa-tion—professional standard, the reasonable person standard, and the subjective standard (Beauchamp et al., 2001). Medical Web sites that disclose information for professionals provide new sources of information for doctors, but are of limited value for the ordinary patient. The sites for ordinary patients are usually written according to a reasonable person standard. These sites can provide the patient with valuable information, helpful for anyone who wants to know more about a disease. Finally, the subjective standard takes the informational needs of the specific patient into consideration. This standard requires an interactive site, which provides the patient with opportunities to enter into a dialogue and to question the information presented. Thus, it seems that medical information via the Internet can be a valuable source for patients wanting to learn more about their disease, provided that there are means to discern which sources are reliable. In this way, the Internet will facilitate the fulfilment of the principle of patient autonomy in healthcare.

From the point of view of both moral and legal responsibility there are problems connected to therapy at a distance via the Internet. Firstly, the doctor might base his or her decision on insufficient information. This is obviously the fact if the diagno-sis is based solely on the patient's own story. If the Internet doctor also has access to the patient's medical records, there is a better basis for diagnosis and therapy. However, the doctor is still lacking information that in ordinary care is received through a personal encounter face to face with a patient, as well as information obtained through a physical examination of the patient's body. Secondly, while lacking a personal encounter, the Internet-doctor is less confident than a regular GP that the patient will follow the recommendations. The possibility of misunder-standing increases the risk that the patient will take the wrong drug or the wrong dosage. Taken together, these factors increase the risk of maltreatment. But it is a risk that the Internet-doctor ought to be conscious about and, thus, he/she is morally responsible for the possible maltreatment.

When we ask about the Internet doctor's legal responsibility in the case of maltreatment we are entering precarious ground. Assuming that the Internet doctor is licensed as a doctor, principles for advisory services should be applied. However, one has to establish in what country the consultation is taking place. Is it in the country of the patient, of the doctor or somewhere between, in cyberspace perhaps? The answer is also decisive for the question, which law that should be applied. According to EU regulations adopted 2001, the law suit should either take place at the court where the harmful event occurred or in the country where the wrongful action was carried out.

Is it possible to apply codes of professional responsibility in the case of maltreatment? If the Internet doctor is a member of the World Medical Association, he or she will be subject to the professional code of the association. This would imply that professional criteria for evaluation and the sanctions for non-compliance would be applied, irrespective of the nationality of the doctor. This is an example of the advantage of an international professional association when dealing with a global technological system.

The possibility to consult doctors on the Internet is of recent date. But, does the Internet-doctor really represent anything new? Have not people always consulted other doctors than their regular ones, for instance a friend or a radio doctor? And what is the difference between using the Internet as a source of information and other media like medical handbooks and encyclopaedias?

There are similarities as well as differences between consulting a friend who is a doctor and consulting an Internet doctor. One similarity is that the patient consults a second doctor and, as a consequence, this doctor becomes involved. A difference is that one important reason to seek help from a friend (i.e., the emotional component of trust) is lacking in the case of the Internet-doctor. And this difference is important. You can count on the friend caring.

There are also similarities between a radio-doctor and a doctor's question and answers column in a magazine on the one hand and the Internet-doctor on the other. In all these cases a sick or worried person gets advice concerning his or her particular worries. And this advice is given without a doctor patient encounter or a personal emotional involvement. One difference, however, is that while the Internet-doctor engages in a particular consultation, the radio- or magazine-doctor usually does not establish a personal doctor to patient interaction. Instead, he/she answers the particular questions in a general way so that anyone interested can take advantage of the recommendation.

There are some obvious similarities between the Internet as a source of medical information and medical handbooks. Both will provide the reader with information about diseases. An advantage with an Internet site is that it can continuously be updated. A possible difference is, as we have noticed, that it is more difficult to control the reliability of the Internet site (i.e., to distinguish a reliable source from a bluff).

Ethics, Technology Assessment, and Introduction of New ICT-Systems

We have noticed that new ICT-systems in healthcare raise important ethical questions. How should these systems be introduced and how can they be part of an ethically based healthcare? By raising these questions I assume that the moral justification of ICT-systems in healthcare is depending on

- How the systems are introduced and who has a say, and, on
- How these systems fit with an ethically based healthcare system.

When the system for patient information was about to be introduced in Swedish healthcare some general practitioners questioned it. The system was then discussed in an ethics committee and the committee formulated some questions about possible risks for privacy violations. As a consequence, a consensus conference with the ethics committee, healthcare professionals and computing personal participating was called together. At this conference, the concerns of the GPs and the committee were discussed and some guidelines for the implementation of the system were formulated.

Is this a way to get acceptance of new technological systems in healthcare? Proponents of what is called "constructive technology assessment" (CTA) or "interactive technology assessment" (iTA) would give an affirmative answer. According to ethicist Schot, social problems surrounding technology must be addressed through a broadening of the design process. This process should then involve more social actors (i.e., stakeholders that are involved and will be affected by the new technology should also exert influence on the designing process). Schot proposes a more ambitious involvement than just one consensus conference. Social actors should according to Schot be involved in the design process as well as in the implementation of a new technology as a regular activity. Technological development is unpredictable and hence, anticipation must be organized as a regular activity (Reuzel, van derWilt, Ten Have, & de Vries, 2001; Schot, 2001).

When asking for inclusion and participation, proponents of CTA are challenging an essentialist view of technology as well as the idea of autonomous technology.

Accordingly, technology should not be understood as autonomous, impossible to influence, and separated from its social context but instead, as the result of social intentions, design decisions etc and these intentions and decisions are not given beforehand but instead possible to influence. The point of assessing new ICT technologies in healthcare from an ethical point of view is to provide arguments for an ICT development in line with basic values of healthcare.

References

Barkham, P. (2000). Is the net healthy for doctors? *The Guardian Online, 8,* 2, June 2000.

Beauchamp, T., & Childress, J. (2001). *Principles of biomedical ethics.* Oxford: Oxford University Press.

Brann, M., & Anderson, J. G. (2002). E-medicine and healthcare consumers: Recognizing current problems and possible resolutions for a safer environment. *Health Care Analysis, 10,* 403-415.

Bruzelius, M. (2004). *Sammanfattning och slutsatser. Patientportalen.* SKILL Studentkompetens AB, (unpublished) Linköping.

Buber, M. (1923). *Ich und Du,* Leipzig, Insel.

Engelhardt, T. (1986). *The foundations of bioethics,* New York: Oxford University Press.

Garpenby, P., & Hisberg, M. (2000) *Hälsoinformation idag och imorgon,* CMT Rapport 2000:3, Linköpings universitet, (unpublished) Linköping

Health on the Net Foundation Code of Conduct, retrieved September 3, 2006 from http://www.hon.ch/HONcode/Conduct.html.

Lucas, J. R. (1995). *Responsibility.* Oxford: Clarendon Press.

McMullin, E. (1983). Introduction. *The Journal of Medicine and Philosophy, 8,* 2-4.

Parent, W.A. (1983). Privacy, morality, and the law. *Philosophy and Public Affairs, 12*(4).

Parker, M., & Muir Gray, J. A. (2001). What is the role of clinical ethics support in the era of e-medicine? *Journal of Medical Ethics,* 2001; 27, suppl I:i, 33-35

Pellegrino, E. D., & Thomasma, D. C. (1981). *A philosophical basis of medical practice.* Oxford: Oxford University Press.

Ramsey, P. (1970). *The patient as person. Explorations in medical ethics.* New Haven, CT: Yale University Press.

Reiser, S. (1978). *Medicine and the reign of technology*. Cambridge: Cambridge University Press.

Reuzel, R. F. P., van derWilt, G. J., Ten Have, H., & de Vries, R. (2001). Interactive technology assessment and wide reflective equilibrium. *Journal of Medicine and Philosophy, 26*(3), 245-261

Ross, S. E., & Lin, C. T. (2003). The effects of promoting patient access to medical records: A review. *Journal of the American Medical Informatics Association, 10*(2).

Schot, J. (2001). Constructive technology assessment as reflexive technology politics. *Technology and Ethics*, eds, Goujon, P. & Heriard Dubreil, B., Leuven, Peeters pp 239-249.

Silberg, W. M., Lundberg, G. D., & Musacchio, R. A. (1997). Assessing, controlling, and assuring the quality of medical information on the Internet. *Journal of American Medical Association, 277*, 1244-1245.

Sundberg, A. (2003). *Nulägesbeskrivning av attityder till patientportalen 2003*, Landstinget i Östergötland, (unpublished),

Sävenstedt, S. (2004) *Telecare of frail elderly – reflections and experiences among health personnel and family members*, Umeå University Medical Dissertations, .

Williams, B. (1993). *Ethics and the limits of philosophy.* London, Fontana Press.

Endnote

[1]   This article draws partly on my article "The Internet doctor and medical ethics", in *Medicine, Health Care and Philosophy*, Vol. 5, No 2, 2002 and my conference papers at Ethicomp 2004, in Syros, Greece, CEPE, 2005 in Enschede, the Netherlands and 7th International Conference on Human Choice and Computers, IFIP, in Maribor, Slovenia 2006.

Section II

Trust, Values, and Healthcare Information Systems

Chapter III

Trust and Clinical Information Systems

Rania Shibl, University of the Sunshine Coast, Australia

Kay Fielden, UNITEC New Zealand, New Zealand

Andy Bissett, Sheffield Hallam University, UK

Den Pain, Massey University, New Zealand

Abstract

Our study of the use of clinical decision support systems by general practitioners in New Zealand reveals the pervasive nature of the issue of trust. "Trust" was a term that spontaneously arose in interviews with end users, technical support person- nel, and system suppliers. Technical definitions of reliability are discussed in our chapter, but the very human dimension of trust seems at least as significant, and we examine what is bound up in this concept. The various parties adopted differ- ent means of handling the trust question, and we explain these. Some paradoxical aspects emerge in the context of modern information systems, both with the question of trust and with the provision of technical or organisational solutions in response to the existence of trust. We conclude by considering what lessons may be drawn, both in terms of the nature of trust and what this might mean in the context of information systems.

Introduction

The use of information technology (IT) in healthcare highlights some issues in the social domain surrounding such technology that might otherwise go unremarked. This chapter discusses the nature of trust and the meanings that this concept might have in the context of computer systems. "Trust" in relation to IT is usually taken to convey an aspect of dependability or security (McDermid, 1991), but it might be that "trust" is both a richer and a more useful concept in relation to some computer systems than in the sense of the narrower, more technical definitions such as "dependability" or "reliability" that software and hardware engineering tend to employ. Trust as a human phenomenon in relation to IT is starting to be discussed, and the concept's use (Raab, 1998) and misuse (de Laat, 2004) have been noted. For the field of computer ethics the term has the advantage that an implicit ethical dimension is captured. We found, when investigating clinical decision support systems (CDSS) in New Zealand, that the term was used unprompted by several different stakeholders when discussing their relationships with other stakeholders and with the technology itself. It seems that trust is an ever-present factor in joint human activity, however technically based that enterprise may initially appear to be.

After a brief discussion of the nature of trust we describe the health sector environment in New Zealand, define clinical decision support systems, introduce the case study, go on to a discussion of our findings, and finally present some conclusions about the meaning of trust in the context of IT.

The Nature of Trust

If, as Bottery (2000) says, "Trust is the cement of human relationships" (p. 71), then we may expect it to feature in the worlds of business and technology as much as in individual relationships. Fukuyama (1996) advances an extensive argument relating the flourishing of business and macro-economic success to the societal prevalence of stable, predictable, trustworthy dealings possible between individual and organisational actors. Echoing this, Bottery remarks how the absence of trust tends to result in, amongst other things: "detailed accountability, exhaustive legal agreements, and extensive litigation … it can mean vastly increased transaction costs, which can have important implications for the efficient use of time and money" (p. 72). O'Neill (2002) takes up these themes of accountability and litigation to develop a broadly Kantian perspective on trust. She argues that, whilst suspicion and mistrust *appear* to be increasing in the developed world, the world of the "audit society" (Power, 1997), nonetheless "We constantly place trust in others, in members of professions and in institutions" (O'Neill, 2002, p. 11). Often we have no ultimate guarantee, and at some point, we have to trust in a chain of information and the judgement that it informs: "Guarantees are useless unless they lead to a trusted source, and a regress of guarantees is no better for being longer unless it ends in a trusted source" (p. 6). O'Neill goes on to note the paradoxical circumstance that the proliferation of sources in the "information society" not only does not make trust redundant; it makes it if anything more problematical. Who should we trust in this world of instantaneous and burgeoning communication? How can we make informed judgements in a world of "information overload" and, sometimes, deliberate misinformation?

O'Neill (2002) offers that trust is needed "because we have to be able to rely on others acting as they say that they will, and because we need others to accept that we will act as we say we will" (p. 4). Borrowing the concept from monetary instruments such as banknotes or coins, some writers have called this ability to accept something (or someone) at face value as "fiduciary," and this fiduciary aspect is no less relevant to the duties of the IT professional, as Gotterbarn (1996) has tellingly argued. Noting that as professions gain in maturity so the nature of their ethical codes change, he writes of maturer professions: "The function of the code is not to protect the profession, but to establish the standards of trust required in a fiduciary relationship ... The fiduciary model is an adequate model of professionalism for computer practitioners" (p. 11). Nearly all definitions of trust share the condition that one party (the truster) must willingly place himself or herself in a position of vulnerability to or risk from another party (the trustee) (Gallivan, 2001; Gotterbarn, 1996). Karahannas and Jones (1999) note that trust is "closely related to risk, since without vulnerability… there is no need for trust" (p. 347). This brings us to our case study, wherein many risks and vulnerabilities are possible.

The New Zealand Health Sector

In the period 1991-2006 New Zealand's health sector has undergone repeated restructuring (Gauld, 2006). The health sector is highly politicised and complex with a history of poorly implemented national ICT systems. In the various restructuring exercises (Gauld, 2006; Wills, 2006) the move, from a public health point of view, has been from a market-oriented approach to a collaborative health service environment upon which managed health IT systems have been a key requirement. This situation of flux, political involvement, and layered complexity has meant that, at the primary health care provider level, primary practitioner trust in ICT has been compromised. On one hand, primary practitioners know they can benefit in a number of ways from ICT supported decision support systems, and on the other hand, the many structural changes have fostered generalised distrust within the health sector.

It is known also that primary practitioners are late adopters of technology (Gauld, 2006) and that voluntary adoption is required for such systems as clinical decision support. Over the last fifteen years, late adoption, together with a public health sector in a continuous state of flux, technologically, has provided a barrier to trust for primary health care decision support systems.

Over this period funded research in health IT systems has been directed at managed systems for public health, not in private practice clinical support. It is as if the political agendas operating during this period have fuelled themselves on one restructure after another, with the political stakeholders rather than the primary care practitioners driving the funding of research in the health sector in New Zealand.

Clinical Decision Support Systems

Within the medical field, there are large amounts of data and information, and the quantities are continuously growing. A general practitioner needs to be kept up to date with this ever-increasing knowledge. Wyatt (1991) estimated that the doubling time of medical knowledge is about 19 years. Using this calculation, during a doctor's professional lifetime medical knowledge will have increased four-fold.

Computer technology can aid with this abundance of knowledge. Information technology used in the area of clinical medicine is known as clinical information systems. Clinical information systems can be divided into four categories (Simpson & Gordon, 1998). These four categories are based on core activities within health-

Table 1. Categories and core activities of clinical information systems

Category	Core Activities	CIS example
Clinical management	Assessment of patient observation and investigation and decision formulation in terms of patient care and management.	Decision support system to aid in clinicians decision making process of diagnosis.
Clinical administration	Scheduling, arranging investigations and appointments, clinical correspondence.	Patient management system for creating appointments and billing.
Clinical services	Support services such as laboratory results, imaging facilities, ward, and theatre management.	
General management	Financial, HR.	Management Information system for payroll, HR.

care: (1) clinical management; (2) clinical administration; (3) clinical services; and (4) general management. Each category has several activities; each of which can be assisted with an information system. Table 1 shows the list of activities for each category and an example of an associated clinical information system (CIS).

The clinical management category is centred around the management of the patient. Clinical information systems in this area often focus on aiding the clinician with the decision making process, hence the use of clinical decision support systems (CDSS).

The main essence of a clinical decision support system is that it should provide the clinician with knowledge, which is patient related and relevant to the current dilemma (Farman, Honeyman, & Kinirons, 2003). Clinical decision support systems are used for a number of purposes. Nevertheless, their use is based on their ability to enhance/improve decisions (Delaney, Fitzmaurice, Riaz, & Hobbs, 1999; Shortliffe, Perreault, Fagan, & Wiederhold, 1990). The role of a CDSS is to improve the clinician's decision without replacing human judgement (Bemmel, 1997).

Clinical decision support systems use artificial intelligence techniques for analysing knowledge and solving problems with that knowledge (Thornett, 2001). They can range from simple systems based on a simple algorithm or complex systems, which draw upon patient data and a database of clinical knowledge and guidelines (Wyatt & Spiegelhalter, 1990). Most clinical decision support systems have been developed for specific medical domains such as diabetes or cardiovascular medicine (Ridderichoff & van Herk, 1997). These medical domains have specific expert knowledge, captured by numerous organisations and codified into knowledge bases. These knowledge bases are the basis of clinical decision support systems and consist of structured and unstructured medical knowledge (Akinyokun & Adeniji, 1991). Typically in a GP's surgery a CDSS might be used to check the amount of paediatric dose (as opposed to adult dose) when making a prescription, or to check on harmful interactions between two or more prescriptions.

The Case Study

This research is a small-scale case study, which examined four groups of people in the healthcare area. In New Zealand the majority of GPs are organised into groups called Independent Practitioner Associations (IPAs). IPAs are now part of "Primary Health Organisations," which provide the first line of health care to a particular geographical area. In addition, IPAs also provide a range of support services including information technology support—and therefore CDSS operation—for their GP members.

The groups were interviewed in depth regarding the use, development, and implementation of a CDSS. The following were the participants of the study:

- Three doctors who would use decision support systems in their work;
- Two practice managers (IPAs);
- One knowledge company who wrote their own software;
- One knowledge company whose data was incorporated into an IS by other organizations (software developers).

It has often been argued that small-scale studies are unlikely to provide general conclusions from a small sample (Bell, 1987; Tellis, 1997). However, it has also been strongly argued (Bassey, 1981; Hamel et al., 1993; Yin, 2003) that the merit of a case study, whatever the size, is the extent to which details are adequate and suitable for someone in a similar situation. Bassey (1981) also states "the relatability of a case is more important than its generalisability" (p. 85). Many related cases in different reports by various researchers can later be used to form an overall idea about a situation (Bassey, 1999). Thus, small cases still have a significant role to play in research.

The interviews were approximately an hour long and were based on open-ended questions. The interviews were not tape-recorded. The original intention of the discussions was to find partners, GPs, IPAs, knowledge companies, and software developers for an in-depth study into the design and use of CDSS in practice. During the interviews, the four parties all indirectly raised the notion of trust with regard to the use and development of clinical decision support systems. The questions in Table 2 were some of those which related to the issue of trust and DSS infrastructure.

The theme of trust arose at different system levels within the investigation and at both sides of the CDSS in question, from the user wanting to place trust in the decisions provided by the system to the database owners wanting enquiries based on their data to be trustworthy.

Trust in a CDSS at the highest level could be the medical practitioner's trust in the CDSS and in turn the patient's trust of the practitioner and CDSS working together successfully. From an information systems perspective, however, it is clear that there are a number of other systems involved, each of which has to work effectively and be trusted by other parties for this top level of trust to be on a sure footing. In particular, consider a CDSS where the data is maintained by one company (often a publishing company) and is presented through application software developed by another, yet all of the associated hardware and software are managed by general practitioner clinics themselves. This is the usual case in New Zealand.

Table 2. Questions used in the interviews which elicited answers related to trust issues

Doctors	Knowledge companies	Knowledge companies (who develop their own software)	Practice managers
Are there any knowledge companies, which you have issues with?	How long have you been in the industry?	How long have you been in the industry?	How many GPs are in your IPA?
What are these issues?	What made you go electronic?	Was your company always into software development?	What degree of authority do the GPs have?
Are there any software developers, which you have issues with?	How do you ensure that your publishing is accurate?	What made you decide to develop your own software?	What role does the IPA have towards the GPs?
What are these issues?	How do you choose software developers to develop your publishing?	What benefits and limitations do you think developing your own software has?	In terms of IT, what role does the IPA have?
	Are there concerns with the software development process?		Who decides which software is to be installed, do the doctors have a say?
	How do you identify errors in the software development process?		
	How do you ensure that minimal errors occur in the software development process?		
	How do you ensure doctors use the correct version of your publications?		

Naturally there are other systems involved, such as the distribution of data updates from the original publishers through to the GP's desktop. Thus a chain or network of trust exists. This concept of needing a network of trust has been recognised in the literature (see Muir (1994), for example).

Trust and Computer Systems: The Technical View

Computer users are more complacent when a system is thought to perform correctly, and if an error occurs, the user's trust in the system will decrease (Muir, 1994). Vries, Midden, and Bouwhuis (2003) found that users who experienced low error rates in a computerised system used the system more than did users who experienced a high error rate. A similar effect was found from a manual system: people displayed a tendency to abstain from use of a manual system with high error rates. However, Vries et al. (2003) found that with the computerised system, the error rates were lower than with the manual system, suggesting that users are more critical of errors occurring with computerised systems and that errors greatly impact the users' trust of the IS.

Several factors underlying trust in automation have been identified, including predictability, reliability, and dependability. Rempel, Holmes, and Zanna (1985) concluded that trust would progress in three stages over time, from predictability to dependability to faith. Muir and Moray (1996) extended these factors and developed a trust model that contains six components: predictability, dependability, faith, competence, responsibility, and reliability. Muir (1987) states that trust is a critical factor in the design of computer systems as trust can impact the use or non-use of computers, and later findings by Vries et al. (2003) confirm this tendency.

Yet it is interesting to note here that trust essentially depends upon the human perceptions of the computer system. Alongside the technical dimension of a computer system and intermingling with it lies the very human question of trust. Whilst the studies above discuss the issue of trust in direct usage of a decision support system, there is a lack of research into trust and the various sub-systems or components that provide the infrastructure of a decision support system used in practice. Each of these components can have an impact on the development, support, and use of the decision support system, and from our research we have seen a number of examples where trust has been a significant factor in the relationship between the various parties involved with different aspects of CDSS infrastructure.

Trust and the Chain of Support

Take the situation, previously outlined, for the infrastructure of a CDDS used in practice. The development of a clinical decision support system involves a number of components. The data used in the clinical decision support system is often created by a knowledge company, the data produced depending on the expertise of the company. This data is then used by the software developer to create a system; in some cases the developer is part of the knowledge company. Once the system is created it is checked by the knowledge company, and then distributed either directly to an independent GP or to a group of GPs through an IPA. It can be seen that there are a number of situations where trust needs to exist between the providers of the components. These are discussed next.

Chain of Support: Knowledge Company and the Software Developer

In order for the developer to use the data to create the system, the knowledge company needs to give the developer the right (often in the form of a license) to use the data, which in its simplest form are tables. It is important for the knowledge company that the developer creates the system correctly, as an error in the development often results in the user not trusting the system as a whole, including the database. With one knowledge company with which we spoke, they were concerned that the representation of their data was not as they expected once the system was developed. This led them initially to employ someone as a systems integrator to ensure that software developers were fully aware of how the data should be handled. Some of the initial problems reported were simple errors in queries, such as only reporting the first match of a drug interaction, rather than showing the full list of interactions held in the data. The second phase of the knowledge company wishing to keep responsibility for its own data has resulted in them changing the format of the data in order to achieve the representation they want. It was reported to us that the software developers also appreciated this situation as they were reluctant to take the responsibility for someone else's data (knowledge base).

In another instance, a knowledge company did not trust any software developer to develop a system with their data, which resulted in them developing their own systems. The main concern with this knowledge company is that other software developers may not produce the end result they are wanting and that it is easier to rely on your own company to get things right. Thus, the issue of trust has caused the knowledge company to act in different ways and take certain actions to ensure that the reliability of their data is maintained.

Chain of Support: Knowledge Company and the GP

With the data produced by the knowledge company, there are always additions or changes that need to be distributed to the end user in order for an accurate and up-to-date decision to be made. It is a concern for the knowledge company that GPs may not regularly install their data upgrades. Although this is a major concern for the knowledge company they are unable to enforce any measure to ensure regular updates. The knowledge company do, however, include a statement that they do not guarantee the data if it is not updated.

The same issue applies between the software developer and the GP. Again, the development of the CDSS software will often require updates and upgrades. Like the knowledge company, the concern for the software developer is that the end user will not install the updates.

There is currently no method or measure to ensure the installation of upgrades, either from the data or the system. Thus both the software developer and the knowledge company must place a degree of trust on the end user, as this aspect is out of their control. It is often the IPAs, acting as a kind of intermediary, that take on the role of ensuring that the systems actually in use are the latest versions of software and data. Here the IPAs are providing responsibility on behalf of the other sub-systems in this DSS infrastructure, and as such can be seen as key players in having the systems used in practice be seen as trustworthy by GPs and patients.

Chain of Support: IPA and Software Developer

The IPA often has the responsibility to choose a preferred software development company. When choosing a preferred company a number of factors are important, and reliability is one of them. This is often expressed in terms of it being essential for the IPA to choose a company that they can trust. Providing updates and upgrades to the system is also important for the IPA. However, the IPA is not concerned that the software developer will not provide timely updates, since it is in the software developer's best interest to provide the updates. On the other hand, the IPA is often concerned that the GPs would not install their updates in a timely manner. However, because the IPA is in a situation of some authority, they often resort to insisting that the updates are installed.

Responses to the Lack of Trust

It can be seen that there are a number of situations where trust needs to exist between the providers of the components. In this section, we identify the types of strategies adopted to deal with the problems of a lack of trust in certain areas. This classification gives us the headings of: creating a new role or job; providing a technical solution; providing an organizational solution; relying on contractual responsibility; and using an agent to manage issues of trust.

Response 1: Creating a New Role or Job

This was the solution adopted by one knowledge company we spoke to who were concerned that the representation of their data was not as expected once the CDSS was developed. The knowledge company created the role of "systems integrator" to ensure that software developers using their data were fully aware of how the data should be correctly handled. This reduced the possibility of errors in the software's logic giving the appearance of a problem with the quality of information.

Response 2: Providing a Technical Solution

This was an additional strategy used in the above scenario. Here some of the query logic was brought back into the knowledge base, thus reducing the responsibility of the software developers when presenting queries in the CDSS. In this situation, we were informed that it was appreciated by the software developers who were uneasy at taking responsibility for information quality in this substantial database, the content of which was out of their domain of expertise. Both of these measures have lead to the knowledge company widening its base of technical skills, which is similar to the next strategy observed.

Response 3: Providing an Organizational Solution

Another knowledge company we talked to felt they could not trust any software developer to develop a CDSS with their data, so they developed their own software.

Response 4: Relying on Contractual Responsibility

In our area of study, healthcare CDSS, a significant aspect is the currency or up-to-date-ness of the data. There are significant trust issues around whether GPs are using and or getting the latest data upgrades. So another element in this complex modern IS is the distribution system for regular data upgrades. The knowledge companies employ the strategy of declining responsibility if the latest data and system upgrades are not used by the end-user, the GP in this case. This of course is quite a negative strategy and places a difficult burden in terms of expertise on the GP. A more positive and possibly more successful strategy is illustrated by our final heading.

Response 5: Using an Agent to Manage Issues of Trust

In our research, the IPA who acted as practice managers for the IT infrastructure of their GPs took on this role of managing issues of trust.

It is often the IPAs who act as a kind of intermediary, and take on the role of ensuring that the systems actually in use are the latest versions of software and data. Here the IPAs are providing responsibility on behalf of the other sub-systems in this CDSS infrastructure and as such can be seen as key players in having the systems used in practice be seen as trustworthy by GPs and patients.

The IPA often has the responsibility to choose a preferred software development company. When choosing a preferred company a number of factors are important, and reliability is one of them. This is often expressed in terms of it being essential for the IPA to choose a company that they can trust. Providing updates and upgrades to the system is also important for the IPA. However, the IPA is not concerned that the software developer will not provide timely updates, since it is in the software developer's best interest to provide the updates. On the other hand, the IPA is often concerned that the GPs will not install their updates in a timely manner. However, because the IPA is in a situation of some authority, it often resorts to insisting that the updates be installed.

Discussion

The factors involved in the trust models mentioned earlier include predictability, dependability, faith, competence, responsibility, and reliability. In our findings, we have come across issues that relate to some of these factors. We found evidence of faulty logic, concern over timeliness, and uncertainty.

The trust between the knowledge company and the software developer has several underlying factors, namely competence, responsibility, and reliability. In order for the knowledge company to proceed with the software developer, they must believe that the software developer has some degree of competence, i.e. that they have the expertise to produce such a system.

Due to the fact that one knowledge company had issues with trust factors, it was unable to trust any other software developer to develop their systems, and thus it decided to begin software development within its own company. The factors that were involved in the decision were those of reliability and competence. This knowledge company was convinced, perhaps from previous experiences, that having control over software development provided it with greater reliability and competence.

In another situation, a knowledge company had issues with dependability and competence of the software developers. However, instead of doing the development themselves, other action was taken. Due to experiences with errors in the display of the data, the knowledge company decided that the software developers were not competent to display the data as was required, causing the knowledge company not to depend on this being fixed in the future. Their course of action was to change the format of the data so as not to give the software developers a chance to err in the future.

The current situation is that the knowledge companies and software developers are able to predict that the GP will install the updates, but as yet there is no mechanism where the trust reaches the level of faith. It is evident, therefore, that the IPA have a continuing role to play to allow the knowledge company and the software developer to trust that their updates will get through to the end user.

With the IPA, there is little concern from their point of view that the knowledge company and the software developer are not reliable in terms of providing the updates, since there is a direct benefit to them in providing timely updates.

In some of the interactions outlined above, the knowledge company and the software developers have little option but to trust the other parties. However, where they can take control and responsibility for themselves, it is clear they are keen to do so.

Trust and "Technical" Responses

O'Neill (2002) presents a strong argument that, where "technical" measures are taken due to a reluctance to place trust, our underlying ethical values should not be forgotten. Such technical responses often include, along with the strategies that we found and summarised in the previous section: service level agreements, audits, quality indicator metrics, benchmarks and so forth. These may all play a helpful role where there is a lack of trust. There is considerable evidence that, within a quality-promoting framework such as a quality management system, such accountability measures as a minimum set a "floor" under quality of service, and if used judiciously are helpful in improving the quality of software based systems (Bissett & Siddiqi, 1995, 1996). They may also, as O'Neill argues, produce further malign effects such as increasing suspicion, and can often introduce "perverse incentives" (O'Neill, 2002, p. viii). An egregious example of the latter appeared in GPs' surgeries in the UK during the summer of 2005. In response to a government target that patients should wait no longer than three days for an appointment with their GP, around a third of GP surgeries refused to make appointments more than three days in advance, an absurd and self-defeating scenario that provoked considerable derision. A reliance on accountability mechanisms on their own is not enough.

This touches upon a debate that has become especially sharp in the public sectors such as healthcare (Exworthy & Halford, 1999). O'Neill argues that professionals should not lose sight of their fundamental values in their efforts to comply with audit systems. We are reminded once again of Gotterbarn's (1996) advocacy of a "new professionalism" for those working in ICT.

Three paradoxical aspects of trust in the "information society" have emerged here. Firstly, as noted in our discussion of the nature of trust, the "information society" of the twenty-first century has by no means eliminated the issue of trust, and secondly, the proliferation of information has made placing trust, if anything, more problematical. The third paradox is that technical measures to address a lack of trust implicitly put trust back on the agenda; without strong guiding ethical values, such measures alone cannot guarantee the successful employment of information systems.

The guarantee that we would really like is that wise, experienced, knowledgeable professionals will conscientiously perform their duties.

Conclusion

The study of CDSS used by GPs in New Zealand shows that the question of trust is never far from the supply, operation, and maintenance of such systems. Responses to a lack of trust were various in nature; adaptive "technical," organisational, or procedural measures were found. Typically these were creating a new role or job; providing a technical solution; providing an organizational solution; relying on contractual responsibility; and using an agent to manage issues of trust. Such strategies can be valuable in the situation studied, where successful use of a CDSS has an immediate impact upon human health. But ultimately the trust issue is difficult to escape; one would expect this human and ethical question to be pre-eminent in other situations where complex information systems have a key role.

References

Akinyokun, O., & Adeniji, O. (1991). Experimental study of intelligent computer aided medical diagnostics and therapy. *AMSE Journal of Modelling, Simulation and Control, 27*(3), 1-20.

Bassey, M. (1999). *Case study research in education settings.* Buckingham, PA: Open University Press

Bassey, M. (1981). Pedagogic research: On the relative merits of search for generalization and study of single events. *Oxford Review of Education, 7*(1), 73-93.

Bell, J. (1987). *Doing your research project*. Philadelphia, PA: Open University Press.

Bemmel, J. (1997). Introduction and overview. In J. Bemmel & M. Musen (Eds.), *Handbook of medical informatics*. Heidelberg: Springer-Verlag.

Bissett, A., & Siddiqi, J. (1996). Deming and software: Strange bedfellows? In M. Bray, M. Ross, & G. Staples (Eds.), *Software quality management IV (SQM'96)* (pp. 23-32). Southampton: Mechanical Engineering Publications Ltd.

Bissett, A., & Siddiqi, J. (1995). How will the CMM fare in Europe? In M. Ross, C. Brebbia, G. Staples, & J. Stapleton (Eds.), *Software quality management III (SQM'95) Vol.1* (pp. 171-182). Southampton: Computational Mechanics Publications.

Bottery, M. (2000). *Education, policy, and ethics*. London: Continuum.

de Laat, P. (2004). Open source software: A case of swift trust? In T. Ward Bynum, N. Pouloudi, S. Rogerson, & T. Spyrou (Eds.), *Proceedings ETHICOMP 2004, Vol. 1* (pp. 250-265). Syros: University of the Aegean.

Delaney, B., Fitzmaurice, D., Riaz, A., & Hobbs, F. (1999). Can computerised decision support systems deliver improved quality in primary care? *British Medical Journal, 319*, 1281.

Exworthy, M., & Halford, S. (1999). *Professionals and the new managerialism in the public sector*. Buckingham UK: Open University Press.

Farman, D., Honeyman, A., & Kinirons, M. (2003). Risk reduction in general practice: The impacts of technology. *International Journal of Healthcare and Quality Assurance, 16*(5), 220-228.

Fukuyama, F. (1996). *Trust: the social virtues and the creation of prosperity*. London: Penguin Books.

Gallivan, M. (2001). Striking a balance between trust and control in a virtual organisation: A content analysis of open source software case studies. *Information Systems Journal* (11), 277-304.

Gauld, R. (2006). The troubled history and complex landscape of information management technology in the New Zealand health sector. *Health Care and Informatics Review Online*, (February). Retrieved November 1, 2006, from http://hcro. enigma.co.nz/index.cfm?fuseaction=articiledisplay&FeatureID=020306

Gotterbarn, D. (1996). Software engineering: A new professionalism. In T. Hall, C. Myers, D. Pitt, & W. Stokes (Eds.). *Proceedings of professional awareness in software engineering* (pp. 1-12). London: University of Westminster.

Hamel, J., Dufour, S., & Fortin, D. (1993). *Case study methods*. Newbury Park, CA: Sage Publications.

Karahannas, M., & Jones, M. (1999). Inter-organisational; systems and trust in strategic alliances. *Proceedings of the International Conference on Information systems* (pp. 346-357). Charlotte, NC.

McDermid, J. A. (1991). *Software engineer's reference book.* London: Butterworth-Heinemann.

Muir, B. M. (1994). Trust in automation, part1: Theoretical issues in the study of trust and human intervention in automated systems. *Ergonomics, 37*(11), 1905-1922.

Muir, B. (1987). Trust between humans and machines and the design of decision aides. *International Journal of Man-Machine Studies,* (27), 527-539.

Muir, B., & Moray, N. (1996). Trust in automation: Part II experimental studies of trust and human intervention in a process control simulation. *Ergonomics, 39*(3), 429-460.

O'Neill, O. (2002). *A question of trust: The BBC Reith lectures.* Cambridge University Press.

Power, M. (1997). *The audit society: Rituals of verification.* Oxford University Press.

Raab, C. (1998). Privacy and trust: Information, government, and ICT. In J. van den Hoven, S. Rogerson, T. Ward Bynum, & D. Gotterbarn (Eds.). *Proceedings ETHICOMP'98* (pp. 565-577). Rotterdam: Erasmus University.

Rempel, J. K., Holmes, J. G., & Zanna, M. P. (1985). Trust in close relationships. *Journal of Personality and Social Psychology,* (49), 95-112.

Ridderichoff, J., & van Herk, E. (1997). A diagnostic support system in general practice: Is it feasible? *International Journal of Medical Informatics, 45*(3), 133-143.

Shortliffe, E., Perreault, L., Fagan, L. & Wiederhold, G. (1990). (Eds). *Medical informatics: Computer applications in health care.* Reading, MA: Addison-Wesley Publishing Company.

Simpson, K., & Gordon, M. (1998). The anatomy of a clinical information system. *British Medical Journal,* (316), 1655-1658.

Tellis, W. (1997). Introduction to case study. *The Qualitative Report, 3*(2), Retrieved November 1, 2006, from www.nova.edu/ssss/QR/QR3-2/tellis1.html

Thornett, A. (2001). Computer decision support systems in general practice. *International Journal of Information Management, 21*(1), 39-47.

Vries, P., Midden, C., & Bouwhuis, D. (2003). The effect of errors on system trust, self confidence, and the allocation of control in route planning. *International journal of Human-Computer Studies,* (58), 719-735.

Wills, M. (2006). Success in health care—making IT work. *Health Care and Informatics Review Online*, (February). Retrieved November 1, 2006, from http://hcro.enigma.co.nz/website/index.cfm?

Wyatt, J. (1991). Uses and sources of medical knowledge. *Lancet,* (338), 1368-72.

Wyatt, J., & Spiegelhalter, D. (1990). Evaluating medical expert systems: What to test and how? *Medical Informatics*, (15), 205-217.

Yin, R. (2003). *Case study research: Design and methods* (3rd ed.). Thousand Oaks, CA: Sage.

Chapter IV

Values of an Electronic Social Record

Karin Hedström, Örebro University, Sweden

Abstract

This chapter analyses the effects of introducing ICT as a support for the social record in elderly care. The effects of the electronic social record are assessed by analysing the different values the electronic social record supports. These values are discussed in terms of "value areas" (values related to administration, integration, professional, and care), which is a categorization of anticipated and experienced effects of using ICT in elderly care. This is a case study where the analysis is a comparison of the social record before and after the introduction of ICT as a support for using the social record. Furthermore, the study also assesses how valuable it is to use "value areas" as an analytical tool when evaluating the effects of ICT.

Introduction

Development of ICT (information and communication technology) systems is a process of making social and technological design choices, with the purpose of serving human interest (Hedström, 2007). This means that development of ICT systems naturally involves moral value judgments (Klein & Hirschheim, 1996, 2001), and neither technology such as ICT systems nor the development process can be seen as value neutral (Klein & Hirschheim, 2001; Mumford, 1981; Winner, 1999). It is therefore important to be aware of the socio-political implications, as well as content, of ICT systems. One example of an ICT system, which in a high degree influences the social, is the electronic record. An electronic record is a medical or social record delivered and used through an ICT-system. ICT systems, such as the electronic record, can be more or less intentionally introduced as a way to change a work practice (see also discussion in Iacono & Kling, 1996). Design and use of records influences how the care is carried out. Introducing new technology, such as ICT systems changes work—and communication routines. These changes may be expected, but often are the effects of ICT difficult to anticipate, with sometimes positive and sometimes negative effects as a consequence.

This chapter analyses the use of a new electronic social record used by nursing assistants and section managers in elderly care, by comparing the use of the social record before and after the introduction of an ICT-supported social record. This article analyses, and discusses, the values of a new electronic social record introduced within elderly care. The social record analysed in this study is one module within a larger application, named SAVA, used for information sharing within elderly care (described in more detail below). The purpose of the social record is to provide documentation of elderly care. Another objective of this chapter is to test the concept of "value areas" (Hedström, 2007) as analytical framework for evaluating the electronic social record. The value of ICT in elderly care can be illustrated by different "value areas," which demonstrates the values that have guided the development process as well as users' experiences of utilizing the ICT system. A value area is classified from the organizational actors' anticipated and experienced effects of introducing and using ICT. These value areas are common values related to the introduction and use of ICT within elderly care (Hedström, 2007) (more discussion on the choice and use of the analytical tool can be found in the section below), such as administration values, integration values, care values, and professional values.

The chapter is organized as follows: section two examines the nature of care work, and section three considers the values of ICT in elderly care. The fourth section describes the case study, followed by the research method in section five. The following and sixth section compares the use of the social record before and after the introduction of SAVA, and section seven analyzes the value of using the electronic social record. The last section in the chapter gives a short conclusion and summarizes the results.

The Social Record

A medical health record supports the interplay and coordination between different actors (Berg & Bowker, 1997). and is therefore important for the production of care services. The record is important for information transfer between care professionals working at a care unit and produces a patient with a history as the record gives a public account of what has happened (Berg & Bowker 1997). Recording is necessary for assuring that the care services are safe and adequate, and as a communication tool for sharing information and experiences about the daily lives and events, as well as actions, related the elderly. The record is dynamic and evolutionary, and can be seen as the hub connecting different care professionals with the elderly, their lives, and needs.

The social record, related to a specific individual, contains the information nursing assistants and section managers decide is important to share with others working with the elderly (an elderly is generally a person of 80 or older, who is entitled to home-care by the municipality). The social record typically contains information on important events and activities related to the production of elderly care, as well as information about the well-being and daily life of the elderly (family, social context, etc.).

The Nature of Elderly Care

Elderly care in Sweden a civil right, and the goal of elderly care in Sweden is to give the elderly the possibility to live such a normal and self-sustaining life as possible. Care services are related to the physical, psychological, and social needs of the elderly. These can be services such as providing food, help with personal hygiene, help to get dressed, medical help, or help to provide a social life. One important goal is to provide support for the elderly so he or she can live in their own home as long as possible This goal is stipulated in the Social Services Act:

The Social Service should, through home-help, out patient care, or other similar social services make it easier for the individual to live at home and be in contact with others.

This means that elderly care services to a large part are provided within someone's private home. Elderly care is therefore something very private, both in terms of types of services provided, and the location of the services carried out.

Conflicting Demands

An important aspect of elderly care work, which influences development and use of ICT, is the complex organization for delivering care services. Elderly care involves many different collaborating and communicating actions and actors, with civil servants, nursing staff, politicians, elderly, and their families as important actors. This complex structure leads to a varied and diverse work practice with many concurrent actors, norms, and actions.

The employees have to address demands not only from the elderly and their families, but have to be loyal to decisions made by politicians and civil servants on different levels in the organization (Silfverberg, 1999). Written documentation is very important due to the communicative and knowledge intense nature of elderly care. A working oral and written information transfer is fundamental for delivering safe and high quality care. Without sufficient information and correct information there is a risk for errors being made, which can, within elderly care, not only lead to inefficiency and irritation, but also become dangerous or even lethal. Development and implementation of ICT systems has to see to the care work's need for communication and knowledge.

In Between the Public and the Private

Working in elderly care means being on the boarder line between the public and the private. The act of caring is fulfilled and created in the meeting between the care giving person and the elderly. To be able to balance the role as a government representative and a caring fellow human being is the big challenge of care work, with sometimes conflicting demands from the dual and concurrent roles. This dilemma is apparent in the care giving actions, when the care giver has to balance the demands from the organization with the elderly's individual needs (Silfverberg, 1999). The employee has to take individual initiatives, and at the same time meet the demands from the organization.

Elderly care work embraces many different dimensions, raising conflicting demands the care givers need to address. It is physical and emotional work, where the action includes moral and ethical judgments. The care giving actions are often concrete and operative. The situations are constantly changing and the precise content in, and experience of, the meeting with the elderly can not be exactly decided beforehand. The care giver exists between the planned and real life, which often means compromising between the planned, and the actual situation at hand. ICT systems within elderly care have to support these varied, and sometimes, conflicting, dimensions of care work.

From Care to Administration

The work of the nursing assistant has changed from being mainly focused on care and the daily lives of the elderly, to include more nurse related work tasks. Concurrent with this is a change with more administrative and managerial work tasks. Politicians and civil servants believe that improved documentation and documentation routines will make elderly care more efficient and improve the quality of information, at the same time, as the work carried out within elderly care will become more visible, and therefore possible to evaluate, manage, and legitimize. These professional shifts coincide, and are made possible, with the use of ICT as a tool for planning, documenting, and evaluating the work in elderly care.

ICT systems within elderly care are often seen, and used as, organizational memories, which holds information that is always available, as well as time-and space resistant. The information can be reached independent of the user's location, or when the information is needed. Related to this is another purpose for using ICT systems in elderly care, which is to make information less private, and hence less vulnerable. This means that the nursing assistant becomes less personally involved which sees as important for developing a professional relation to the elderly, and minimizes the dependency on certain individuals.

The Value of ICT in Elderly Care

Care rationality and care related values are, according to many care researchers, based in praxis and experience (Eliasson, 1992; Sørensen, 1991), meaning that care rationality often is seen as colliding with the administrative and economic rationality commonly symbolized by ICT systems (Beck, 1997; Berg 1999).

Underlying this view on ICT systems care work is a view on the work practice of elderly care and care rationality as non-administrative. But delivering safe and advanced elderly care requires accurate, adequate, and sufficient information as well as safe work routines, which can be supported by well functioning ICT systems developed with attention to the nature of elderly care.

ICT systems embody the interests and values of the people taking part in the development process. Values have a role in the evaluation of ICT systems, as the evaluation of the effects of ICT systems is influenced by the evaluator's own interests and values (for a discussion on the politics of evaluation (see e.g., Wilson & Howcraft, 2000). Values guide the development process towards the anticipated effects (Mumford, 1981), and determine how we value the effects that we experience when we use the implemented ICT system.

Values can be defined as an individual's principles that decide what to prioritize and which actions to take (Kluckhohn, 1951; Rescher, 1969). ICT systems are developed through peoples' actions where every alternative reflects a specific standpoint. The values we hold guide our attention, decide our actions, and influence how we value what we experience. Values are, consequently, related to the driving forces of ICT (c.f. Klein and Hirschheim, 2001), as well as to its effects (c.f. Wilson & Howcraft, 2000). Anticipated and experienced effects can thus be seen as illustrations of values. Anticipated effects are possible to identify through the effects that different actors hope that the future ICT system will contribute with. The anticipated effects include the intended and designed future effects as well as anticipated effects not explicitly included in the design. This can be compared with design ideals, which can be described as the underlying rationality that legitimize and support design decisions (Klein & Hirschheim, 2001). Our values influence which effects we perceive and wish to support. Values are, therefore, also identified through an individual's experience of the effects developing, implementing, and using ICT systems has had on their work practice.

Four Value Areas of ICT

The values of an electronic social record within elderly care, is in this case investigated using the concept of "value areas." This is a categorization of various actors' anticipated and experienced effects of developing, implementing, and using ICT for administrative and communicative purposes in elderly care (Hedström, 2007).

The value areas consist of administration values, integration values, care values, and professional values (see Figure 1). *Administration values* are related to effects on the administration and management of elderly care. Here, I include effects related to increased efficiency, cost reduction, administrative support, quality assurance, and information security. *Integration values* focus on the use of ICT as a means for cooperation, mutual perspectives, and work routines, as well as increased understanding of other professional groups. *Care values* are related to the content of elderly care. An ICT system for care values is a support to increase the quality of care, and a support in the meeting between the elderly and the care professionals. Care values include effects relating to correct care, continuous care, and safe care, as well as increased time with the elderly and legal rights for the elderly. *Professional values* depict in what ways ICT systems can be used to strengthen the professional work in elderly care. These include ICT as a tool for modernization and increased status, knowledge development and support for national, organizational, and local norms, as well as developing the role of nursing assistants and giving care work higher visibility.

Figure 1. The four value areas of ICT in elderly care (Hedström, 2007)

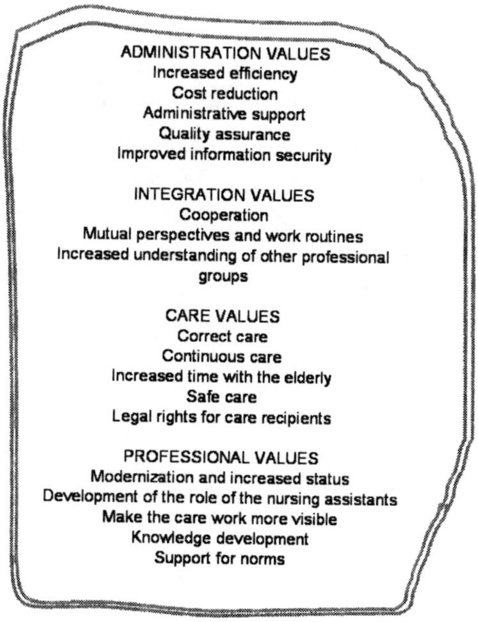

ADMINISTRATION VALUES
Increased efficiency
Cost reduction
Administrative support
Quality assurance
Improved information security

INTEGRATION VALUES
Cooperation
Mutual perspectives and work routines
Increased understanding of other professional
groups

CARE VALUES
Correct care
Continuous care
Increased time with the elderly
Safe care
Legal rights for care recipients

PROFESSIONAL VALUES
Modernization and increased status
Development of the role of the nursing assistants
Make the care work more visible
Knowledge development
Support for norms

Case Study: SAVA

SAVA was developed as a communication tool with the purpose of supporting individualization and quality assurance in elderly care, as put forward in the Social Services Act and by the National Board of Health and Welfare. The objectives with SAVA was to develop an ICT system that could ensure that the elderly would attain the contracted and necessary care services for securing a good everyday life, and that the care service were carried out in a safe and secure manner with the possibility for evaluation. One major goal was to improve knowledge transfer between care employees as one way of ensuring safe and adequate care. Another aim with developing SAVA was to make routines possible to observe and therefore improve, while taking different actors' values and norms into consideration. SAVA was developed as an action research project (Kemmis & McTaggert, 2000; Mumford, 2001), in collaboration with researchers and care professionals (nursing assistants and section managers) at one rural care unit located at different places in Linköping municipality. The care unit serves approximate 350-400 clients, and employs approximate 120 nursing assistants, section managers, and administrative staff.

Description of SAVA

SAVA supports communication between care professionals about the elderly, their needs, circumstances, as well as events and actions related to the life of the elderly and the work practice of caring. It means that SAVA supports the planning, carrying out, and following up of the nursing assistants' work with the elderly (Cronholm & Goldkuhl, 2006). SAVA includes modules such as case management and planning, following up, records, archive, and administration (see Figure 2). The development of SAVA started in 1999, and the system was introduced in 2002, and is now used daily as part of the working routines by nursing assistants, administrative staff, and section managers.

The Electronic Social Record

The electronic social record in SAVA is extensively used by the nursing assistants and their managers. I will briefly describe one electronic document that is central in the record module. This is the document "searching for events" (see Figure 3),

Figure 2. First page of SAVA

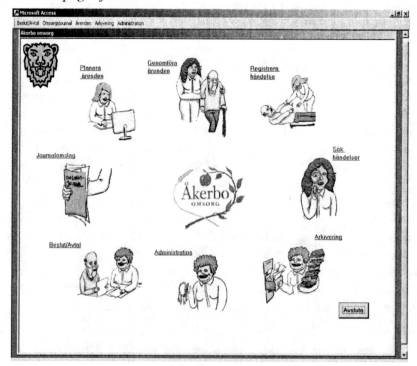

Figure 3. Document "searching for events" as part of the record module in SAVA

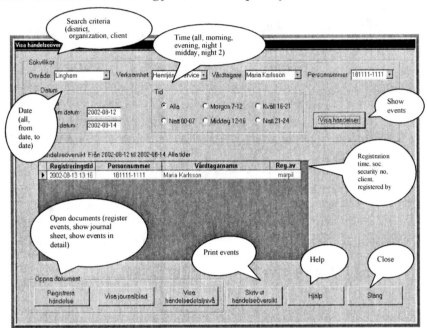

which shows that an event has been registered (i.e., events related to the elderly could be medical or social events) and considered important enough to communicate and save) registered by nursing assistants or their managers. Events related to the elderly are registered together with actions taken, time, and registering user (see Figure 3).

It is possible to search for events and related actions on three different levels: general for the whole unit (district), organization within the district (organization), and a specific individual (client) belonging to an organization within a district (see Figure 3). It is also possible to search for events using dates and time as denominators (see Figure 3).

If a user wants to have more detailed information about the event, including information about actions taken, the user has to open another document ("show record sheet"). It is not possible to change an entry after it has been saved. If the user notices an error after saving, it is necessary to make another entry.

The first thing the nursing assistants do when they come in to work is to log on to SAVA and check the record to see if anything had happened since the last time they worked. As a nursing assistant said concerning the use of SAVA:

We use SAVA for records when we register a new client and when we search for family members. [We use it] several times every day. It is the first thing we do in the morning. To know what has happened since last time we worked. It is our report, naturally we check it.

Development of SAVA

SAVA was developed as part of an action research project where research questions and the needs of the practice were mutually developed (Mumford, 2001). The system was developed as a result of a collaboration between section managers, nursing assistants, and researchers at one elderly care unit. The nursing assistants and section managers and their questions and requirements were the main basis for development, whereas the researchers contributed with critical questions about the work practice and ideas on how ICT could be used in order to improve the work in elderly care.

SAVA was developed using four design principles. The first design principle is the principle of dialogue, the second design principle is the principle of using existing documents as a basis for analysis and reconstruction, the third design principle is the principle of shifting between the abstract and the concrete, and fourth and last design principle is the principle of development based on comparison and learning.

The principle of dialogue means having an open dialogue paired with critical questions and discussions, and has been central for understanding, analysing, and developing the practice of elderly care. This way of working was a fundament when we started to design SAVA. Ideas as well as more or less evolved prototypes were tried, discussed, analysed, and evaluated from its use in and effects on the work practice. The second principle focuses the use of existing documents as a basis for analysis and reconstructions, as the information they include communicate something of importance. Elderly care has a rich amount of local documents as well as documents used in the entire organization. These are used for communication and information transfer between different organizational actors. Using documents was also a way to meet and make dialogue and discussion possible. Actors knowing very little about elderly care can ask relevant questions based on the documents, at the same time as novice users find it easier to criticize and comment on suggested design solutions when using documents as a basis for discussion (Cronholm & Goldkuhl, 2006). One important document for study has been, of course, the social record. In order to penetrate the needs a future electronic version of the social record should meet we used the hand-written social record currently in use (see Table 1) as a starting point for discussion. We asked question such as (Cronholm & Goldkuhl, 2006):

- What is the social record used for?
- Who uses the social record?
- When is the social record used?
- Is any information missing?
- What information is necessary?
- How is the social record used?
- What does the information in the current social record mean and stand for?
- Who uses this information?
- Who sees the information as necessary?
- Is there any information missing?

The knowledge developed from penetrating the social record was then used as a basis for designing, jointly by researchers, nursing assistants, and care managers, a new electronic version of the social record.

Closely related to the principle of using existing documents, is the third principle, which means shifting between the abstract and the concrete. Design suggestions and questions about the work practice were based on earlier theoretical work (see e.g., Goldkuhl & Ågerfalk, 2002), and discussed on a more abstract level. But at the same time made the practical nature of care work, together with the care professionals´ very limited experience of using and developing ICT systems, it necessary to work with concrete design suggestions. Using the concrete, in forms of documents or design suggestions as a basis, it was possible to analyze and discuss the work practice and ICT's role in elderly care. The fourth and last principle, development based on comparison and learning, included using other similar work practices as a basis for developing SAVA and the social record further. We started to develop SAVA for one specific work group, but spread its use, as well as evaluated the use and adapted SAVA, to other work groups in the same elderly care unit.

Table 1. The hand-written social record (one patient's) (the record notes are not related to a real person) as it was used at the case site

Date	Action/problem/observation (notes in the journal has to been signed)
020206	Anna's leg was hurting today. I gave her two Panodil (painkillers) / Astrid
020306	Anna has been to the hospital today with a meeting with the doctor about her leg. If it doesn't improve, we shall call again/ Emma
020406	Anna fell today in the morning /Annika

Research Approach and Methodology

This is a case study (Yin, 1994), with a focus on the values of using an electronic social record. SAVA was selected as an example of an electronic social record as it provides interesting comparison between the use of the social record before and after the introduction of an ICT system. Another objective with this study is to validate whether the concept, and content of, "value areas," is valuable for analysing the use of ICT systems within an organization. As this test is an important objective of the study it was important that the case study and the analytical framework matched (i.e., I wanted the case (the social electronic record in SAVA) to correspond to the types of systems used for developing the analytical framework) (for a description of the cases see Hedström, 2007). This match ensures the validity of the analytical model.

The use of SAVA as a social record, and its effects, has been studied through a combination of interviews and document studies (e.g., data triangulation) (Patton, 1990). I have conducted interviews with managers and nursing assistants using SAVA. The interviews for evaluating the use of SAVA were carried out during 2003 and 2005. The first set of interviews were carried out in relation to the implementation of SAVA, while the second set of interviews were carried out when SAVA had been in use for two years. The interviews lasted approximate one hour and were semi-structured. The questions asked were related to how, when, and by whom SAVA was used as a support for information transfer in the work practice. I also asked questions more specifically related to the use of SAVA as a recording system, and whether and how the introduction of an electronic social record had changed the work practice.

Another very important source of data for understanding how the practice of using a social record has changed has been the content of the social record. By having access to entries from the social record, before and after the introduction of ICT, I could compare the effects of introducing an electronic social record. The interviews were complemented with empirical data in the form of transcripts from the social records used in the elderly care unit before and after the introduction of SAVA. The content of the hand-written social record was compared with the electronic version of the social record implemented in SAVA. The comparison focused on how the record keeping was conducted, who was responsible for making notes, what type of information that was recorded, and changes in the work practice.

Result: A Change in Using the Social Record

The use of SAVA, in combination with a changed attitude of how, and why, to use a social record related to patient care, has changed the use of social records at this elderly care unit. With SAVA, the recorded information has become much more contextual and holistic. Implementation of a new ICT system for documentation concurred with training on how to document and why. The nursing assistants have also been trained in how to use computers, and have started to use e-mail as part of their everyday activities. They were earlier total novices in using ICT. One section manager stresses that she sees it as very important to include the context when making entries in the social record. What seem as unimportant observations can in a later stage, be of utmost importance. She points out that it is very important to view documentation as evolutionary and dynamic. She also stresses that SAVA should be used as the main tool for communication.

Information in the social records, before the introduction of an ICT system, was mainly related to medical events. The use of SAVA has changed that. The current documentation serves many different interests, where exchange of medical information is only one part. The records now include information on work routines, goals related to patients' well-being, and information about the atmosphere at the patients' homes. One example on work routines and goals related to the patient gives the following note from the electronic social record. *"We will train [the patient] to walk at least once a day. When we work with [the patient] we walk either from the bedroom to the toilet or the other way around. We use the walking buck and the red belt, at the same time as one of us walks behind the wheelchair."* The notes are now richer with references to the patient's daily mood, and if considered important, notes on relatives' moods and disposition. *"[The patient] was silent and a bit sad when we arrived in the evening. [Her husband] was drunk."* The writings are often in form of dialogues. There are also greetings from patients to the nursing staff as well as notes directed to other members of the staff. *"Hello night staff! Don't forget to clean the toilet bucket after emptying, it smells so bad."* Other changes, compared to the manual records, are related to the elderly care unit's district. As the staff work from different locations, the use of SAVA has made communication more efficient, more convenient, as well as improved quality of the written information. Records were earlier stored at one place, with no means of access from other locations. Now everyone can access the records, irrespective of location. SAVA has erased the border of space and time. Managers use the record as a way to communicate with nursing assistants. They save time and the information is easy accessible, not changing, and durable.

The way the records are used has also changed in terms of structure. As the ICT system supports a more structural approach to recording, it is easier to distinguish occurrences related to patients, and if relevant, actions taken as a consequence. When SAVA fails to support the needs of its users, or they find the system unnecessary complicated, they work around it. The users invent new usage patterns. Such as using the record for many different purposes and sometimes registering "XXXXX" instead of actions taken when reporting on events as a way to illustrate that he or she has been aware that he or she should write in that column, but chooses not to.

This means that communication has been canalized into one main medium, SAVA, and the number of loose, and sometimes dislocated, notes has decreased. There is less discussion during break about work related activates. Discussions during the daily morning report use the text in SAVA as a starting point and are of a more practical nature. It is assumed that information in SAVA is common knowledge, and questions and discussions use the recorded information as a starting point for discussions.

It can be viewed as a problem that the social record in SAVA includes social as well as medical entries. All entries are saved, and it is perhaps not necessary, and sometimes not even appropriate to save entries not directly related to the clients and their history. One example is entries directed to other employees (such as "Hello night! Don't forget to empty the night bucket"). The communication pattern between care services employees in the elderly care unit has changed. It is not even accurate to call it a record anymore; a more correct term would be a communication system. The record in SAVA is a combination of record, diary, and dialogue. This illustrates the need for a more holistic and multifaceted system for dialogue and communication.

Analysis: The Value of the Electronic Social Record

If we relate the results of using the social record in SAVA to the value areas, we find that SAVA, in varying degree, supports all value areas. Most support can be found for administrative and integration values.

The social record in SAVA supports the administrative values. Information transfer has become more efficient, mainly due to a mutual organizational memory, where information is stored at one shared place. SAVA is an administrative support, and makes it possible to access information irrespective of time and place. Using SAVA has improved the possibility to inform oneself and inform others, without having to travel or use the telephone. There is also support for documentation, as the implemented record provides a structure for registration of information. Information security is another area, which has improved with SAVA. Information is more secure than before, as the number of miscellaneous notes has decreased, and users have to log in to view or enter information. Using ICT has improved information quality as information no longer is documented by hand, which makes it more accessible as writing by hand is less illegible. As SAVA supports different search functions and different ways of structuring information, the possibility for follow up and quality assurance has improved. SAVA is used as an organizational memory for documenting, sharing, and following up care related activities.

The integration values focus ICT's role as a tool for collaboration, development of shared documentation, and mutual work routines. The social record in SAVA is in a high degree seen and used as an organisational memory with shared, lasting, and easily available information. Information will stay in the organisation irrespective of changes in the work force or illness. Record keeping is no longer a private affair, but is instead a matter of cooperation with, and criticisms of, colleagues (see also Berg, 1999). Support for communication between nursing assistants and nursing assistants and section managers is a major reason why SAVA is seen as a success. This might be especially important at this care unit as the nursing assistants and section managers work from different geographical locations. Another area that has improved is communication and information transfer between night and day staff. This was earlier a problem, but using SAVA has improved information transfer between these two groups. Another implication of using a common ICT system is the development of mutual work routines, as the process of developing, implementing, and using a new ICT system unifies work routines. Using a mutual tool for communication and documentation stresses the importance of similar ways of working.

An ICT system supporting care values is seen as an instrument for improving the meeting between the elderly and care professionals, as well as the client's experience of being an elderly care recipient. In what degree the social record in SAVA supports care values is difficult to assess as no interviews have been conducted with the recipients of the care services—the elderly. But hopefully will the support SAVA provides improve the production of care services. SAVA is viewed as a communication and knowledge tool, where access to information increases the possibility to deliver accurate, individualized, and safe care. Improved knowledge about patients and their needs increases the possibility to offer tailored and personalized care, which takes the patient's current disposition and home situation into account. It becomes easier to introduce new staff to the clients as information is collected at one place. Another important contribution is the section manager who uses SAVA as a tool for communicating with the nursing assistants. This increases the knowledge about patients and how to work in order to sustain and improve their health.

Professional values are related to SAVA as the introduction of a computerized social record, requires a development in documentation and ICT competence, as well as modernizes the work with the elderly. The professional values are mostly related to changes and developments in areas such as ICT competence and competence developing and using documentation. The use of SAVA has made the content of care work more visible, which is important for legitimizing care work, and improves the knowledge of the elderly and their needs. As the work tasks become more visible, they also become possible to criticize and manage (see also Berg, 1999). Visibility of care work is important for increasing the status of the care work.

Conclusion

This chapter had two purposes—to evaluate the use of a new electronic social record in elderly care, and to test an analytical framework using the concept of "value area" and its content as a guide in the evaluation process.

The chapter illustrates how the introduction of a new electronic social record has transformed the reasons for using, and the usage of social records within elderly care. It is evident that different practices of reading and writing the record has evolved (Berg, 1997). These changes concern changes in communication patterns, and documentation routines as a consequence of using a new electronic social record.

The introduction of SAVA coincided with training on how to use computers as well as discussions and training about documentation routines. Another very important aspect influencing the usage of SAVA is the section manager responsible for development of documentation routines and training who stressed the importance of recording in context, and using SAVA as *the* instrument for communication between employers. This, together with lack of support for a "general" communication space, has contributed to make the record SAVA multifunctional with records not only on medical matters, but also records such as diary notes, reminders, and greetings. The social record in SAVA contains medical as well as social and physiotherapeutic related information.

It is clear that the introduction of a new computerized social record changes the way social records are used, and the rational for using them. This as technology, such as ICT, includes the social as well as the technical. Implementation of new work systems and instruments invariably involves making decision about communication patterns and routines—elements that are by its very nature social.

The social record in SAVA has mainly influenced and supported the administrative and integrative value areas as the record in SAVA is seen and used as an organizational memory supporting communication, coordination, and documentation. The use of SAVA should also contribute to better care as the nursing assistants and managers experience SAVA as a valuable tool that has improved transfer and access of information about the elderly. This is however difficult to assess, as there is lack of data from the elderly and their experience of how SAVA is related to care values.

It has been valuable to use "value areas" for evaluating and analyzing the use of a new computerized social record. By using such a theoretical lens, focus is drawn to what can be considered as important aspects for administrative ICT systems within elderly care. One drawback can naturally be that important aspects, not covered by the value areas, are missed.

Acknowledgment

I wish to thank all staff at Linkoping municipality who so generously invited us to their work place. I have learned a lot from their expertise and experience. Thank you. I would also like to thank the anonymous reviewers for their helpful comments.

References

Berg, M. (1999). Patient care information systems and health care work: A sociotechnical approach. *International Journal of Medical Informatics, 55*(2), 87-101.

Berg, M., & Bowker. (1997). The multiple bodies of the medical record: Towards a sociology of an artefact. *The Sociological Quarterly, 38*(3), 513-527.

Cronholm, S., & Goldkuhl, G. (2006). Involving novice users in document-driven system requirements analysis. *Journal of Information, Information Technology, and Organizations, 1*, 131-149.

Eliasson, R. (1992). Omsorg och rationalitet. In R. Eliasson (Ed.), *Egenheter och allmänheter. En antologi om omsorg och omsorgens villkor.* Lund: Arkiv förlag.

Goldkuhl, G., & Ågerfalk, P. (2002). Actability: A way to understand information systems pragmatics. In K. Liu & M. Fl. (Eds.), *Coordination and communication using signs: studies in organisational semiotics* (Vol. 2, pp. 85-113). Boston: Kluwer Academic Publishers.

Hedström, K. (2007). The values of IT in elderly care. *Information Technology & People, 20*(1), 72-84.

Iacono, S., & Kling, R. (1996). Computerization, office routines, and changes in clerical work. In R. Kling (Ed.), *Computerization and controversy. Value conflicts and social choices* (Vol. 2, pp. 309-315). San Diego: Academic Press.

Kemmis, S., & McTaggert, R. (2000). Participatory action research. In N. K. Denzin & Y. S. Lincoln (Eds.), *Handbook of qualitative research.* Thousand Oaks, CA: Sage Publications, Inc.

Klein, H. K., & Hirschheim, R. (2001). Choosing between competing design ideals in information systems development. *Information Systems Frontiers, 3*(1), 75-90.

Klein, H. K., & Hirschheim, R. (1996). The rationality of value choices in information systems development. *Foundations of Information Systems, September 26.*

Kluckhohn, C. (1951). Values and value-orientations in the theory of action: An exploration in definition and classification. In T. Parsons & E. A. Shils (Eds.), *Toward a general theory of action. Theoretical foundations for the social sciences*. New York: Harper & Row.

Mumford, E. (1981). *Values, technology, and work*. The Hague/Boston/London: Martinus Nijhoff Publishers.

Mumford, E. (2001). Advice for an action researcher. *Information Technology & People, 14*(1), 12-27.

Patton, M. Q. (1990). *Qualitative evaluation and research methods* (2 ed.). Newbury Park, CA: Sage Publications.

Rescher, N. (1969). *Introduction to value theory*. Englewood Cliffs, CA: Prentice-Hall.

Silfverberg, G. (1999). *Praktisk klokhet. Om dialogens och dygdens betydelse för yrkesskicklighet och socialpolitik*. Stockholm: Brutus Östlings förlag Symposion.

Sørensen, K. H. (1991). Mot en omsorgspreget teknologi? Om likestillingspolitikkens muligheter og begrensningar på et mannsdominert område. In R. Haukaa (Ed.), *Nye kvinner, nya menn* (pp. 207-227). Oslo: Ad Notam.

Wilson, M., & Howcraft, D. (2000). *The politics of IS evaluation: A social shaping perspective*. Paper presented at the 21st International Conference on Information Systems, Brisbane, Australia.

Winner, L. (1999). Do artifacts have politics? In D. MacKenzie & J. Wajcman (Eds.), *The social shaping of technology* (2nd ed., pp. 28-40). Buckingham: Open University Press.

Yin, R. K. (1994). *Case study research. Design and methods* (2nd ed.). Thousand Oaks, CA: Sage Publications.

Section III

Responsibility and Healthcare Information Systems

Chapter V

Are Agency and Responsibility Still Solely Ascribable to Humans?
The Case of Medical Decision Support Systems

Hannah H. Gröndahl, Formerly of CTE Centre for Applied Ethics,
Linköpings Universitet, Sweden

Abstract

Are agency and responsibility solely ascribable to humans? This chapter explores the question from legal and ethical perspectives. In addition to presenting important theories, the chapter uses arguments, counterarguments, and scenarios to clarify both the actual and the hypothetical ethical and legal situations governing a very particular type of advanced computer system: medical decision support systems (MDSS) that feature AI in their system design. The author argues that today's MDSS must be categorized by more than just type and function even to begin ascribing some level of moral or legal responsibility. As the scenarios demonstrate, various U.S. and UK legal doctrines appear to allow for the possibility of assigning specific types of agency—and thus specific types of legal responsibility—to some types of MDSS. The author concludes that strong arguments for assigning moral agency and responsibility are still lacking, however.

Introduction: Why MDSS Deserve a Closer Look

Are agency and responsibility solely ascribable to humans? The advent of artificial intelligence (AI) appears to be chipping away at the traditional foundations of moral agency and responsibility. Despite the increasing attention of many philosophers and ethicists to AI, there continues to exist a fair amount of conceptual muddle on the conditions for assigning agency and responsibility to such systems, from both legal and ethical perspectives.

*In contexts where the requirements for attributing responsibility are not met, we are mistaken if we assign responsibility to machines. In such cases, we need to make it clear to those designing and employing the machines that responsibility rests on them. Since my argument has the conclusion that currently available computer systems do not meet the conditions for being responsible agents (although some will come close to meeting the conditions), it has an implication that **for now** issues concerning responsibility must be directed at those designing and using the machines.* (Bechtel, 1985, p. 297, Bechtel's own emphasis)

Bechtel wrote the previous passage over twenty years ago. Have things changed since then? This chapter explores the possibility that the answer could now be affirmative:

*Now it can be shown that there is an increasing class of machine actions, where the traditional ways of responsibility ascription are not compatible with our sense of justice and the moral framework of society because nobody has enough **control** over the machine's actions to be able to assume the responsibility for them. These cases constitute what we will call the **responsibility gap**.* (Matthias, 2004, p. 177, Matthias's own emphasis)

Roadmap of the Chapter

The first section of this chapter introduces the various types of advanced medical decision support systems (MDSS) and AI that are the focus of this analysis. It also outlines the moral and legal issues that drive the study. The second section presents important non-mainstream arguments and counterarguments for ascribing moral agency and responsibility to such systems. The third section, in addition to providing some background to the relevant legal principles, explores the potential current and future legal ramifications of MDSS, through the use of informed legal conjecturing and scenarios.[1]

Introduction to Advanced MDSS: Types, Applications, & Functions

Should you ever require treatment at a reasonably advanced hospital, your treatment probably will either be monitored by an advanced MDSS or monitored by a healthcare professional who uses such a system to diagnosis your condition or to plan the next step in your treatment. Doctors, trainees, nurses, and other healthcare professionals often rely to various degrees on advanced MDSS for diagnosis, treatment routes, education, or a combination of these. GIDEON, Help, and Iliad are just a few examples of AI systems in routine use in primary care and point of care (Coiera). MDSS are used often in the diagnosis and treatment of diabetes, for example (Collste, 2000). Quick Medical Reference (QMR), which itself grew out of the INTERNIST-1 project, is yet another MDSS used for consulting and diagnosis (Miller & Masarie, 1990).

Miller and Goodman (1998) point out that MDSS can perform a variety of different roles—anything from reminder systems, to consultation systems, to education systems, to diagnostic and treatment systems. In a review of clinical trials of MDSS, Garg et al. (2005) suggest slightly different categories: systems for diagnosis, reminder systems for prevention, systems for disease management, and systems for drug dosing and/or drug prescribing. This chapter argues that it is possible—and necessary—to distinguish types and levels of responsibility assigned to MDSS, depending on whether it is used for reminding, consultation or education, and also whether the system merely "supports" the user's autonomous decision-making, or whether it instead autonomously "replaces" some of the user's decisions and, possibly, actions. The distinction between support and replacement is not always a sharp one and so requires that one analyze the entire environment in which the MDSS is used.

The design and operation of these systems pose a number of potentially problematic issues of human-computer interaction at the level of the user or operator. For example, MDSS can restrict the doctor's treatment or diagnostic options to only those options programmed into the system at its conception. In addition, the architecture of the system's reasoning and logic paths is seldom transparent, which means that the doctor might not be able to understand why the MDSS reached its decision. In short, the MDSS affects the doctor or healthcare professional's decision-making process, to various degrees. Here, the verb "affect" necessarily has multiple and ambivalent connotations, with positive meanings (i.e., to improve, to enhance, to support), negative meanings (to limit, to hurt), and neutral ones (to frame, to shape, to mediate, to set the conditions for). The scope of this "affecting" is itself determined by the role the MDSS plays and the MDSS's design. This, as will be shown, in certain cases requires that one assign a degree and type of responsibility to such systems.

The Three Dimensions of MDSS Use

This chapter classifies the consequences of MDSS into three different dimensions, each of which has ethical implications.

The *patient's health* dimension concerns primarily questions of patient well-being and patient outcomes, which in turn can be interpreted either as receiving the best possible care or as receiving successful, effective treatment, or both.

The *doctor-patient relationship* dimension primarily concerns questions about the effects of MDSS on this relationship, which, for example, the Hippocratic Oath and the deontological duty of beneficence require that the doctor uphold. Within this dimension there is a concern that the time the doctor spends operating and consulting the system draws away from the time he or she could have spent speaking to and consulting the patient, who is the ultimate receiver of the MDSS's operations.

The *doctor-only* dimension touches most fully upon questions of responsibility for knowledge and decision-making. Whether one views the MDSS primarily as a medical tool, or as a "partner" in decision-making (King, Garibaldi, & Rogerson, 2002), in most situations the MDSS stores, filters, or even analyzes medical knowledge and, in some cases, patient data. Each of these actions serves to reduce the doctor's knowledge burden to know the patient's exact data and medical history; yet simultaneously, each also serves to increase the doctor's knowledge burden to understand the basic functioning and operation of the MDSS. The state of the system's knowledge base is of primary importance to the doctor. Because the MDSS is a potentially safety-critical system, the doctor needs also to have faith in its analytical and reasoning "abilities" and accuracy of information. The ability to recognize "faulty reasoning" that is not immediately obvious (such as an incorrect diagnosis that does not stem from incorrect patient data but rather from faulty analysis), requires that the doctor understand, to a degree, the way the system works.

Systems that Learn

This chapter focuses primarily on intelligent systems because their unique system design enables greater capacities and wider applications, which, this chapter argues, may accord them a degree of agency and responsibility for their decisions. Here, "intelligent computer system" does not mean intelligent in the Turing test sense, as it is not really based on overt behavior; rather, "intelligent" here means that the system features AI in its design. In simplistic terms, AI allows it to assess its environment, to react to it, and to learn from this interaction. AI can itself be divided into categories and degrees of complexity (similar to "degrees of intelligence").

Matthias (2004) categorizes "learning automata" (AI systems) into four types: symbolic systems, connectionism and neural nets, genetic algorithms, and autonomous agents (p. 178-181). Most MDSS are symbolic systems. "A system built along these lines contains long sequences of axioms and derivation rules that are usually expressed in some kind of predicate calculus. The system is either able to derive conclusions from the facts stored in its database [what many in the field call its "knowledge base"], or else to extend this database by adding new rules and facts to it (which is what constitutes learning)" (p. 178). This learning process usually occurs when the system interacts with its user/operator or creator, who can usually correct "faulty" or incomplete knowledge, or incorrect "reasoning," or inappropriate "behavior." Indeed, the term "AI" may sometimes be applied to an MDSS more as a selling point or marketing ploy than as an accurate description of the MDSS. If unsure, one should examine the technical specifications of an MDSS before deciding conclusively whether or not it incorporates AI in its system design.

As the term is used in this chapter, the intelligence of the intelligent system is determined less by its outward behavior than by its internal system design. When it comes to determining agency and responsibility, however, judgment is determined largely by the system's outward behavior, because these are inextricably tied to its role in its overall environment. Indeed, when judging whether or not an agent is morally or legally "responsible," one is not always required to assess the agent's internal (or mental) condition. For example, causal responsibility, like strict liability in the law, can be assigned irrespective of mental condition. A strict interpretation of role responsibility, for example, does not necessarily refer to the mental or psychological conditions of the agent. As Snapper (1998) notes, "[m]uch of the process for assessing [legal] responsibility does not depend on the human features of the agent, only on the nature of judgment" including, presumably, the appropriateness and correctness of that judgment (p. 48).

As an alternative to traditional and contemporary accounts of moral agency and responsibility that refer to human action and human intent, this chapter proposes an analysis that is similar to the Turing test, in that it does not consider how internally complex the computer system is but rather how it mediates its interaction with its environment, which here includes humans. Such an analytical approach—which focuses on the actual role the technology plays, its current functioning and application in today's healthcare environment—is in theory able to avoid getting trapped in endless and fruitless debates about an intelligent system's ability or inability to replicate human cognition and reasoning, and whether or not such ability constitutes a capacity for rational thinking and responsible action. While this behavioral and situational approach also examines the design and operation of these systems, it focuses more on the user: the way the user operates and navigates the system, and interprets and applies the information or decisions it provides. This chapter argues for a middle road position that considers both system design and behavior. This may force one to abandon, in some cases, traditional ethical and legal doctrines of agency and responsibility.

Ascribing Agency and Responsibility: Unique Ethical Perspectives

One could argue that all legal and ethical accounts seem to share one basic assumption: that agency comes before responsibility. Or, to put it another way: agency entails responsibility, provided that certain other conditions are met. For this reason it is appropriate to discuss moral and legal agency first, before moving on to moral and legal responsibility, which this chapter treats as natural outgrowths of agency.

Moral Agency has Aspect

In most accounts of moral agency, a moral agent exhibits aspect, much in the same way that languages do; thus, one can speak of first-person aspect and third-person aspect, or first- and third-person "perspective." According to the first-person perspective, a moral agent "pursues personal desires and interests based on his or her beliefs about the world, and morality is a constraint on how those interests can be pursued, especially in light of the interests of others" (Johnson & Powers, 2004, p. 423). According to the third-person perspective, a moral agent can sometimes act to further the wishes or beliefs of another party, called either the "client" or the "principal" (*Ibid.*). When acting from—or in the service of—the third-person point of view, the agent is not free of morality but is "still being constrained [...] in the guise of such notions as duty, right, and responsibility," although the exact content of these notions will be determined by the role the agent plays in this agent-client or agent-principal relationship (*Ibid.*). When humans act as moral agents from this third-person perspective, the type of agency in question is often called "human surrogate agency," as further discussed below.

Argument for Considering Computers as Intentional Systems

Dennett (1978), whose argument has been extended by Bechtel (1985), has identified—perhaps unintentionally—an intriguing way to tie computers to accountability and responsibility: via his "intentional system" theory. From the outset it must be noted that Dennett's account of intention and rationality does not correspond to everyday, colloquial accounts of intention and rationality. As Bechtel also points out, Dennett's original theory did not explicitly foresee its application to assigning some version of responsibility or accountability to a computer program, as the theory actual refers no more to a computer system than to an alien life form in another galaxy. Nonetheless, Bechtel's extension of the concept to moral responsibility theories has opened new doors, some of which this chapter walks through and re-examines, now that Bechtel's writings are over two decades old.

One can apply the intentional system label under some conditions to something in order to predict its behavior. According to Dennett, an intentional system exhibits three primary features: (1) it has beliefs, (2) it has desires or goals, and (3) it responds to its environment. Dennett writes, "One predicts behavior in such a case by ascribing to the system *the possession of certain information*, and supposing it to be *directed by certain goals*, and then by working out the most reasonable or appropriate action on the basis of these ascriptions and suppositions. It is a small step to calling the information possessed the computer's *beliefs*, its goals and subgoals its *desires*" (p. 6, Dennett's own emphasis). Here, possessing information or misinformation means not only simply storing the information but also actually using and acting upon that information (p. 7). From an epistemological perspective, it is not important to know or be able to prove that the computer actually "believes" in the same sense as, say, a human might; rather, the important point is that someone who has adopted the intentional stance, can predict or explain its behavior by ascribing beliefs to it. While the intentional approach does, by Dennett's own admission, suffer from a mild case of mentalism, Dennett has ready a response to critiques of this sort: "All that has been claimed is that on occasion, a purely physical system can be so complex, and yet so organized, that we find it convenient, explanatory, pragmatically necessary for prediction, to treat it as if it had beliefs and desires and was rational. The chess-playing computer is just that, a machine for playing chess, which no man or animal is; and hence its 'rationality' is pinched and artificial" (p. 7-8). To related critiques that the intentional stance serves to anthropomorphize its subject, Dennett counters that one only ascribes to the system a limited account of rationality, which here corresponds to its having justified beliefs, or beliefs in logical truths. This account of rationality does not exclusively apply to humans, as other animals may exhibit logical behavior.

Bechtel (1985) agrees with Snapper that any attribution of responsibility to computer systems must be shared with humans. He also suggests that one reason to consider partially attributing responsibility to computers is that humans are unable to bear the responsibility that currently rests on them when they design or use the computers (p. 297). Here one can refer to another philosopher's writings on the inability of humans to bear full responsibility when they use computers: Moor, who writes of varieties of an "invisibility factor" (Johnson & Nissenbaum, 1995b, p.14-15) that require that the computer user's degree of responsibility be reduced. Moor's *invisible programming values* are what the programmer decides to include and to omit from the program's specifications, which in turn mediates the entire user experience. *Invisible complex calculation* occurs when a computer program makes calculations that humans may be unable to comprehend. "The invisibility factor presents us with a dilemma. [...] In terms of efficiency the invisibility factor is a blessing. But it is just this invisibility that makes us vulnerable [...] [and] open to invisible abuse or invisible programming of inappropriate values or invisible miscalculation." (p. 15).

The Black Box and Epistemic Enslavement

Analogous to a "black box," these invisibility factors are an unavoidable aspect of computing. One would severely retard computing capacity if one did away with complex calculation, or required that it be visible. Invisibility factors may also imply that the moral responsibility of the user be reduced, according to van den Hoven (2001) and Matthias (2004). Van den Hoven argues that users of MDSS are subjected to "epistemic enslavement" because they are not able to control the acquisition of their beliefs (here, the beliefs or conclusions they reach as a result of the MDSS's recommendations). A plausible counterargument to this view is to assert that the user is always able to choose not to believe the MDSS's decision. Van den Hoven responds that, once the user has seen the decision, "once the user has given in, she is unable to provide good reasons to opt out [to not believe]…If a user is epistemically enslaved vis-à-vis system S, then non-compliance with the system's output constitutes a form of moral risk taking [which] the user cannot justify, at the moment of non-compliance" (p. 6).

If one removes some degree of responsibility from the system's creator or operator, to what would one add the now "unassigned" moral responsibility? Bechtel (1985) would argue that, under limited conditions, one may assign it to the computer system. He first establishes his conditions for assigning responsibility via Aristotle: "that the decision stem from the agent and be within the agent's control" (p. 298). But to claim that control stems from the ability of the agent to do otherwise, which is the "free will" or "free choice" argument, and "is thought to require freedom from causal determination," would imply that one must show that computers also possess a sort of free will or free choice (Ibid.). Bechtel responds that probabilistic and random events also appear to be free from causal determination. Instead, moral responsibility rests on whether or not the outcome was caused "in the proper way" (Ibid.). Even though computers perform what they are programmed to perform and thus do not possess a "free will," the criterion for assigning moral responsibility is not dependent upon a "violation of causal determination of events," and is thus a non-issue (Ibid.). Bechtel then looks for a type of causal determination "that is compatible with a decision stemming from an agent and being within the agent's control," for which he finds argumentative evidence if one views a computer system from Dennett's intentional perspective, in which it possess beliefs, desires, and the ability to respond and adapt to its environment (even, Bechtel says, to have beliefs and desires about its environment). While Bechtel's argument rests, at least in part, on a simplified understanding of the internal system design of the computer system, it nonetheless rests primarily on the external environment. "[A]n intentional system must both have the right kind of relationship to the environment and have an internal configuration that permits such a relationship" (p. 300).

Argument for Artificial Moral Agency

Floridi and Saunders (2004) argue that there is yet another way to locate some computer systems in the realm of morality: through ascribing to them "artificial agency," as defined in a way different to the artificial legal agency of Chopra and White (described below). Floridi and Saunder's "artificial agency" rests upon a distinction between moral agents ("as entities that can perform actions…for good or evil") and moral patients ("as entities that can be acted upon for good or evil") (p. 349). Essentially the distinction comes down to "sources" (agents) vs. "recipients" (patients) of moral action (p. 349-50).

They argue that focusing only on the mental and psychological capacities for agency and responsibility—and adopting an anthropomorphic stance, which ascribes such capacities solely to humans—is "worryingly dogmatic. Surely more conceptual analysis is needed here: what has happened morally when a child is deemed to enter adulthood, or when an adult is deemed to have lost moral autonomy, or when an animal is deemed to hold it?" (*Ibid.*, p. 374). Underlying these remarks is the concern voiced throughout this chapter: that it is likely impossible and of little practical help to determine the precise mental and psychological conditions of moral behavior. Ignoring the fact that non-humans can be both the sources and receivers of immoral action results in a narrow and absolute view of morality, which itself ignores the often dual or shared nature of morality. An artificial moral agency approach is more appropriate. As described shortly, U.S. and UK law recognize such artificial legal agency, in certain circumstances, and grant such agents legal rights and obligations.

Argument for Surrogate Agency and Beyond

Johnson et al. (2004) argue that advanced MDSS are not mere "tools" but rather are able to mediate and influence the decisions that operator makes. "To think that only human designers are subject to morality is to fail to recognize that technology and computer systems shape what humans do" (p. 434). This shaping power of computer systems is indicative of their possessing "a kind of intentionality" (a lower-order, not higher-order intentionality) (*Ibid.*). Surrogate agency is a useful model for explaining and predicting the effects of certain types of computer system's shaping or mediating power, but not all computer systems, nor all behaviors of those systems, fit the analogy of surrogate agency. "The best computer surrogate agents, then, are likely to be expert systems, or perhaps even 'artificially' intelligent computers, that can advise clients or users through a maze of complex rules, laws, and guidelines" (p. 432).

In human surrogate agency, the agent acts as "an agent of a third party—a client. The surrogate agent acts from the point of view that can be characterized as a 'third-person perspective.' […] consider[ing] not what he or she wants, but what the client wants. […] The morality constraining surrogate agents is role morality, a system of conventions and expectations associated with a role" (p. 423). Third-person agency is currently the only type of agency a computer system can express (p. 427). But "while computer systems do not have first-order desires and interests, they are designed in ways that represent interests, interests about the interests of users" (*Ibid.*). Users indicate their interests through requesting the system to perform certain tasks, and they have an expectation that the system will accurately and correctly perform those tasks. Assuming it is designed to fulfill requests (as opposed to ignore them, act duplicitously, or otherwise "misbehave"), then the system "adopts" the user's interests as its own.

- **Counterargument 1:** MDSS is simply a tool that supports human decision-making and action. In that supporting role, and being a computing technology, the design of the MDSS will necessarily result in some loss of user control, some limiting of user's scope for decision making. For example, of the treatment options suggested by the MDSS, there will also be options left out. Any tool, however, mediates the user's experience. This, in and of itself, simply pushes the matter into the realm of ethical deliberation. It does not, however, necessarily mean that the system also assumes responsibility.

- **Counterargument 2:** Most counterarguments to the surrogate agent model focus not on the feasibility of extending the model but rather on any attempt to ascribe agency and moral responsibility to non-human actors, regardless of the type of agency or responsibility. The current mainstream accounts of action, actors, and agency—particularly their requirements of anthropocentric and corporeal action—appear not to allow room for digital actions. Most accounts also require the requirement of intentionality. The type required for moral deliberation—what Dennett calls "higher-order intentionality" (1997, p. 354)—is itself an outgrowth of empathy, perceptual input, and complex interaction with one's environment. As of 1997, Dennett finds higher-order intentionality lacking in any AI system.

Argument for Legal Liability on Utilitarian-Consequentialist Grounds

Snapper (in Goodman [ed.], 1985, 1998) argues that continued use and future uptake of safety-critical technologies might be encouraged if some degree of responsibility or accountability were assigned to the intelligent computer system. Although his argument is here referring explicitly to intelligent computer systems, it is not a stretch to conclude that it applies to intelligent MDSS, which themselves are a type of computer system. Snapper's main arguments are that MDSS perform a necessary role both in the immediate doctor-patient interaction and in the overall healthcare environment, and that they function as "borrowed servants" of the hospital (1998, p. 49). Advanced MDSS are able to perform tasks "better" than, or at least faster than, the humans who operate them. In order to provide the best possible care, healthcare professionals must then use them, constituting a new standard of care.

- **Counterargument 1:** Not all MDSS play such a role. The creators of a consultation MDSS intend their system to be used for just that—consultation—but nothing more. The attending physician or healthcare professional may consider the recommendations, but nonetheless retains full autonomy (and thus full responsibility) in reaching decisions. This counterargument, however, ignores the mediating power of the technology.

- **Counterargument 2:** Where are the data? A study by Garg et al. (2005) indicated that data on practitioner performance only demonstrated overall improved practitioner performance (such as helping a doctor detect high blood pressure) in 64% of the cases studied (p. 1223). Of the 52 trials that assessed at least one patient outcome, only seven reported an improvement in outcomes (such as achieving lower or better-controlled blood pressure) (Ibid.). A relative dearth of data across a large population and time period makes it difficult for anyone to verify claims as to the prevalence, use, and effectiveness of MDSS. As previously noted, such claims often find their way into utilitarian-based arguments for assigning responsibility to MDSS on both moral and legal grounds, such as the "standard of care" argument. Some data do exist, however.

Argument that Uncertainty in Law Hinders Uptake

Snapper (1998) also argues that uptake of MDSS will be hindered by uncertainty in the moral and legal arenas. Some doctors will morally object to relinquishing some decision-making control to a computer system. Other doctors will be reluctant to use MDSS due to uncertainty of the legal consequences that could come to bear on their use.

- **Counterargument:** This argument is more of a cluster of assumptions than an argument, in the sense that the statements are largely unverifiable (it is far from clear how, for example, a social scientist would go about empirically testing that "uncertainty" would negatively impact the future use of MDSS).

That said, it is not entirely unthinkable, and it appeals to one's intuition. As for uncertainty in the legal situation: this uncertainty is a constant feature (some might call it an asset) in any legal system in which doctrine can be set and broken by precedent, or case law. While it can be valuable to venture predictions about which legal doctrines would plausibly apply in a particular case, in the end the only definitive answers come from either a legislature's lawmaking or a judge's ruling.

Argument for Shared Responsibility Due to Unpredictability

Nearly 20 years after the comment by Bechtel, which appears at the beginning of this chapter, Matthias (2004) claims that a responsibility gap has arisen. Advanced MDSS perform not only invisible complex calculation but also unpredictable, uncontrollable complex calculation. It is not morally defensible to hold either the system designer or the operator responsible for behavior they cannot conceivably control.

- **Counterargument 1:** This depends on the type of AI used by the MDSS. The system operator of a symbolic system-based MDSS can almost always edit the system's knowledge base to update facts or correct errors, so a great deal of control is possible.

- **Counterargument 2:** Matthias has not defined "responsible." The term is more nuanced than his usage would suggest. Responsibility—particularly causal responsibility—is hardly confined only to the area of blameworthiness. It also includes praise and recognition, as in "the aid agency was responsible for saving the lives of thousands of refugees." Here it can mean that the agency has a role responsibility, to see to it that lives are saved. It can also mean that the agency's actions (or omissions or failures to act) are causally responsible for saving lives.

Argument that MDSS Constitute New Standard of Care

What to do if advanced MDSS form the *de facto* standard of care, bestowing a moral responsibility on healthcare professionals to use them? Many argue that, when used properly, expert systems may lead to improved health, increased efficiency, cost savings, and overall increased welfare for both healthcare professionals and patients.

- **Counterargument 1:** Again, where are the data to back up such an assumption of improved patient outcomes and increased efficiency, not to mention the claim to improved "well-being," however defined? Hard data are hard to come by. As discussed earlier, Garg et al. (2005) conclude, in their review of 100 clinical trials of MDSS, that the majority of MDSS do improve practitioner performance, but that the current lack and low quality of data preclude the conclusion that MDSS use also improves patient outcomes. Success rates varied significantly across system application areas (diagnosis vs. drug prescribing, for example).

- **Counterargument 2:** MDSS negatively impact the doctor-patient relationship, by decreasing "face time" when the doctor is updating the system, operating it, or considering its decision. This argument is of the more general "technology encroachment" type.

- **Counterargument 3:** Even if this assumption could be verified independently, it still smacks of utilitarianism. Just because a technology is used now, does not mean that it should be used. One must move from the "is" to the "ought."

Ascribing Agency and Responsibility: Unique Legal Perspectives

What is a Legal Agent?

One might assume that the ethical perspectives on agency usually inform the legal ones, and also that there exists a sort of feedback mechanism by which the legal perspectives reinforce and sometimes influence the original ethical ones (although not all laws concern expressly moral issues, nor do they always concern positive or negative rights; some are simply rules about procedure). Some might take issue with this assumption, to which one could respond that the question, "which comes first: ethics or the law?" is a bit like the "chicken or the egg" conundrum, and, ultimately, does not serve to advance any meaningful discussion.

Upon further examination, however, legal perspectives on agents and agency have seemingly little to do with ethical perspectives—at least, not in some important aspects. Although it may seem counterintuitive at first glance, the law actually does not function solely upon humans. For example, non-human entities that may enter into contracts and be both subject and object in a liability case include immaterial things (such as organizations and corporations) and, sometimes, material things (such as ships). Although these things, on their own, cannot perform actions (they can only do so through agents), they are commonly said to have legal "personality" or "personhood." Potentially confusingly, the term is often used interchangeably with legal "agency." But one would not want to overstate the amount, type, and occurrence of legal agency currently ascribed to such entities. Legal agency derives its nature, in turn, from the precise nature of a relationship, as explained below. Indeed, humans, or human-made decisions and actions, are not far removed from either corporations or other material things that are given legal agency or legal personality. For example, humans create and manage a corporation; thus, one could argue that human brains and brawn are largely behind the actions of a corporation.

In law the terms "agent" and "agency" usually arise only in the context of the relationship between an agent and a principal (the legal definitions employed in this chapter are common to both the U.S. and UK legal systems and can be found in nearly any legal dictionary, and the terms are essentially the same in both jurisdictions, regardless of the area of state or federal law). Simply put, an agent acts on behalf of a principal. Depending on the relationship, agent and principal can be people or entities, in singular or plural form, or a combination of all of these (such as a company's board of directors [the agent or agents] vs. the company shareholders [the principal or principals]).

In addition, U.S. and UK law is generally silent when it comes to defining "action," as in, "what does it mean for an agent 'to act'?" To view it another way, the law adopts an open definition, which ensures the law's applicability to potential current and future situations, where the definition of "action" might not include any physical or bodily manifestation or produce any physical effect. This way the law can be stretched to cover digital and electronic actions. When it comes to considering MDSS as legal agents (with the attendant rights and obligations), the law lags behind, however, as it is created by humans and for humans, with little exception (remember corporations?). Thus, when discussing MDSS, current U.S. and UK law explicitly regulates the humans that develop, build, or use the system. At this stage in U.S. and UK law, MDSS use (or non-use, refusal to use) falls most likely under the various doctrines of tort law, particularly negligence, products liability, and strict liability. At present the author is unaware of any cases in the U.S. state, U.S. federal or UK courts that involve MDSS use and questions of agency. Given this lack of precedent, the following discussion is necessarily exploratory.

Whatever the name—legal "agency," "personhood," or "personality"—the concept entails rights and obligations, including the obligation of responsible action. Both legislation and case law in the U.S. and UK lag behind the reality of DSS usage today.

MDSS as Artificial Agents

If one adopts the agency theories presented earlier—surrogate agency, artificial agency—it would seem possible legally to apply agency to computer systems. Most relevant to this study is the legal status of non-living, non-human entities, such as digital or electronic "artificial agents." Today, the commonest approach is to treat such electronic agents as "mere tools" or "mere means of communication" (Chopra et al., 2004, p. 636). This approach creates the possibility that the designer, manufacturer, or vendor could be held liable for any damage, injury, or mistakes that result from the agent's actions, whether in the area of tort law or contract law. This approach also would prevent liability from being assigned directly to the artificial agent; as stated, liability rather bounces back to humans or the corporations for which they work.

Interestingly, many seemingly commonsensical notions about moral agency fail to find their complement in legal theory. Ethical perspectives on agency and responsibility often originate in a list of criteria required for assigning moral agency and responsibility. Often on the list are criteria such as autonomy, the mental capacity to make decisions, the ability to perform cognitive tasks, self-awareness, existence in physical bodily form, and so on (this list is not exhaustive). Not surprisingly, many philosophers adopt a similar approach when refuting the ascription of moral agency and liability to non-human agents: comparing such agents to the preceding grocery list of criteria, and marking where artificial agents fall short.

Chopra et al. raise the point—as does this chapter—that debates on the mental capacities and intelligence of any agent, human or otherwise, inevitably reduce to irresolvable debates about the validity of unverifiable assumptions about mental and physical processes. Such discussions often dissolve into semantic debates (such as on the meaning of "cognitive processes," and whether the algorithmic and electrical functioning of a computer system can be classified as cognition, even though they are synthetic). Instead, Chopra et al. advocate a pragmatic approach (which often finds its purest form in legal theory) that adopts Dennett's intentional stance and focuses on an agent's behavior, rather than the mental and physical processes that led to the behavior. They write,

[i]t is not clear, however, whether a legal system would deny an agent [legal] personality on the basis simply of its internal architecture, as opposed to whether it engaged in the right kinds of behavior, because its behavior is what will regulate its social interactions. Note, too, that the distinction made above assumes that we know what the actual features of mentality are. (Ibid., p. 638)

By "the right kinds of behavior," Chopra et al. do not appear to mean "right" in any normative sense, as in "good" or "proper"; rather, they refer to rightness as those types of behavior governed by law.

This is a good point at which to deal quickly with some oft-heard legal arguments against ascribing legal personality to artificial agents:

1. Some argue that **artificial agents are not their own "person," and so cannot enter into contracts.** In U.S.-UK legal systems, however, no contract is necessary to establish a relationship between a principal and agent that will have the force of law.

2. Some argue that **artificial agents do not exhibit the required mental capacity of a human adult.** This argument compares the artificial agent's internal system design, not behavior, to the assumed mental and psychological makeup of a human. But here again, possessing the mental capacity of a human adult is not a requirement for entering into a contract. Many jurisdictions rely instead on a "sound mind" for agency, which usually "means that the agent must understand the nature of the act being performed" (*Ibid.*, p. 637), although there may be debate as to exactly what is involved in understanding the nature of an act (for example, does it require recognizing the internal logic of an act, or just anticipating the consequences of an act, or does it mean judging—ethically or morally—the environment and conditions in which the act is to be performed? All of these seem plausible interpretations).

3. Some argue that **some degree of consciousness is necessary for legal agency and responsibility.** But "[t]he [U.S.-UK] legal system has not seen consciousness as a necessary or sufficient condition of legal personality. Historically, many categories of fully conscious humans—such as married women, slaves and children—have been denied legal personhood. Conversely, persons in comas or asleep [...] are not denied legal personality on that basis [...]" (*Ibid.*, p. 638).

There does exist an important criterion for assigning agents legal personality: their ability to control money. Obviously, this criterion arose out of tort law's *raison d'être*: to award financial compensation for injury and damage. It also makes only non-human entities that have money—such as corporations—able to compensate for their actions (although it must be noted that the corporation itself cannot handle or dispense money; agents must act on its behalf). In the case of computer systems, this means that compensation currently falls to the humans who designed, built, or sold the system, or even to the user who incorrectly used or applied the system, as further discussed next.

Many artificial agents are able to act autonomously and remain within legal boundaries. "Autonomy" is allowed for in many agency relationships, such as general agency, where the agent carries out actions on behalf of the principal in all matters in furtherance of the principal's particular business. In most legal contexts, "[a]utonomous action takes place without the knowledge (at least contemporaneously and of the specific transaction) of the principal" (*Ibid.*, p. 636). Autonomous action does not necessarily equal unpredictable, erratic action, however. Indeed, unpredictable or

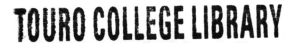

unforeseeable behavior could be the limit up to which the autonomy standard holds: if behavior is unpredictable (as Matthias claims it can be, or almost always is), then the standard could fail. But this is not necessarily the case.

Legal Definitions of Agency

The law distinguishes between more types of agency than just the artificial vs. the actual type. *Express agency* exists when the principal, either in writing or by speech, authorizes the agent to act on the principal's behalf (note that the principal may state the exact nature of the agent's authority, but does not have to). *Implied agency* exists when the principal, by nature of her actions (including the non-verbal and non-written), reasonably signals her intent to forge an agency relationship with the agent. *Special agency* specifies the exact acts that the agent may carry out—such as when, where, and how. *General agency* describes an agency relationship in which the agent carries out actions on behalf of the principal in all matters in furtherance of the principal's particular business.

Legal Definition of Action

The law (here, U.S. state and federal law, UK local and national law) is generally silent when it comes to defining "action," as in, "what does it mean for an agent 'to act'?" To view it another way, the law adopts an open definition, which ensures the law's applicability to all potential current and future situations, where the definition of "action" might not include any physical or bodily manifestation or produce any physical effect. This way the law can be stretched to cover digital and electronic actions.

Legal Responsibility and Liability

HLA Hart wrote extensively on responsibility, and his work appears to form the backbone of current U.S.-UK legal philosophy.[2] It can be difficult to divorce the terms "agency" and "responsibility," particularly when speaking about legal perspectives, because the law often views agency and responsibility as two sides of the same coin. When a human reaches "legal age," he or she is usually deemed to possess the conditions for agency. Much of the same argument can be made about moral agency: that it is required for responsibility.

Categorization of the types and elements of responsibility serves to clarify an important point: that responsibility does not necessarily entail liability. Often, legal liability is created in situations where there exists some sort of moral blameworthi-

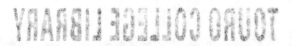

ness. But this is not always the case. The U.S.-UK doctrine of *respondeat superior* (lit. "may the superior give answer") arises only in tort law and, even then, usually only in employment contexts, where the employee is the agent and the employer is the principal. In a tort law situation, where the agent's actions have caused injury or damage, *respondeat superior* holds that the principal can be legally liable for those actions, regardless of whether they stemmed from the principal's direct orders (such as in special agency relationships), or whether they are reasonably deemed merely similar to the actions the principal herself would have made (such as in general agency relationships). The concept of *respondeat superior* falls under the more general term *vicarious liability* (note that the author is not aware of any continental legal systems that recognize vicarious liability of this or any sort).

By the same token, an actor can be causally responsible for an outcome of his actions (such as setting in motion a series of events), without being legally liable, because many doctrines require that the actor fulfill a series of psychological criteria, such as awareness of the law, awareness of consequences of action, and ability to control action. But there are exceptions to this, too: if the standard applied is that of strict liability, for example, the actor's psychological state is immaterial to establishing liability.

Courts' Treatment of Liability

When speaking of legal responsibility, the courts usually refer to legal liability.[3] Liability arises in instances of defect, damage, or harm, and involves a duty to remedy or compensate said defect, damage or harm. Harm can be physical or mental, tangible or intangible (such as economic harm), and can affect humans, non-humans, property, and intangibles (such as reputation, or brand). In this regard there is an explicit connection between the law and morality: the injurer, who by virtue of his obligation of care to the injured, also has a duty to remedy injury that is the direct and foreseeable consequence of the injurer's actions (although note that, in most types of negligence, such as UK's negligent misstatement law, there must be a degree of proximity in the relationship between the injurer and the injured, to establish a reasonable standard of the accused party's ability to foresee and prevent harm, as well as reasonably to contemplate the potential people or things to which they might be liable). This duty to remedy harm usually manifests itself in economic terms, whereby the liable party compensates the injured party with money or other financial instrument. It can also manifest itself in punitive damages, whereby the liable party is punished—by paying fees, by performing community service, by losing a professional accreditation, and so on.

Liability is also not an absolute quality, insofar as it can be held to various degrees, where some types of law are concerned. The idea that liability can be shared *and* quantified (*i.e.*, a dollar amount can be assigned to it, which may increase or decrease with respect to the number of parties to the suit, or the degree to which each party is deemed liable) is the primary driver behind the monetary awards given in a liability suit. In some liability doctrines, however, the injured party's contribution to her own injury is a bar to compensation.

In clinical medicine, liability arises usually in cases where a healthcare professional's actions or failures to act have caused injury or harm to a patient. Such liability suits are usually referred to as medical malpractice cases, where "malpractice" implies that there is some generally agreed-upon standard of care in the profession, which has not been upheld. Where this study is concerned, liability suits can arise when the healthcare professional uses (or fails to use) any variety of medical tools, potentially including intelligent computer systems such as MDSS, if the use of MDSS is deemed the standard of care, as discussed throughout this chapter. Many MDSS (particularly those used for diagnosis and treatment) are termed "safety-critical" because they regulate or affect life-critical processes. As will be discussed more below, in the U.S. and UK, purchasers and users of defective or damaging hardware or software can find remedy through both the civil law (contract and tort law), and, in some cases, the criminal law.

As this chapter has already hinted, when it comes to tort law, it is also relevant whether the computer system (here, hardware plus software) is a product or a service. In most cases involving computer systems, however, the lines are blurred; most computer systems, particularly those used in clinical medicine, exhibit properties of both products and services. Hardware on its own is a product, whereas software is often classified as a service. Which doctrines of tort law that can apply will depend on which aspect of the system is claimed to be defective.

In order to fall under the protection and control of contract law, the purchaser of the software must also be the aggrieved or harmed party. On the other hand, invoking tort law, which concerns civil wrongs, does not depend on the existence of a contract between parties, and so is more likely to be the appropriate type of law in most cases involving clinical medicine, doctors, and their patients. U.S. and UK tort law includes the law of negligence, negligent misstatement, and products liability.

While products and services—both of which are non-human, one of which is intangible—may be deemed faulty and defective, in both everyday speech and legal proceedings, they in and of themselves cannot provide remedy to the injured party.[4] The express purposes of tort law, for example, are to provide remedy to the injured party (usually by offering economic compensation), to ensure the proper application of products and services (by punishing people who incorrectly use a product and thus cause a harm), or to deter the appearance of faulty products and services on the market (by punishing careless or negligent designers, manufacturers or vendors). In most cases, a product, on its own, cannot provide compensation (it has no money, nor can it be punished), but its manufacturer or developer can. The manufacturer may be in the legally-recognized form of a corporation, or it may be a person. So, while the courts might in theory locate the direct and proximate cause of an injury in a defective product or service, in practice they will look to human, or to a money-possessing entity, to provide compensation.

A number of legal principles (pragmatically termed "laws") govern contract and tort law cases involving safety-critical computer systems:

- *Negligence* forms the basis of medical malpractice suits (Miller, 1989). It can be invoked only if three conditions are met: (1) that the relationship between the injured party and the defendant involved a duty of care; (2) that the duty of care was breached; (3) and that damage (to persons or property), injury (to persons or property), or other loss (mental, physical, or economic) occurred as the direct and reasonable result of that breach (Bainbridge, 2000).[5]

- In the U.S., a case of *negligence per se* (also called "negligence *res ipsa loquitor*," lit. "the thing speaks for itself") does not require a trier of fact to prove the exact acts of negligence that led to injury, because the circumstances and degree of injury are such that it is obvious that there was negligence (for example, a doctor leaves a medical instrument inside a patient after surgery). *Gross negligence* occurs when the defendant did not exercise any regard whatsoever for the safety of others; gross negligence can also bring criminal charges. In some instances, *contributory negligence* (whereby the injured party has to some degree contributed to his or her injury, possibly including implied risk) is a bar to compensation.

- The law of *negligent misstatement* (in the UK also called "tortuous liability for negligent advice") is of particular relevance to intelligent expert systems, such as MDSS. [6] No contractual relationship is necessary in order to this doctrine to apply; rather, the defendant must simply present himself (and be understood as such) as an expert and give "advice which is intended to be taken seriously and acted upon" (*Ibid.*, p. 188). If the recipient of the expert advice suffers injury, damage, or loss as a direct and proximate result of the advice, then he or she may have legal recourse to seek compensation from the designer or manufacturer of the system. At present, UK law has:

[…] the effect of making the persons and organizations responsible for the creation of expert systems liable to the ultimate consumers of the advice generated. The experts who provided the rules and facts used by the system, the knowledge engineers who formalized the knowledge, the programmers and analysts responsible for designing the inferencing and interface programs could find themselves liable if the advice generated by use of the system is incorrect. (Ibid., p. 189)

There are at least two defenses possible to this in today's UK law: there was no duty of care (either the damage was not foreseeable, the relationship between system developer and recipient of information was too attenuated, or the information was used for a purpose unknown to or reasonably unintended by the system designer), or a reasonable disclaimer, exemption clause, or limitation clause existed which limited or absolved the creators of the system of liability (*Ibid.*). That said, no disclaimer absolves of liability in cases of product liability or malpractice that lead to death or personal injury (*Ibid.*). The potential implications of applying various negligence claims to cases involving MDSS is presented next.

Products liability allows the consumer to sue the designer, manufacturer, or vendor of a defective product without having to prove negligence and without having to prove a contractual relationship.[7] Of course, products liability can refer to negligence law, but does not have to. In the U.S., products liability often takes the shape of strict liability (described below). It can also involve claims on warranty of fitness. All products liability cases center on a claim or claims of fault or defect in one (or more) of the following areas: design, manufacturing, or marketing. Locating the defect can be incredibly difficult in cases involving hardware and software.

The most important and effective defense to products liability suits in the UK is that of "state of the art," whereby the defendant need only prove that "the state of scientific and technical knowledge at the relevant time was not such that a producer of products of the same description of the product in question might be expected to have discovered the defect if it had existed in his products while they were under his control" (*Ibid.*, p. 195). Once a product has left the factory floor, however, "control" by the manufacturer is largely no longer possible.

The doctrine of *strict liability* (which operates primarily on manufacturers and vendors of products) requires that the injured party demonstrate that the faulty or damaging product is the direct and proximate cause of injury. For strict liability to hold, the causal pathway may not be too attenuated between injured party and faulty product, nor may the injured party have in any way and of own volition contributed to the injury. Not important, however, is whether or not the defendant exercised care in preventing the injury; carefulness does not even enter the picture. Strict liability is, thus, a special type of liability that recognizes causal responsibility, regardless of intent. In other words, someone may be held strictly liable for an event or outcome if it can be shown that that person's actions directly and causally led to the outcome.

The initiator of an accident, or of unintended consequences, can come under this doctrine. As mentioned above, the establishment of a clear, limited causal pathway between agent and outcome is sufficient to assign strict liability; but establishing causal or strict liability is quite different from establishing moral responsibility, which sets the bar at a higher level. Should the doctrine be applied often to cases involving harm or damage due to MDSS use, it could effectively curtail research and development of future systems, as manufacturers and vendors would be held legally responsible to create systems of an impossible (and undesirable) standard: the error-free system (Miller, 1989). The potential implications of applying products liability or strict liability to cases involving MDSS is presented next.

Potential Legal Scenarios

While this chapter has primarily focused on the possibility of assigning some level of legal responsibility to advanced MDSS, the chapter has also noted that current liability and negligence law already acts upon the users of MDSS (usually, the medical professional) and the objects of MDSS use (usually, the patients and sometimes the medical professionals, too, if they are using the system in order to increase their knowledge).

The legal issues that arise with the use of MDSS most often involve questions of liability for harm or damage caused. The law of negligence—as invoked in medical malpractice suits—turns in part on the "standard of care" due the patient. The future-proof standard is always evaluated with reference to the field in question, and so will differ by medical area, geographical location, and time. At some point it may no longer be possible for medical professionals—and the hospitals that employ them—to avoid using MDSS; indeed, they will have a duty to use them, both legally (to uphold the standard of care and thus avoid malpractice) and ethically (to uphold the principle of beneficence, to provide the best possible care to patients).[8] Once this happens, and assuming that intelligent systems continue to develop so-called intelligent capabilities, one could even argue that advanced MDSS move from being mere tools in decision making, to being partners in decision making, perhaps partners in healthcare. From this perspective it would appear imperative that some degree of legal liability be assigned to the intelligent system.

- **Strict Liability Scenario 1:** Should strict liability be applied often to cases involving harm or damage due to MDSS use, it could effectively curtail research and development of future systems, as manufacturers and vendors would be held legally responsible to create systems of an impossible (and undesirable) standard: the error-free system (Miller, 1989, p. 76). Because of the potentially exorbitant costs to physicians and hospitals to purchase products liability insurance for using MDSS, Miller argues that judges are not likely to apply strict liability except in the most clear-cut and extreme of cases.
- **Strict Liability Scenario 2:** What Miller did not consider in 1989, however, is that today's systems that feature AI in their system design are unable to function entirely error-free, as committing mistakes is part of the way in which they "learn." This makes strict liability an even more prohibitive doctrine to

apply (as it would stifle development) and more difficult legally to justify (as it relies on a clear connection between human error in design, manufacturing, or marketing, and damage or injury to the defendant).

- **Products Liability Scenario 1:** The designer of a controllable system that aids or replaces human decision-making can be held liable (under products liability) for the damage the system creates only if the product has functioned or performed incorrectly due to its design, manufacturing or marketing, all of which are determined prior to the product leaving the factory floor. For products liability, the type of MDSS is of little issue, so long as its incorrect or damage-causing behavior can be traced back to human error.

- **Products Liability Scenario 2:** The designer of a system that performs outside of human control (outside of human predictability) is likely not liable for the above situation, under products liability, because the incorrect or damage-causing behavior cannot necessarily be traced back to human error. To do so would effectively end the development of all learning automata.

- **Negligence Scenario 1:** If a healthcare professional uses a system that functions as aiding, but not replacing, decision-making, the operator retains ultimate control of, and legal liability for, the application of the MDSS' advice, under negligence law. If a patient is injured as a result of the operator's decision (even though it was partially informed by the MDSS), and not as well by the patient's own accord (as contributory negligence is a bar to recovery in many jurisdictions), then the patient has the right to seek recovery via negligence law.

- **Negligence Scenario 2:** If the use of MDSS is claimed to form the standard of care, then a healthcare professional's decision not to use it could bring negligence claims. In legal systems that recognize vicarious liability, the employer of the healthcare professional (usually a hospital) is potentially also open to negligence claims.

- **Negligent Misstatement Scenario 1:** Insofar as an MDSS is considered an expert system by users, the person or persons who create, edit, or update the MDSS's knowledge base are likely to be held responsible for the accuracy of that information, as they have a duty of care to the receiver of such expertise.

- **Negligent Misstatement Scenario 2:** But where the MDSS "learns" from iterated interaction with the user, and in the process makes mistakes and adjusts behavior, it is less clear that a person or persons would be held liable for the accuracy of such statements, as it is far less clear who holds the duty of care. An analogous situation: licensed physicians graduate from medical school, where they receive much of their ground education, which is later supplemented by interning at medical facility. If a physician's actions cause damage or injury to a patient, neither the medical school nor the medical facility where the physician received his or her practical training, is open to liability under negligent misstatement, although it could be argued that the physician bases his or her actions on the "statements" or expertise offered by, and gained at, the medical school and the medical facility. One could thus draw an analogy with the duty-of-care status of the person(s) who supply and edit the MDSS's knowledge base.

One important theoretical reason why negligence (including negligent misstatement) claims might still operate only on humans (as opposed to the system) is that, where a healthcare professional owns and operates an expert system, he or she could be held partially liable for the misapplication or misinterpretation of the expert system's advice. This is because "[p]ossible existence of errors in communication may make it difficult to establish the product as the direct cause of the patient's injury" (Miller, 1989, p. 79). Errors in communication could stem from the user interpreting commands and prompts differently than that system (or, the system designer) intended. Unfortunately, the user would necessarily discover communication errors *post facto*, after acting upon information provided by the MDSS and noticing harm or damage to the patient (because, before that point, the communication cannot be deemed to be incorrect or faulty but must be considered correct).

Conclusion

Responsibility Differs by MDSS Type and Usage

The arguments and theories summarized in this chapter generally subscribe to one of essentially two ways of viewing MDSS:

1. As a black box, where "users are unable to monitor what is going on in the system as a matter of fact (inaccessibility) and secondly, even if they could monitor what was going on, they would not be able to keep track of it (intractability)" (van den Hoven, 2001, p. 2); or

2. As a complex internal system, the behavior of which can ultimately be controlled and predicted.

To determine which view to adopt, one should assess the MDSS' behavior and usage environment. Is it used (or to be used) as an *aid* or a *substitute* for human decision-making?[9] The arguments and counterarguments presented herein for assigning a least three types of agency to computer systems are all dependent upon the classification of the MDSS as an aid/supporting system, or a replacement/substitute for human decision-making. Nearly all such arguments eventually rest upon role responsibility: surrogate agency, borrowed-servant agency, artificial legal agency (via Chopra & White), and artificial moral agency (via Floridi and Saunders). Where an MDSS actually actions a course of treatment, causal responsibility can be assigned. The causal pathway is less clear for an MDSS that is used in a primarily support position.

Legal Agency and Liability are Most Viable

This chapter's exploration of the relevant legal doctrines of tort law indicates that the easiest way to assign agency and responsibility is to do so via the law. In this respect, there appears to be a significant divergence between moral and legal philosophy, which usually overlap to a high degree.

Chopra and White are correct to point out that the law does not yet preclude the possibility of applying artificial agency to non-human actors, as legal agency and legal personhood do not rely necessarily on consciousness, adult mental capacity, or the presence of a contract between agent and principal, all of which are oft-voiced barriers to granting legal personhood. If one argues that an MDSS fulfills the conditions for legal personhood via artificial legal agency, this comes with rights and obligations, including the possibility of liability under both negligence and strict liability law.

This chapter also notes that current liability and negligence law already applies to users of MDSS and the objects of MDSS use, which are usually patients but can also be the medical professionals if they are using the system for increasing their knowledge. Some might argue that to hold the system designer or operator liable for the to-some-degree-unpredictable statements of a computer system would serve to stifle development in the industry.

The legal issues discussed in this chapter most often involve questions of liability for harm or damage caused. The law of negligence—as it is invoked in medical malpractice suits—turns in part on the standard of care due the patient. Goodman (1998) writes: "The future of the health professions is computational," (p. 1), potentially implying that MDSS uptake will increase until it becomes the norm: "Suppose the use of medical computers evolves to the point that half of all practitioners employ them to good effect. Are those who do *not* use computers then providing substandard care? [...] It will not be obvious when we cross such a Rubicon" (p. 7, Goodman's own emphasis). Standard of care is a future-proof legal concept, insofar as it changes in step with developments in technology. The standard is always evaluated with reference to the field in question, and so will differ from field to field, country to country.

The legal discussion herein is intended to highlight some of the potential legal consequences of MDSS use. As there is a dearth of actual precedent (in both the case law and legislative law) upon which to base them, the scenarios presented herein are necessarily hypothetical and exploratory. Uncertainty in the law is a constant feature in any legal system in which doctrine can be set and broken by precedent. As stated earlier, it can be valuable to venture predictions about which legal doctrines would plausibly apply in a particular case, but in the end the only definitive answers come from either a legislature's lawmaking or a judge's ruling, but at the same time, not forgetting that matters of law are often matters of interpretation.

Greater Capacities, Wider Applications

The scope of the issues raised by learning automata extends beyond the immediate world of healthcare. Healthcare is an industry in which the technology is gaining a firm foothold and in which the use of decision support systems is often safety-critical, which it is not often in other areas in which decision support systems are sometimes employed. The reality today is that decision support systems are used in many aspects of modern life. For example, if you buy shares in a mutual fund, the fund manager's decision when to buy or sell stock is almost certainly informed (if not actioned) by a computer program, which crunches large amounts of market data to identify the optimal conditions—arbitrage situations—for executing a trade. If you apply for private, non-federal health insurance in some countries, your medical, financial, genealogical history— and even geographical location—may all be analyzed by a computer program to calculate the premium you pay, or the amount of the claim you may seek, each of which itself is assessed by calculation of the risk that you will draw on the insurance at a certain time, for certain amounts.

There is little reason to suspect that the use of intelligent or advanced decision support systems will not extend into yet other areas of society, commerce, and science in the future. But blind faith in the advantages and capabilities of an advanced decision support system can be just as harmful as irrational fear of the technology. It is time to begin thinking of potentially novel ways to deal with the moral and legal consequences of their use. MDSS technology continues to develop and evolve; so, too, should the debate.

References

Bainbridge, D. (2000). *Introduction to computer law* (4th ed.). Harlow, UK: Pearson Education.

Beauchamp, T., & Childress, J. (1989). *Principles of biomedical ethics* (3rd ed.). Oxford: Oxford University Press.

Bechtel, W. (1985). Attributing responsibility to computer systems. *Metaphilosophy, 16*(4), 296-306.

Chopra, S., & White, L. (2004). Artificial agents—Personhood in law and Philosophy. *Proceedings of the European Conference on Artificial Intelligence 2004.* Retrieved April 15, 2005, from http://grimpeur.tamu.edu/~colin/Papers/ama.text.html

Collste, G. (2000). Ethical aspects on decision support systems in diabetes care. In Collste (ed.), *Ethics in the age of information technology. Studies in applied ethics* (Vol. 7, pp. 181-194). Linköping: bpt-TRYCK AB.

Coiera, E., & Open Clinical (eds.). *Open clinical directory of DSS in healthcare.* Retrieved January 2, 2005, from http://www.openclinical.org/aisinpractice.html

Dennett, D. (1997). When HAL kills, who's to blame? Computer ethics. In D. Stork (ed.), *HAL's legacy: 2001's Computer as Dream and Reality* (pp. 351-365). London: MIT Press.

Dennett, D. (1978). *Brainstorms.* Hassocks (Sussex): Harvester Press.

Floridi, L., & Saunders, J. W. (2004). On the morality of artificial agents. *Minds and Machine, 14,* 349-379.

Garg, A. X., Adhikari, N. K. J., McDonald, H., Rosas-Arellano, M. P., Devereaux, P.J., Beyene, J., Sam, J. & Haynes, R. B. (2005). Effects of computerized clinical decision support systems on practitioner performance and patient outcomes. *Journal of the American Medical Association, 293* (10), 1223-1238.

Goodman, K. W. (1998). *Ethics, computing, and medicine.* Cambridge: Cambridge University Press (CUP).

Johnson, D. G., & Nissenbaum, H. (1995). *Computers, ethics, & social values.* Upper Saddle River, NJ: Prentice Hall.

Johnson, D. G., & Powers, T. (2004). Computers as surrogate agents. *Proceedings of ETHICOMP 04 The 7th ETHICOMP International Conference on the Social and Ethical Impacts of Information and Communication Technologies: Challenges for the Citizen of the Information Society, 1* (pp. 422-35). University of the Aegean, Syros, Greece, April 14-16, 2004.

King, H., Garibaldi, J., & Rogerson, S. (2002). Intelligent medical systems: Partner or tool? *Proceedings of ETHICOMP 02 The 6th ETHICOMP International Conference on the Social and Ethical Impacts of Information and Communication Technologies: The Transformation of Organisations in the Information Age, 1.* Universidade Lusiada, Lisbon, Portugal, November 13-15, 2002.

King, H., & Rogerson, S. (2004). Ethical analysis of the behaviour of clinicians using expert systems. *Proceedings of ETHICOMP 04 The 7th ETHICOMP International Conference on the Social and Ethical Impacts of Information and Communication Technologies: Challenges for the Citizen of the Information Society, 1* (pp. 508-519). University of the Aegean, Syros, Greece, April 14-16, 2004.

Matthias, A. (2004). The responsibility gap: Ascribing responsibility for the actions of learning automata. *Ethics and Information Technology, 6*, 175-183.

Miller, R. A. (1989). Legal issues related to medical decision support systems. *International Journal of Clinical Monitoring, 6*, 75-80.

Miller, R. A., & Goodman, K. W. (1998). Ethical challenges in the use of decision-support software in clinical practice. In K. W. Goodman (ed.), *Ethics, computing, and medicine* (pp. 102-114). Cambridge: CUP.

Miller, R. A., & Masarie, F. E. (1990). The demise of the "Greek oracle" model for medical diagnostic systems. *Methods of Information in Medicine, 29*, **1-2.**

Moor, J. (1995a). Is ethics computable? *Metaphilosophy, 26*, 1-21.

Moor, J. (1995b). What is computer ethics? In D. Johnson & H. Nissenbaum (eds.), *Computers, ethics, & social values* (pp. 7-15). Upper Saddle River, NJ: Prentice Hall.

Snapper, J. (1985). Responsibility for computer-based errors. *Metaphilosophy, 16*, 289-295.

Snapper, J. (1998). Responsibility for computer-based decisions in healthcare. In K. W. Goodman (ed.), *Ethics, computing, and medicine* (pp. 43-56). Cambridge: CUP.

van den Hoven. (2001). Moral responsibility and information technology. In In T. W. Bynum, H. Krawczyk, S. Rogerson, S. Szejko, & B. Wizniewski (eds.), *ETHICOMP 01: Proceedings of the 5th ETHICOMP International Conference on the Social and Ethical Impacts of Information and Communication Technologies: Systems of the Information Society.* Technical University of Gdansk, Poland, June 18-20, 2001. Published by Leicester: DeMontfort University. CD-ROM only.

Endnotes

[1]   This chapter is a condensed and significantly revised version of part of a published Master's thesis: Haviland, H. *"The Machine Made Me Do It!": An Exploration of Ascribing Agency and Responsibility to Decision Support Systems,* available on-line at: http://urn.kb.se/resolve?urn=urn:nbn:se:liu:diva-2922

(retrieved on 2007-09-19) to which I would refer any readers interested in a fuller treatment of the ethical and legal theories presented so briefly here.

2   See, for example, HLA Hart (1994 edition), *The Concept of Law*.

3   Hart writes, "[...] though in certain general contexts legal responsibility and legal liability have the same meaning, to say that a man is legally responsible for some act or harm is to state that his connexion [sic] with the act or harm is sufficient according to law for liability. Because responsibility and liability are distinguishable in this way, it will make sense to say that because a person is legally responsible for some action he is liable to be punished for it." (*Ibid.*, p. 521).

4   Although if the injured party seeks compensation in the form of ensuring that the product is removed from the market and no longer poses a threat, then the product's removal could be a form of compensation—albeit intangible, mental compensation. But there again, it is a person or persons who actually remove the product from the market. The product cannot do so itself.

5   According to Bainbridge (2000), the UK law of negligence has its origins in *Donoghue* v. *Stevenson* [1932] AC 562, which is a generally uncontested assumption. I have yet been unable to determine the exact case law origins of US negligence law.

6   UK law of negligent misstatement has its origins in *Hedley Byrne & Co Ltd.* v. *Heller & Partners Ltd* [1964] AC 465, according to Bainbridge (2000, p. 188). *Hedley Byrne* has since been stretched to cover negligent provision of a service (*Ibid.*, p. 193), which theoretically brings it into the domain of expert systems based on software *per se*.

7   In the UK, products negligence law stems from the *Consumer Protection Act 1987*. In the US, products negligence law stems from various state statutes, some of which are based on the *Model Uniform Products Liability Act* and the Uniform Commercial Code. No federal products liability statutes exist in the US.

8   One could potentially go so far, invoking King and Rogerson's (2004) study of ethical principles, to argue that the patient's right to equality (here, equal care and treatment) requires the use of MDSS.

9   I first heard the terms "aid versus substitute" used in this context during conversations with Simon Rogerson, May 2005.

Chapter VI

Responsibility in Electronic Health: What Muddles the Picture?

Janne Lahtiranta, University of Turku, Finland

Kai. K. Kimppa, University of Turku, Finland

Abstract

In this chapter, we look into the potential problems arising from the use of information and communication technology (ICT) artifacts in electronic health. We focus on issues such as liabilities and responsibilities and discuss these issues on the basis of patient-physician relationship, negligence, agentization, and anthropomorphism. We conclude the chapter with recommendations originating from different fields of industry. These recommendations are applied to the field of electronic health in order to make users more aware of the nature and use of ICT artifacts in various health care situations.

Introduction

In electronic health, care is mediated using different ICT artifacts, sometimes over geographical and organizational barriers. The technology provides an extension to health care processes, which are traditionally interpersonal by nature. Ideally, the introduction of technology should not negatively affect the quality of care. However, the constantly advancing technology and ever increasing demand of cost deductions can lead to a situation where less attention is given to ethical issues. Many of the solutions of electronic health exist today only to serve the purposes of better profit and decreased costs of operations. While these reasons are undoubtedly valid, they should not be pursued at the expense of ethics, which is the foundation of all medical practice.

When ethical, legal and risk issues in electronic health in general are considered, the following issues are typically raised (see, e.g., Rodrigues, 2000; Stanberry, 2001; Wagner, 1999):

- Confidentiality
- Security
- Consent
- Responsibility
- Liability

While confidentiality and security are vital aspects in electronic health, in this chapter we focus on the issue of responsibility, to which issues of consent and liability are closely tied. Our emphasis is within the context of the issue of the implementation of the technologies, giving less attention to technological details such as the standardization of communication protocols for example.

While our sole focus is not in the technology *per se*, we must acknowledge that its rapid advance has had a tremendous impact on the health care processes and practices. The rapid adoption of different artifacts of information and communication technology (ICT) in health care has created a concern about a patient's ability to identify where the responsibilities lie when these artifacts are used. The patient does not necessarily know when an actual doctor-patient relationship is formed or with whom it is formed. ICT intensifies this problem since in electronic health the technology not only enables information exchange with physicians or other professionals of health care; it also enables the use of different information systems or devices in the decision making process related to the actual care. This is problematic especially in a situation where the patient is not aware that the interaction originates from a device or a system, not from a clinician.

Issues such as agentization and anthropomorphism further muddle the picture since the artifacts used in ICT mediated health care may contain characteristics which are intended to create an illusion of life where there is none. This can be particularly problematic in a situation when the user is not familiar with the technology they are using, or where they have a decline of mental or cognitive capability that may have an effect on their user experience. This may be especially relevant given the current trend of creating ubiquitous or "invisible" solutions in the field of home care.

The lack of ethical procedures, guidelines, and standards in the field of electronic health could easily be blamed on the speed of technological development. This view, however, is flawed since many of the legal and ethical issues related to electronic health are common to health care in general (Stanberry, 2001). Such issues simply emerge in a different fashion when they are considered in the context of electronic health. In general, the change has been so rapid that legislation and standardization have not been able to keep up with the changing context.

This is particularly the case in electronic health where the legislation is inconsistent and ranges from a light "reasonable" approach to the very strict (Wachter, 2002), and where professional guidelines, standards and regulations are either inadequate or do not exist (Stanberry, 2001). Due to this rapid development of technology, standardization, and legislation tend to be reactive, rather than proactive. This has resulted in a situation where rules and regulations specific to the field of electronic health come into force after the technical applications and associated systems are already in production. However, in order to ensure the successful and seamless adoption of electronic health, consideration on how they should be adopted and integrated into the health care system in general must be made beforehand, not at the production stage.

Models of Patient-Physician Relationship

Throughout history, ethics has always played an important role in (western) medicine. Until the emergence of modern medicine around 1800, philosophy and medicine enjoyed a rather close partnership (Svenaeus, 2001). For example, the Hippocratic Oath founded by Hippocrates around 400 BC still captures the essential responsibilities and duties of physicians today. Even though the speed of technological advance today is almost impossible to comprehend, the practice of medicine should still be about patients, not just about science and technology.

Patients and their relationship with their physician has been one of the central aspects of medical ethics ever since the early days of the Greek and Roman philosophers. In the spirit of these ancient philosophers, this relationship has been characterized as a form of friendship, which was the focal point of the moral life at that time (see e.g., Plato 380 BC, Aristotle 350 BC). Much later, particularly in Spain, this friendship between the patient and the physician has been known as "medical philia" (Svenaeus, 2001), which emphasizes and even idealizes the special relationship between the two.

Childress and Siegler (1984) further characterize this relationship using five different models. The first model, paternalism, describes the relationship as akin to a relationship between a parent and an infant. According to this model, the relationship is by nature asymmetrical and hierarchical, and the doctor has a moral authority over the patient. If we consider the empowerment of patients enabled by the increased and ever increasing access to different medical information sources made available via the Internet, this model is now under heavy dispute. For example, the pharmaceutical companies advertise their products more directly to patients (via email for example), creating a potential conflict between the demands of the empowered patient and knowledge of the physicians. Nowadays it is not unheard of that the patients challenge the authority of their "parents" (i.e., physicians) by demanding a certain type of treatment or medication.

The second model, partnership, emphasizes collaboration and association between the patient and the physician creating a covenant of a sort. In this model, the two parties together strive to pursue the shared value of patient's health. In contrast to the paternalistic model, this one perceives the patient more as an equal, or as an adult, and respects the personal autonomy of the patient. In partnership, the physician does not automatically "know" what is best for the patient and the physician considers the patient as an indispensable source of information, that must be taken into consideration when planning their health care.

The partnership model is a step closer to the third model, which is known as rational contractors, in which the care is perceived as a contract between two parties. Like the second model, this describes the relationship between the two parties in terms of equality and autonomy. In this model, the parties agree to exchange goods and services according to contracts, which are often subject to governmental sanctions. The sequential nature of these contracts largely forms what we understand as patient trajectory. It can be argued that this kind of model promotes mutual trust, but it fails in many areas. For example, the model neglects the fact that some sick and elderly people with declining mental and cognitive abilities are unable to act as full partners. As described by Childress et al. (1984), the model also neglects virtues of care and compassion, which are present in the previous two models.

The fourth attempt to describe the relationship between the patient and the physician is called the friendship model, which in practice captures the spirit of "medical philia" discussed earlier. Distinct from the medical partnership, which emphasizes the limited scope of the relationship and emotional reserve related to it, the medical friendship stresses the intensity of the relationship applying ingredients from more personal models into the mix. This friendship model is probably the closest one to the arguments made by Post (1994) who states that in order to recover trust physicians must demonstrate personal care and compassion to their patients.

While the first four models create plausible models for the relationship between the patient and physician, Childress et al. (1984) consider the final model as the most unrealistic and undesirable. This final model—known as the technician model—perceives the physician as an engineer, who provides a technical service to patients who are consumers. In this model, the physician simply describes the facts of the condition thus handing the autonomy, and largely the responsibility, over to the patient. In her article, Cohn (2004) compares the physician in this model to an automobile mechanic. Similarly to a mechanic, the physician assesses the problem, provides available options, and is obligated to provide the treatment selected by the patient. In this model, there is no real two-way relationship between the parties and it is hard to point to where the moral responsibility lies. While Childress et al. (1984) consider this model as the most unrealistic of the five, we argue that this model captures some of the worst elements of electronic health, creating a potential to multiply risk issues. Like Post (1994) we argue that the pressures of technology, as well as those of time and money, work against the kind of care that promotes personal care and compassion.

Defining Electronic Health

To give a comprehensive definition of electronic health is difficult. The concept of using ICT artifacts in health care has many faces and many names. In literature the concept is known variously as "telecare," "telehealth," and "telemedicine" (amongst other), which all give a special notion on the use of technology. One of the concepts that capture certain key elements of electronic health is "telemedicine," which literally means "medicine at distance." A more formal definition for telemedicine is provided by the European Commission (1993): "Rapid access to shared and remote medical expertise by means of telecommunications and information technologies, no matter where the patient or relevant information is located." This term draws its power from a vision of providing care to those who need it, disregarding all barriers. What this definition itself does not explicitly state is the nature of medical expertise; does it originate from "the man or the machine"?

Amongst others, electronic health has applications in basic health care (diagnostics and treatment), health education, health informatics, self-care, and research. Especially in (western) industrial countries, there are only a few, if any, domains in health care in which ICT artifacts are not used. Due to its wide spectrum, electronic health is considered in this chapter as an inclusive term, which covers all health care professionals and different customers of health care services. Fundamentally, the term is about providing best health care possible to those who need it.

Using ICT in health care has a long and interesting history. If electronic health is considered in a broad sense, it came about with the introduction of telephone when Dr. Alexander Bell called "Watson come here, I want to see you" on March 10, 1876 because he inadvertently spilled acid on himself (Hodson, 2003). Today, medical practitioners around the world are starting to realize the potential of ICT in health care. Powered by modern telecommunication technologies, it is possible to interact with colleagues and patients around the globe. This possibility to overcome geographical distance is considered as the major technical novelty in electronic health (Raes, 1997). While overcoming geographical distances might be just a matter of technology, a more challenging obstacle lies in the organizations that employ ICT in health care processes. In order to fully utilize ICT in day-to-day operations of health care, organizational (including legislative) and social barriers (such as user resistance to change) must be leveled as well.

Example applications in use today include: remote consulting, transfer of images and health data on patients, data mining of patient records for use in medical education and training, intelligent medical systems (see e.g., Coiera, 2003; King, Garibaldi, & Rogerson, 2002), and interaction with medical hardware such as diagnostic instruments or the remote monitoring of a patient either by a clinician or by a system or a device.

Defining Anthropomorphism

Anthropomorphism, which commonly means endowing human characteristics to nonhuman objects or forces, arose initially in the context of theology, where the question was how to understand the nature of God. In the context of ICT anthropomorphism is commonly attributed towards artificial intelligence, robotics, or user interfaces (see e.g., Carrier, 1990). According to Takeuchi and Naito (1995) through intentionally designing anthropomorphic interfaces even experts, let alone laymen, are easily led to act as if the computer software was a social actor, in regard to computers and software such as the patients or physicians might use.

Anthropomorphism has intentional and unintentional dimensions. Intentional, or planned, anthropomorphism exists when human-like attributes are purposefully introduced to electronic services and applications in order to provide natural and comfortable interaction, and conversational communication (Marsh & Meech 2000; Takeuchi & Nagao 1993). Non-intentional anthropomorphism occurs when people humanize the inhuman for example, by attributing human-like attributes to computers and other media, treating them like people (Heckman & Wobbrock 2000). According to Heckman & Wobbrock (2000): "With surprising ease, overly trusting consumers may be persuaded to interact with anthropomorphic agents in a way that endangers them" (p. 435). This is even more the case in electronic health, where the possible danger is direct and ever-present due to the nature of the situation. In the field of electronic health, intentional anthropomorphism exists for example in applications and systems of telepresence, and in electronic services for the aging. For example, a Japanese nursing home has used ifbot 620, a robot that can sing, express emotions and give trivia quizzes, in their elderly care (Reuters, 2007).

Regardless of the potential benefits of intentional anthropomorphism there are some possible risks—especially in the matters of authenticity, trust, and credibility (Dowling, 2001). Users must be able to discriminate between real and unreal. As Dowling suggests, the inability to make a distinction between human-originated and machine-originated data is of importance; but the authors want to stress the importance particularly in electronic health, since in such a critical area people must be able to effectively utilize and judge the information they receive. If the information is of dubious value, it is unlikely to be incorporated into the individual's decision-making (Bengtsson, Burgoon, Cederberg, Bonito, & Lundberg, 1999) but if the information received from an intentionally or unintentionally humanized interface is taken uncritically, then relevant questions will not even arise.

In electronic health, anthropomorphism has taken extreme forms in the teaching and training of medical skills. While we all are probably aware of using the Resusci ® Anne CPR training manikin for the training of resuscitation skills, far more advanced artifacts are used. For example, in the UNAM University in Mexico City and Royal North Shore Hospital in New South Wales, amongst others. These facilities

Figure 1. Gaumard ® Noelle ® birthing simulator (Figure courtesy of Gaumard Scientific Company, Inc.) Used with permission.

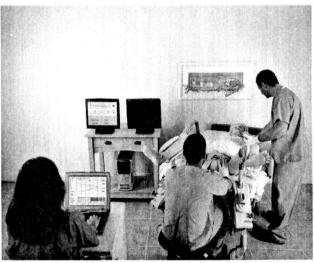

employ extremely anthropomorphized artifacts in patient care and in training for midwifery (Lahtiranta & Kimppa, 2006a). One of the companies, which provide highly anthropomorphized manikins to the field of medical training, is Gaumard Scientific Company, Inc. (www.gaumard.com). Their products, such as the Noelle ® birthing simulator (Figure 1) are used for training of medical students in most of the Kaiser Permanente's 30 hospitals in the United States (Elias, 2006).

The Noelle ® is a programmable, full-size simulator, designed to reproduce different births, including those with such complications as caesarean sections and breach deliveries, in real time or accelerated speed. The simulator is equipped with an interactive female model with one birthing baby and one interactive neonate. With the simulator, the students can have a safe environment in which to learn about effective work in a real world clinical situation.

Defining Agentization

The advent of different self-diagnostics and online solutions has given birth to a different kind of problem, which is closely related to the technician model by Childress et al. (1984). In addition to anthropomorphism, a different kind of phenomenon is emerging, namely agentization of ICT artifacts. While anthropomorphism by its definition is about giving human characteristics to nonhuman objects and forces, agentization is about imposing human-like activity on non-human objects. In future studies, agentization also contains a notion of independence and existing independently of the human. Agentization, like anthropomorphism, is something we use and encounter on a daily basis. Probably every one of us remembers more than one situation in which we wonder what our computer does all by itself. In those infuriating moments, it almost feels like "it" (the computer) has a will of its own.

Like anthropomorphism, agentization can be considered as a way of handling uncertainties. It is easier to imagine that an ICT artifact acts like a human thereby allowing the opportunity of predicting its operation. For example, when a computer is under a heavy workload and the pointer on the screen turns into an hourglass (or similar), some users refer to the action as "thinking" (i.e., the computer is thinking what it is going to do next). In electronic health, agentization can be considered as a way of shifting responsibilities or even distancing oneself from the patient. A physician, or a patient, can use agentization as a defense mechanism and a utility of the technician model by referring to a computer as an authority. The computer users can also use an ICT artifact as their base of power, as a way of justifying their actions (i.e., it "said" that certain conditions are met, therefore specific actions "must" be taken). This kind of attributing of human action onto a computer may lead to a gradual erosion of control as the users create a habit of misplacing trust on to the

ICT artifacts. By giving away a part of their autonomy to these artifacts, and by extension to their authors (e.g., programmers, etc.) they will eventually pick up a habit of considering ICT artifacts as actors, not as the tools that they should be. For a more thorough insight into this issue, see Chapter V by Gröndahl in this book.

Defining Ubiquitous

In 1991 Mark Weiser, a man considered today as the father of ubiquitous computing (Yu, 2005), wrote his seminal article in which he declared, "The most profound technologies are those that disappear. They weave themselves into the fabric of everyday life until they are indistinguishable from it." (Weiser, 1991). After this first declaration of what today can be considered as ubiquitous we have witnessed the slow evolution of his vision.

At first, Weiser's (1991) vision was brought to reality in the form of mobile technologies and slowly as the technology advanced, more multiform technologies came into play. Surrounding the concept various projects were launched in universities and companies around the world, some of the most famous ones being Xerox's Smart Media Spaces and Microsoft's Easy Living (cf. Ma et al., 2005; Yu, 2005). The purpose of these projects was to create a dynamically adaptable environment for multiform (ICT) devices in order to create a single, coherent, user experience where the devices communicate seamlessly with each other and with the users.

Weiser's (1991) vision has also given rise to other closely related, or even overlapping, concepts such as ambient and pervasive technologies. For example, European Union's Information Society Technologies Program Advisory Group (ISTAG) defined the concept of ambient intelligence as a situation in which people are surrounded by intelligent intuitive interfaces that are embedded in all kinds of real-world objects producing an environment which is capable of recognizing and responding to the different individuals in seamless and unobtrusive way (cf. Ducatel, Bogdanowicz, Scapolo, Leijten, & Burgelman, 2001). Regardless of the actual term, all of these concepts share the same notion presented by Ludwig Wittgenstein in his Philosophical Investigations (1968): "The aspects of things that are most important for us are hidden because of their simplicity and familiarity (one is unable to notice something—because it is always before one's eyes)." In the spirit of this notion, ubiquitous, ambient and pervasive technologies are similarly inconspicuous, sharing the following basic requirements: they need to be contextualized, responsive, (inter)connected, and invisible.

In electronic health, ubiquitous solutions have become abundant during the last few years. Particularly with regard to home care for the elderly ubiquitous solutions are considered as a partial solution to the imminent and large-scale demographic change in which the proportionate amount of the elderly is forecast to increase rapidly. For example, the European Union has allocated significant funds in its Framework Programmes to projects such as CAALYX (http://caalyx.eu) which aims to answer the needs of the ageing population through the implementation of ubiquitous systems.

Consent

Consent is one of the key issues when ethical, legal, and risk aspects in electronic health are considered. Consent is about the acceptance of, and the need for, the patient to give fully informed approval for a physical examination, other health care procedures, and also to the use of electronic data, which contains personal identifiable health data.

In general, two types of consent can be identified—implied and expressed. Implied consent is behavioral (for example, the patient undresses for the examination). Express consent is explicit; the patient gives permission verbally or in writing (Machin, 2003). Consent can never be regarded as a paper exercise or mere process. It is essential that the patient knows what the consent is about and what they are agreeing to (i.e., the patient is informed). Without knowing what the consent is referring to and what the consequences of it are, the patient cannot make sound judgments, and therefore the validity of the consent is questionable. In addition to being informed, the consent must be valid before the law; the patient must be competent as defined by law and the consent must be given freely. The fourth issue raised by Machin (2003) is a requirement that the consent is appropriate (for example, consent to sterilization does not include bilateral salpingectomy, that is, the removal of both fallopian tubes in a woman).

Informed consent originated from common law principles of non-disclosure. Since then it has developed from various interpretations by the courts and legislatures into a patient's right to participate in the decision-making process regarding to the type of treatment the patient is about to undergo (American Association of Endodontists 1997). In the majority of western countries the patient's right of informed consent is protected by the legislation. Furthermore, the contents and structure of the informed consent documents and process are defined in a detailed level (for example: Connelly, 2000). Despite the legislation, due to the number and type of different actors potentially involved in the care and because of different interpretations on the contents of the consent form, it can be difficult to ensure that the patient has given consent, informed or otherwise.

Different parties related to the care of patients exchange, require and contain different information in such amounts that a complete picture of the information flow between the parties can be hard to control—or even to understand. As communication with different parties outside the sphere of health care is required to a greater extent, the complexity of information that is being exchanged grows even more. For example, in the case of a chronically ill elderly patient the chain of service might require interaction with transportation, laboratory, general practitioner, specialist, nurses, and so on (Lehto, 2000). All of these actors require different information on the patient and they interpret the information they receive in their own unique ways.

This kind of cross-referring between and within different actors might cause distortion of the health information that has been exchanged especially when information is conveyed by a human actor between different ICT artifacts, or when the information exchanged is converted to meet the requirements of different channels and standards used in the communication between the ICT artifacts. Distortion, or even corruption, of the health information can go unnoticed especially if the clinician or patient does not feel the need to question the validity or the reliability of the information conveyed by some ICT artifact. Distortion and uncritical views towards ICT mediated health information has direct implications for consent and care. If the physician presents the information from an ICT artifact to the patient or to the colleague as facts without verifying the validity and origin of the information the rationale behind the informed consent becomes flawed. Therefore the patient and the physician should always be aware of the origin of the information and of the possible effect of the information exchange standard or mediating channel used.

Distancing

Generally, distancing can be defined as declaring oneself to be unconnected or unsympathetic towards something or someone. In practice, this means that individuals, or groups of individuals, create emotional or physical barriers between themselves and the objects they perceive in negative fashion (fear, loathing, even awe). Lott (2002) approaches this social phenomenon by dividing it into two categories, cognitive and institutional, according to its function.

Cognitive distancing occurs when individuals emotionally separate themselves from other individuals, or groups of individuals. This phenomenon typically relies heavily on stereotypes, creating a distinct view of two different groups, "us" and "them." For example, this kind of separation can be made on the basis of social status (economic, occupational, or educational), religion, or ethnic background.

Lott (2002) also describes institutional distancing, which is the more tangible and direct of the two categories. Effectively, institutional distancing is implemented by creating barriers of societal participation and it can be realized, for example, via education, legal advice, and health care. It is not unknown that those with low social status, are often forced to attend to state owned schools, or they have to rely on public health services, which usually suffer from lack of resources and may be of lower quality.

While these two forms of distancing stem from individuals, from their values, morals and education, effectively defining discrimination, and thus separating "us" from "them," we must consider the phenomenon both ways. In addition of being devalued by an individual, or a group, the target of this phenomenon can suffer from more tangible exclusion as well. Alienation, or forcible disconnection from the people, values, or things, which are important for an individual can be viewed as a similar mechanism of social distance as that of distancing, with one distinctive difference; this forcible separation is typically enforced by external factors, such as for example the prevailing views of the general public.

Particularly in the case of home care, where different solutions of ubiquitous technology are emerging, potential effects of distancing must be taken into account. For example, if patients are forced to interact primarily (or solely) with their care provider by using a technological medium (such as a computer or a digital television), they may be prone to institutional distancing. The patients may feel discriminated against, or separated, perhaps even not worthy of the "normal" face-to-face health care they are used to. For elderly people in particular, the visit to the physician can have a significant social meaning, potentially superseding the significance of the care itself. If this social interaction is diminished, or completely removed due to an ICT artifact, the effect of institutional distancing may be even stronger. In situations in which the information exchange goes unnoticed, via some ubiquitous solution, the patient may especially feel stripped of all emotion and compassion—as described in the first four patient-physician models by Childress et al. (1984).

In addition to institutional distancing, interaction that primarily (or solely) is based on some electronic medium can also make the patient and the care provider prone to the effects of cognitive distancing. The risk of this effect is particularly increased where the technology is used to encapsulate certain ethnic or demographic groups. For example, if ubiquitous solutions for home care become abundant amongst elderly people who live assisted lives alone at their homes, the technology can be used to separate, and potentially alienate, this group from other patients and groups.

Patient-Physician Relationship in Electronic Health

Rapid advancement of ICT combined with organizational and social innovation has brought applications of electronic health from the context of health centers and hospitals to the layman. This move from a process or patient centered health care delivered by professionally trained staff towards consumer health care has created new business models, introduced new service providers and given room for new and alternative treatment methods. As applications of electronic health become commonplace and multiform, they give rise to new forms of the chain of care where the patient-physician relationship is more difficult to construct and, if constructed, it is in general inferior to the non-mediated interactions between patient and physician (Bauer, 2004). The change in the relationship and in the duty that follows from the relationship has created a situation where the practice of electronic health has intensified liability and risk issues, which are already inherent in conventional medical practice.

The purpose of electronic health is to assist in the delivery of health care regardless of the location of patient, health care provider and relevant information. In practice, this means that the patient can access not only their family doctor in the same town or cardiologist in the same country, but also some other health care professional anywhere in the globe. Or, by the nature of electronic health, the patient can access all three of them. This means that there can be any number of professionals involved in the care of a single patient and these professionals can consult any number of other professionals anytime anywhere in the world during the period of care. The number and geographical distribution of the physicians potentially participating in the care of a single patient has created a situation where the patient does not always know if and what kind of patient-physician relationship is created.

The relationship between patient and physician is further blurred with the use of technology, which by definition plays a central role in electronic health. This means that information exchange and communication, and even decisions on how and what kind of care is provided to the patient can be based on different computer applications or information systems. Due to rapid advances in technology, applications and information systems used in electronic health care can range from inexpensive hand-held devices to email or telephone, or even to large and complex expert systems of health care. In Figure 2, we have provided an illustrative example of a potential network of communicating actors and artifacts that can all be related to the care of a single patient.

This complicated Web of different technologies and actors has already had an impact on the patient-physician relationship. When the patient and the physician meet face-to-face, they are generally in a situation where both parties are aware of the professional relationship and respect it. In electronic health this mutuality is usually not present and the relationship can be formed on the basis of distant interaction without actual (physical) examination of the patient. In this situation information on the patients or of their condition does not necessarily originate from the patient themselves but indirectly from another source, such as the devices and applications used in electronic health. While in a face-to-face situation, the relationship can be regarded as one conforming to the partnership or friendship model described by Childress et al. (1984), a complex Web of different ICT artifacts can easily lead to the technician model in which the physician merely dictates the results and hands

Figure 2. Example of potential actors and artifacts related to the care of a single patient

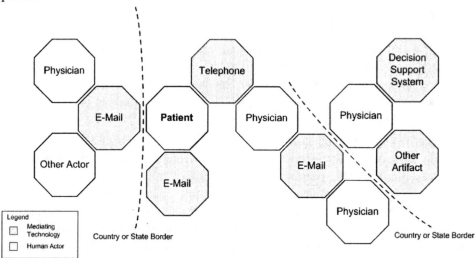

over the responsibility of care to the patient. The risk of employing this kind of model is also present in different self-diagnostic utilities and online services.

Services and solutions where the patient-physician relationship is not formed or maintained in a traditional face-to-face manner are abundant in the Internet environment. Different counseling and guidance services in particular have become common during the last few years—for example, the interactive symptom checker offered by WebMD (http://www.webmd.com/), one of the pioneering companies offering health information and online health management tools. The symptom checker uses interactive Internet technologies to analyze what an individual's symptoms may mean. First, the user provides background information related to his or her current physical condition (such as gender and age). Then, they select the symptoms that apply to their ailment. Following a step-by-step process the user is able to review possible conditions and is provided with instructions as to when they should seek medical care. In such cases, which typically require immediate action, the system instructs the user to seek prompt medical attention.

As part of their online services, the WebMD also provides a centralized health record service in which the users can store and maintain their personal health history. With the service, the users can manage and share their health information with other users, such as authorized care providers. When combined with the WebMD risk assessment, the users can compare their personal health score to their peers and track their progress against a predefined health plan. Furthermore, a personalized health report, containing potential health risks, is provided to the user by the system for discussions with the health care provider.

Another example where the traditional patient-physician relationship is affected by introducing an ICT artifact to the chain of care is a device, which provides (semi) automatic care for patients suffering from diabetes. The device is a product of Medtronic MiniMed Inc. (http://www.minimed.com) and is approved by the Food and Drug Administration (FDA). The device interprets the metabolic situation of the patient and automatically calculates the correct quantity of insulin for the insulin pump to use. The dose is not automatically injected and the product is not intended for every-day use but it would seem that approval of the device by the Food and Drug Administration (FDA) can be considered as a prelude to a future where adaptable control loop systems are commonplace to self care. A similar device for personal diabetes treatment has also been researched in the EU-project ADICOL, which ended in 2002 (Information Society Technologies 2003). In the EU Framework Program 6 (IST) the technology developed in ADICOL project was further refined into CLINICIP system (http://www.clinicip.org), which is a glucose monitoring system intended to be used in intensive care units.

At the moment physicians are generally aware of the source of their information regarding patients. As the applications and systems of electronic health are developed incorporating more or less anthropomorphic features, the line between human-originated and machine-originated diagnosis becomes faint. One example of an anthropomorphic interface that mixes real and virtual data—potentially altering engagements between patient and physician (Bauer, 2003)—is telepresence. This has a unique place in the field of electronic health. For example, at the moment applications of telepresence are utilized in the advanced casualty treatment procedures of battlefield electronic health (Riva & Gamberini, 2000).

In the situations previously described, distancing is also taking place. If the interaction between the user and artifact forms into a complex Web of different ICT artifacts, the health care professionals are easily distanced from the patients. When the professionals use the artifact for inputting health related information, or recover the information from it, they can be seen as sole mediators of the information, or human extensions to a technological artifact. This kind of interpretation can be further emphasized when the health care professionals use artifacts during the face-to-face patient visit changing a relationship, which is bilateral and deeply personal by its very nature, into something else. Distancing may also occur in very special health care conditions, such as in the battlefield when the nature of the care becomes more a case of preserving warfighters' efficiency, or when the health related information is used for justifying actions in a crisis area (Lahtiranta & Kimppa, 2005).

Where Does the Responsibility Fall?

Liability and responsibility issues in electronic health and in health care in general are intertwined with the concepts of malpractice and acts of negligence. Health care professionals have duties that are specific to their field of expertise. In addition, professionals must follow certain standards of health care in order to help their patients. If the professionals neglect their duties or breach standards of care, they commit negligent acts (Ashley, 2002). Some of these duties and standards are common to all in the profession. Some of them are dependent on the legislation. In electronic health, the patient and the physicians in the care of the patient can all reside in geographically different locations to the extent of being in different nation states. Therefore it can be difficult to decide which standards and laws apply.

The role of technology in electronic health creates an interesting aspect with regard to liability and responsibility issues. It is according to the spirit of electronic health that a device or system can be used for self-care or self-diagnostics, for example in diabetes. A physician may further use the information from the device or system and base the diagnosis or recommendation on care for the patient solely on that information. If the physician—when using a device or system—acts in accordance with a practice supported by a responsible body of medical practitioners experienced in the relevant specialty and causes direct or indirect harm to the patient, who can be held liable? The answer could be (For other examples, see e.g., McCarthy, 2001; Tremblay, 1997):

- Equipment manufacturer
- Equipment seller
- Equipment operator
- Maintenance provider
- Telecommunications company (or other service provider)
- Sponsoring hospital or similar party, such as some governmental institute
- Patient
- Health care provider at either or both ends of the chain of care for
  - Decision to use or not to use
  - Inadequate training
  - Misuse
  - Misinterpretation of data

In general, proving malpractice can be laborious. Before a physician or other health care professional can be blamed for such an act, it must be proven. In addition, the act must meet the criteria for malpractice or negligence in the legislation, which can vary regionally. Proving such an act can be particularly difficult since those who are accused are typically the ones who write the medical records and take a central part in the paper trail, which forms the basis of accusation. This can be even more difficult in ICT mediated health care where the actual paper trail might not exist, except in the computer log files of the different parties (if there are any). Even if malpractice can be proven, it should not have occurred because of ICT use in health care. Any such potential situation should have been resolved proactively before the related ICT artifact(s) had been put into practical use.

First, a patient-physician relationship—which is the prerequisite for the subsequent duty—must be proven. The court may decide that the relationship is formed if some kind of advice has been provided. Then, it must be proven that the following duty has been breached. And finally, the harm caused by the breach must be pointed out (U.S. Congress 1994). If these three issues can be pointed out, the juridical basis for further actions is relatively solid. In electronic health, these issues become murkier, especially due to the lack of appropriate case law (Erickson & Sederstrom 2004) and due to the mosaic or Web-like structure of different actors involved in the care of a single patient. For example, in the following scenario proving patient-physician relationship, duty and harm can be difficult: the physician remotely diagnoses a patient on the basis of feedback from different devices and systems. Then the physician consults a number of different colleagues and expert systems for advice and second opinion. As a result of the diagnosis the patient must be treated. The treatment is provided by a group of physicians and other personnel using robotic surgery. Afterwards, different devices and systems are used to control the condition of the patient. Some or all of the care provided after the patient has been discharged is given by using approved instruments and systems of self-care and self-diagnostics. Who is responsible in the case of malpractice or negligent act, how can such an act and its consequences be pointed out afterwards?

Certain information systems of health care keep extensive logs on what information has been accessed and altered, who has made changes, as well as the original record. The paper trail and medical records are replaced with digital counterparts and access to the information is monitored. In this case, it is not easy to alter or hide information afterwards. However, in general the logging only provides information about the data that has been accessed and altered. It does not necessarily provide sufficient information on the act itself; what has been done and by whom; or moreover, what is thought to have been done and whether the act was intentional or not. The interpretation of the action still remains with the actors themselves.

Distancing occurs outside the agentization phenomenon as well. When the health care professionals interact with the patients from behind layers of technology, sometimes even asynchronously, they can effectively insulate themselves from the patients, removing the more personal elements such as care and compassion from the relationship. While certain mediated care provided by (asynchronous) ICT artifacts can be seen to promote medical partnership, for example due to more exact collection of personal health information, the "medical philia" (medical friendship) can be diminished. The lack of a personal touch in electronic health care can also lead to a situation where the patients feel alienated and even unimportant.

Proposed Solutions and Discussion

Legislation and International Cooperation

The role of different standards, guidelines and recommendations has increased, and will increase, in working life. Different companies apply different standards and protocols in order to ensure the high quality and efficiency of their products and processes. Especially in health care these instructions are plentiful, yet most of them are not applicable, or are not applied, to electronic health in particular. The scarcity of different recommendations and instructions, which are specific to the field of electronic health, suggests that it has not yet become routinely used and therefore can be regarded as immature (Loane & Wootton, 2002). As electronic health is commonly considered to be one of the most significant ways of providing high quality care for the increasing amount of elderly people, the need for developing these standards, guidelines and recommendations in global cooperation is immediate—not when different devices and systems of electronic health are in production and routine use.

As long as legislature is not violated, organizations and individuals related to the care of a single patient can craft their own private agreements on responsibility and liability matters. Therefore, especially in the field of electronic health, responsible partnering must be employed. Responsible in such a manner that partnering agreements are formed only with organizations and individuals who comply with the relevant standards, guidelines and recommendations of good practice. An issue closely related to responsible partnering is transparency. Transparency in partnering and funding is needed in order for each partner to demonstrate capability, and a commitment to assess its own dependencies and interests. Principles of responsible partnering, informed consent and privacy, amongst others, are included in the eight principles of the eHealth Code of Ethics, which was introduced by the Internet Healthcare Coalition (IHC) in the spring of 2000 (Carey, 2001).

It is particularly problematic when information systems or devices of electronic health are unintentionally anthropomorphized, or they are ubiquitous by nature. This hinders the ability to treat the applications with the required objectivity. In order to prevent a potentially distorted interpretation about the participating identity (actor or artifact), its role and credentials must be clearly established. Both the patient and the health care professional must be aware when they are using an artifact and not consulting directly with another person. On top of this, they must understand limitations of the artifact and not to trust it as they would trust a person with a complete picture of the situation at hand. This could be done with technical means by removing the unnecessary intentional anthropomorphism from systems and devices, by defining distinct means for separating human-oriented information from machine-oriented information, and by avoiding the placing of artifacts behind a veil of invisibility (i.e. making them ubiquitous) without a proper justification.

Applying E-Commerce Solutions

We agree to a large degree with the danger reducing suggestions made by Heckman et al. (2000) in regard to anthropomorphic agent design, and we are confident that these suggestions can be applied to the field of electronic health. When applied to electronic health the design suggestions can assist in limiting threats to the consumers and users of the devices and systems of electronic health. Heckman et al. (2000) present five different suggestions:

- Create transparent agents
- Create humble agents
- Avoid unnecessary realism
- Carefully consider agent-mediated persuasion
- Facilitate user goals

The suggestions can be elaborated to fit the field of electronic health in the following manner.

Create transparent agents. In the anthropomorphic agent design this principle suggests that the agent should not be a "black box," which presents apparently intelligent thoughts and behaviors. Instead, the agent should inform the user of their intentions and when needed, explain their actions. Similarly, the principle of transparency should be adapted to the devices or systems of electronic health. The decision making criteria, as well as the utilized health information (or other data) and its origin, should be clearly presented to the user. Furthermore, the device or system should be able to present the rationale behind the use of certain analysis method or algorithm. This kind of transparency should lessen the illusion of the infallibility of ICT, and should also assist in decision-making since the origins of the decision provided by the device or application are presented.

Create humble agents. Anthropomorphic agents should be designed in such fashion that they do not strive to maintain the illusion of life by pursuing a life-like dialogue unnecessarily (for example by turning around an unanswerable question). We suggest that the agent should rather inform the users of the boundaries of the agent. In electronic health the awareness of the limitations and boundaries of the artifact in question is of utmost importance, since the information provided by them can be utilized in a critical decision making process with regard to the health and care of the patients. When the device or system of electronic health provides results to the user, it should be able to present the error margins and risk factors related to the results. In addition, if the system recommends certain treatment on the basis of the results, it should be able to reflect the error margins and risk factors to the potential risks emerging from applying the suggested treatment. This view is also supported by Don, Brennan, Laurel, and Shneiderman (1992) who consider that systems, which are capable of behaving as interactive partners, should be able to present their limitations frankly. By combining the principles of creating transparent and humble agents, the user should be sufficiently informed about the potential risks related to the use of the artifact, and if the user should transfer this knowledge forward, for example to a patient, it should promote aspects related to making an informed consent. The question about the boundaries and limitations of an artifact is a particularly tricky one in the case of ubiquitous systems. Presenting their limitations and making the system in question transparent in terms of decision making typically requires stripping it, at least partially, of the very properties that make it ubiquitous.

Avoid unnecessary realism. In many areas of user interface design realism is used to provide a better user experience. However, there is no clear indication that realism should result in better user experience. For example, there are various arguments for and against anthropomorphism in ICT. While some argue that the introduction of human-like features into ICT artifacts creates unpredictability and vagueness (Nass & Moon, 2000; Schneiderman, 1988), others claim that anthropomorphism ensures better user acceptance and creates better user acceptance (Cassell et al., 1999; Gong, 2002). The principle of avoiding unnecessary realism should be applied when a device or system of electronic health is designed. By avoiding unnecessary realism the unnecessary anthropomorphism of the artifact can be reduced. In this regard the impact of the anthropomorphism and agentization which could affect the way we interact with the ICT artifacts can be, at least partially, removed from the decision making process. Again, the ubiquitous systems are problematic in this regard since when they are implemented according to their essence, they are gracefully integrated to daily activities of human society (Yu, 2005). In this regard, avoiding unnecessary realism means making systems less ubiquitous.

Carefully consider agent-mediated persuasion. In e-commerce and in electronic health the use of persuasion is a delicate matter. However, the use of illusion to affect the attitudes and behavior of the user may result in user injury and designer liability. Especially in electronic health the use of persuasion may have dire consequences on the patient and on the liability of the physician. Therefore, applications and systems of electronic health care should not persuade the users but merely state the necessary facts that can be deciphered from the situation. In this area, if ubiquitous systems are implemented in such fashion that they are truly indistinguishable from everyday life, this principle is typically already in place since such systems are in a sense submissive to real human processes, in leisure and work. However, if the systems steer human processes, slowly altering them to meet the visions of those who implemented the system in first place, this aspect is more valid.

Facilitate user goals. The facilitation of user goals should be one of the goals in anthropomorphic agent design, and in the design of devices and systems of electronic health. This facilitation should not be employed at the cost of user safety nor should it have a negative impact on the definitive judgment of the user. As an aspect specific to the field of electronic health, the facilitation of user goals should not muddle informed consent of the patient and it should not impact negatively on the decision making. The facilitation features of the device or system (ubiquitous or not) should follow the principle of careful consideration presented above, and therefore the manifestation of the features should be carefully considered.

In addition to the recommendations by Heckman et al. (2000) we would like to recommend the following actions to be taken when anthropomorphic applications and systems of electronic health are designed:

- Enable the use of an ombudsman.
- Make a clear distinction between actors and artifacts.

Enable the use of an ombudsman. Particularly in a situation in which the degree of user's capabilities are lowered or unknown, use of an ombudsman, or similar practice, may be in order (Lahtiranta & Kimppa, 2006b). The purpose of the ombudsman is to support the user's actions and ward off one of the potential risks of the ICT mediated transactions. Especially in the field of electronic health, the need for such a mediator may arise due to the terminology and concepts used, or due to the potential differences between the health care practitioners. When considering the use of ubiquitous or anthropomorphized ICT artifacts, an ombudsman may be needed to point out the differences between the artifacts and actual human actors. It might also fall to the ombudsman's realm of responsibilities to convey the instructions and care, mediated by different ICT artifacts, in such a way that the human touch, the personal care and compassion, are not lost to the patient, thus mitigating the distancing effect. Furthermore, considering that one of the key aspects of electronic health is to overcome organizational and geographical boundaries, a mediator who understands the differences, for example in licensing and reimbursement, may be a requirement.

Make a clear distinction between actors and artifacts. In the literature there is an ongoing debate about the potential benefits and disadvantages of anthropomorphic user interfaces. We would like to recognize the possible scenarios in which highly anthropomorphic interfaces may be irreplaceable. However, we recommend that in such situations, such as in teaching and training of medical skills, the artifacts are clearly marked in order to make a clear distinction between an artifact and an actor (Lahtiranta & Kimppa, 2006a).

Conclusion

We have introduced the application field of electronic health, discussed consent, patient-physician relationship, and responsibility issues and arrived at some conclusions as to what is necessary to be done in the field of electronic health. The proposed solutions of this chapter are related to legal, international treaty and technical solutions, the last of these three arising from existing solutions from the field of e-commerce. National legislation must be put in place for the clinicians to be able to know who is responsible and to be able to inform their clients on this. International treaties must at least try to harmonize the field so that the individual clinicians can trust the application of electronic health to be somewhat similar in other states and countries as it is in theirs. Solutions from e-commerce will hopefully make the use of electronic health more transparent and remind the clinician or the patient of the potential problems with the automated health care they are applying or receiving.

When health care professionals are consulting each other, they must be aware of all sources of the information used in the decision making process. The same applies to the health care professionals' conduct with the patients. The patients must also be able to know the source of the information, especially if the health care professionals are not physically present. Uncritical reliance on computer generated information for health care issues might bias the information processing, and the decision making might thus be based on false premises.

The direct consequences of trusting applications and devices of electronic health always fall to the patient, but the responsibilities and liabilities of those consequences can be difficult to determine.

References

American Association of Endodontists. (1997). *Informed consent guidelines*. Retrieved May 15, 2007, from http://www.aae.org/NR/rdonlyres/87C213CB-ED33-4ADB-94AE- 0C22B2BCE099/0/informedconsent.pdf

Aristotle. (350 BC). *Nicomachean ethics*. In W. D. Ross (Ed.), Clarendon Press, 1908. Retrieved May 15, 2007, from http://classics.mit.edu/Aristotle/nicom-achaen.html

Ashley, R. C. (2002). Telemedicine: Legal, ethical, and liability considerations. *Journal of the American Dietetic Association, 102*(2), 267-269.

Bauer, K. A. (2004). Cybermedicine and the moral integrity of the physician-patient relationship. *Ethics and Information Technology, 6*(2), 83-91.

Bengtsson, B., Burgoon, J. K., Cederberg, C., Bonito, J. A., & Lundberg, M. (1999). The impact of anthropomorphic interfaces on influence, understanding, and credibility. In R. H. Sprague, Jr. (Ed.) *Proceedings of the 32nd Annual Hawaii International Conference on System Sciences* (Vol. 1, pp. 1051). Los Alamitos, CA: IEEE Computer Society.

Carey, M. A. (2001). The Internet healthcare coalition: eHealth ethics initiative. *Journal of American Dietetic Association, 101*(8), 878.

Carrier, H. D. (1990). Artificial intelligence and metaphor making: Some philosophic considerations. *Knowledge and Policy: The International Journal of Knowledge Transfer and Utilization, 3*(1), 46-61.

Cassell, J., Bickmore, T., Billinghurst, M., Campbell, L., Chang, K., Vilhjailmsson, H., & Yan, H. (1999). Embodiment in conversational interfaces: Rea. *Proceedings ACM SIGCHI '99* (pp. 520-527). Pittsburgh, PA: ACM Press.

Childress, J. F., & Siegler, M. (1984). Metaphors and models of doctor-patient relationships: Their implications for autonomy. *Theoretical Medicine and Bioethics, 5*(1), 17-30.

Cohn, F. (2004). Addressing paternalism with patients' rights: Unintended consequences. *Americal Medical Association Journal of Ethics, 6*(2). Retrieved May 15, 2007, from http://www.ama-assn.org/ama/pub/category/11849.html

Coiera, E. (2003). *The guide to health informatics* (2nd ed.). Arnold, London.

Connelly, C. M. (2000). *Guidelines for informed consent*. Retrieved May 15, 2007, from http://www.hms.harvard.edu/orsp/doc/informed_consent.PDF

Don, A., Brennan, S., Laurel, B., & Shneiderman, B. (1992). Anthropomorphism: From Eliza to Terminator 2. In P. Bauersfeld, J. Bennett, & G. Lynch (Ed.), *Proceedings of the SIGCHI'92 Conference on Human Factors in Computing Systems*. (pp. 67-70). Monterey, CA: ACM Press.

Dowling, C. (2001). Intelligent agents: Some ethical issues and dilemmas. In J. Weckert (Ed.), *ACM International Conference Proceeding Series: Vol 7, Selected papers from the 2nd Australian Institute Conference on Computer Ethics* (pp. 28-32). Canberra, Australia: Australian Computer Society, Inc.

Ducatel, K., Bogdanowicz, M., Scapolo, F., Leijten, J., & Burgelman, J-C. (2001). *Scenarios for ambient intelligence in 2010*. European Commission.

Elias, P. (2006, April 15). *Robot birth simulator gaining in popularity*. Associated Press. Retrieved February 14, 2008, from http://www.usatoday.com/news/health/2006-04-15-robot_x.htm

Erickson & Sederstrom (2004). What you need to know about telemedicine. *Practical Health Law Newsletter, March/April 2004*, 2-3. Retrieved May 15, 2007, from http://www.eslaw.com/Uploads/HealthLaw/March-April-2004HealthLawNewsletter.pdf

European Commission. (1993). Directorate general XIII, research and technology development on telematics systems in health care, Advanced Informatics in Medicine (AIM) programme. *Annual Technical Report on RTD: Health Care*, 18.

Gong, L. (2002). Towards a theory of social intelligence for interface agents. In *Workshop on Virtual Conversational Characters: Applications, Methods, and Research Challenges Conjunction with the Human Factors. Conference*. Melbourne, Australia.

Heckman, C. E., & Wobbrock, J. O. (2000). Put your best face forward: Anthropomorphic agents, e-commerce consumers, and the law. *Proceedings of the 4th International Conference on Autonomous Agents* (pp. 435-442). New York: ACM Press.

Hodson, P. B. (2003). Telemedicine: A new frontier. *BICSI News, 24*(3). Retrieved May 17, 2007 from http://www.bicsi.org/Content/Files/PDF/News07_03.pdf

Information Society Technologies. (2003). *Applications Relating to Health, Fifth Research and Development Framework Programme 1998-2002, Final Report, April 2003 Edition*, 30.

King, H., Garibaldi, J., & Rogerson, S. (2002). Intelligent medical systems: Partner or tool? In I. Alvarez et al. (Eds.), *Proceedings of the 6th ETHICOMP International Conference on the Social and Ethical Impacts of Information and Communication Technologies* (pp. 181-190).

Lahtiranta, J., & Kimppa, K. (2005). Some ethical problems related to the near-future use of telemedicine in the armed forces. In G. Collste, S. O. Hansson, S. Rogerson, & T. W. Bynum (Eds.), *Looking back to the future: Ethicomp 2005*.

Lahtiranta, J., & Kimppa, K. (2006a). The use of extremely anthropomorphized artefacts in medicine. *International Review of Information Ethics, 5*(1), 13-18.

Lahtiranta, J., & Kimppa, K. (2006b). Elderly people and emerging threats of the Internet and new media. In R. Suomi, R. Cabral, J. F. Hampe, A. Heikkilä, J. Järveläinen, & E. Koskivaara (Eds.), *Project E-Society: Building Bricks, 6th IFIP Conference on e-Commerce, e-Business and e-Government (I3E 2006)*. Springer.

Lehto, J. (2000). Saumaton palveluketju mosaiikkimaisessa järjestelmässä. *Hyvin-vointivaltion palveluketjut*, (pp. 33-48). Helsinki: Tammi.

Loane, M., & Wootton, R. (2002). A review of guidelines and standards for telemedicine. *Journal of Telemedicine and Telecare, 8*(2), 63-71.

Lott, B. (2002). Cognitive and behavioral distancing of the poor. *American Psychologist, 57*(2), 100-110.

Ma, J., Yang, L. T., Apduhan, B. O., Huang, R., Barolli, L., & Takizawa, M. (2005). Towards a smart world and ubiquitous intelligence: A walkthrough from smart things to smart hyperspaces and UbicKids. *International Journal of Pervasive Computing and Communications, 1*(1), 53-68.

Machin, V. (2003). *Churchill's medicolegal pocketbook*. Edinburgh and London: Churchill Livingstone.

Marsh, S., & Meech, J. (2000). Trust in design. *Proceedings of CHI 2000 Development Consortium, CHI 2000 Extended Abstracts* (pp. 45-46).

McCarthy, S. M. (2001). Practicing telemedicine and ohio's new telemedicine licensure law. *Health Care Commentaries, 9*(4).

Nass, C., & Moon, Y. (2000). Machines and mindlessness: Social responses to computers. *Journal of Social Issues, 56*(1), 81-103

Plato. (380BC). *Lysis*. Jowett, B (Tr.), Scribner's Sons, 1871. Retrieved May 15, 2007, from http://classics.mit.edu/Plato/lysis.html

Post, S. G. (1994). Beyond adversity: Physician and patient as friends. *The Journal of Medical Humanities, 14*(1), 1994, 23-29.

Raes, K. (1997). Ethical aspects of telesurgery and telediagnostics. *Annales Medicinae Militaris Belgicae, 197*(11), 188-189.

Reuters. (2007). Robots turn off senior citizens in aging Japan. *Reuters News, September 20, 2007*. Retrieved September 24, 2007, from http://www.reuters.com/article/scienceNews/idUST29547120070920

Riva, G., & Gamberini, L. (2000). Virtual reality in telemedicine. *Telemedicine Journal and e-Health, 6*(3), 327-340.

Rodrigues, R. J. (2000). Ethical and legal issues in interactive health communications: A call for international cooperation. *Journal of Medical Internet Research, 2*(1), e8. Retrieved May 15, 2007, from http://www.jmir.org/2000/1/e8

Shneiderman, B. (1988). A nonanthropomorphic style guide: Overcoming the humpty-dumpty syndrome. *The Computer Teacher, 16*(7), 9-10.

Stanberry, B. (2001). Legal ethical and risk issues in telemedicine. *Computer Methods and Programs in Biomedicine, 64*(3), 225-233.

Svenaeus, F. (2001). *The hermeneutics of medicine and phenomenology of health: Steps towards a philosophy of medical practice*. Springer.

Takeuchi, A., & Nagao, K. (1993). Communicative facial displays as a new conversational modality. *Proceedings of the SIGCHI Conference on Human Factors in Computing Systems* (pp. 187-193).

Takeuchi, A., & Naito, T. (1995). Situated facial displays: Towards social interaction. *Proceedings of the SIGCHI Conference on Human Factors in Computing Systems* (pp. 450-455).

Tremblay, M. (1997) *Telemedicine: Legal issues.* Amersham: Rainmaker Publications.

U.S. Congress, Office of Technology Assesment. (1994). *Defensive medicine and medical malpractice.* Washington, DC: U.S. Government Printing Office.

Wachter, G. W. (2002). Telemedicine liability: The uncharted waters of medical risk. *Telehealth Practice Report, 7*(3), 6-7. Retrieved May 15, 2007, from http://tie. telemed.org/legal/other/malpractice0702.pdf

Wagner, I. (1999). Ethical issues of healthcare in the information society. *Opinion of the European Group on Ethics in Science and New Technologies to the European Commission.* Retrieved May 15, 2007, from http://ec.europa.eu/ european_group_ethics/docs/avis13_en.pdf

Wittgenstein, L. (1968). *Philosophical investigations.* London: Oxford University Press.

Weiser, M. (1991). The computer for the twenty-first century. *Scientific American, Sept. 1991*, 94-104.

Yu, Y. (2005). *Systematic design of ubiquitous systems.* Turku, Finland: Turku Centre for Computer Science.

Section IV

Quality Management in Healthcare Information Systems

Chapter VII

Compliance and Creativity in Grid Computing[1]

Anthony E. Solomonides, University of the West of England, Bristol, UK

Abstract

Grid computing is a new technology enhancing services already offered by the Internet offering rapid computation, large-scale data storage, and flexible collaboration by harnessing together the power of a large number of commodity computers or clusters of basic machines. The grid has been used in a number of ambitious medical and healthcare applications. While these have been restricted to the research domain, there is a great deal of interest in real applications. There is some tension between the spirit of the grid paradigm and the requirements of healthcare applications. The grid maximises its flexibility and minimises its overheads by requesting computations to be carried out at the most appropriate node in the network; it stores data at the most convenient node according to performance criteria. A healthcare organization is required to maintain control of its patient data and be accountable for its use at all times. Despite this apparent conflict, certain characteristics of grids help to resolve the problem: "grid services" may provide a solution by negotiating ethical, legal, and regulatory compliance according to agreed policy.

Introduction: The Computing Context

This chapter will develop an argument concerning "healthgrid," the application of grid computing to biomedical research and healthcare. The issues that will concern us arise in the first place from a number of exemplar projects and research prototypes in the field.

Let us first consider the concept of grid computing. "Distributed computer systems" predate even the Internet and the World Wide Web ("the Web"). By means of a network of interconnections, computers are able to share a workload that would ordinarily be beyond the capacity of any one of them; they may also distribute data to different locations according to need or frequency of use. On the other hand, since the explosion of the Web in every conceivable statistic—users, nodes, volume of information—we are familiar with its ability to serve information and misinformation in equal measure. The grid combines the technical features of distributed systems and the Web, but efforts are also being made to ensure that it is not beset by the same problems of abuse, misuse and contamination as the Web has been.

The ideal grid, envisaged as a servant of a new paradigm of scientific research called "e-science," would provide transparent processing power, storage capacity and communication channels for scientists who may from time to time join the grid, do some work and then leave, so that the alliances they form in their scientific endeavours might be described as "virtual organizations" or VOs for short. Different sciences have different needs, and the grid concept has become differentiated: particle physics generates enormous amounts of data which must be kept, but not necessarily instantly processed; on the other hand, data in bioinformatics is not large by comparison—it is, of course, in plain terms, large—but requires intensive processing.

In extending the application of grid computing to biomedical and healthcare applications, another feature becomes pre-eminently necessary: that of collaboration. Indeed, from the outset, grid computing has been associated with smoothing the process, or "workflow," in data- and computation-intensive science; this is the notion, which led to the term e-science. Were it not that the term "e-health" was already in use and generally accepted to mean something at once broader and narrower—"health services and information delivered or enhanced through the Internet" (Oh, Rizo, Enkin, & Jadad, 2005)—the term "healthgrid" would not have had to be invented.

An important consequence of the fluidity of collaboration in grid computing has been in the choice of "architecture" for grid systems. "Architecture" is used loosely in computer systems to describe the manner in which hardware and software have been assembled together to achieve a desired goal. Favoured also in the commercial application of the Web, the so-called "service-oriented architecture" (SOA) has been widely adopted in grid applications. In effect, it means that needed services—software applications—once constructed, are provided with a description in an agreed language and made available to be "discovered" by other services that need them. A "service economy" is thus created in which both *ad hoc* and systematic collaborations can take place. It may almost be objected that SOA is no architecture at all, since the assembly of services (its "components") takes place as and when required.

Compared with data from physics or astronomy, medical data is less voluminous, but requires much more careful handling. Among the services it therefore calls for are "fine grained" access control (e.g., through levels of authorization and authentication of users) and privacy protection through anonymization or pseudonymization of individual data or privacy enhancing technologies, such as "outlier" detection and disguise in statistical data. There are, of course, many more specialist medical services, as our examples below reveal. It is a current requirement in the United States, for example, that if head images are communicated outside the team immediately caring for a patient, all facial features, which might identify the patient, must be removed. Thus a three-dimensional image created for radiotherapy planning, say, should not depict so much of the face that the patient is recognizable. (Conversely, programs that are used to recreate facial features from skeletal data, for example, to identify murder victims, pose a risk to this method of "de-identification.")

Breast Cancer and MammoGrid

Breast cancer is arguably the most pressing threat to women's health. For example, in the UK, more than one in four female cancers occur in the breast and these account for 18% of deaths from cancer in women. Coupled with the statistic that about one in four deaths in general are due to cancer, this suggests that nearly 5% of female deaths are due to breast cancer. While risk of breast cancer to age 50 is 1 in 50, risk to age 70 increases to 1 in 15 and lifetime risk has been calculated as 1 in 9. The problem of breast cancer is best illustrated through comparison with lung cancer, which also accounted for 18% of female cancer deaths in 1999. In recent years, almost three times as many women have been diagnosed with breast cancer as with lung cancer. However, the five-year survival rate from breast cancer stands at 73%, while the lung cancer figure is 5%. While this reflects the perniciousness of lung cancer, it is also testament to the effectiveness of modern treatments against breast cancer, provided it is diagnosed sufficiently early. These statistics are echoed in other countries. The lifetime risk of breast cancer in the USA has been estimated as 1 in 8. Here also incidence has increased but mortality decreased in the past twenty years. Twenty years ago, breast cancer was almost unknown in Japan but its incidence now approaches Western levels (Ahmedin, Ward, & Thun, 2007; Cancer Research UK 2005).

The statistics of breast cancer diagnosis and survival appear to be a powerful argument in favour of a universal screening programme. However, a number of issues of efficacy and cost effectiveness limit the scope of most screening programmes. The method of choice in breast cancer screening is mammography (breast X-ray); for precise location of lesions and "staging" (establishing how advanced the disease is) ultrasound and MRI may be used. A significant difficulty lies in the typical composition of the female breast, which changes dramatically over the lifetime of a woman, with the most drastic change taking place around the menopause. In younger women, the breast consists of around 80% glandular tissue, which is dense and largely X-ray opaque. The remaining 20% is mainly fat. In the years leading up to menopause, this ratio is typically reversed. Thus in women under 50, signs of malignancy are far more difficult to discern in mammograms than they are in post-menopausal women. Consequently, most screening programmes, including the UK"s, only apply to women over 50.[2]

The increasing use of electronic formats for radiological images, including mammography, together with the fast, secure transmission of images and patient data, potentially enables many hospitals and imaging centres throughout Europe to be linked together to form a single grid-based "virtual organization." The full range of advantages that may accrue to radiologists working in such virtual organizations is not yet fully understood, since the technological possibilities are co-evolving with an appreciation of potential uses. One that is generally agreed is the creation of large, broad-based, "federated" databases of mammograms, which appear to the user to be a single database, but are in fact retained and curated in the centres that generated them. Each image in such a database would have linked to it a large set of relevant information, known as metadata, about the woman whose mammogram it is. Levels of access to the images and metadata in the database would vary among authorized users according to their "certificated rights": healthcare professionals might have access to essentially all of it, whereas, for example, administrators, epidemiologists, and researchers would have limited access protecting patient privacy and in accordance with European legislation.

The Fifth Framework EU-funded MammoGrid project (2002-05) (European Commission 2001a) aimed to apply the grid concept to mammography, including services for the standardization of mammograms, computer-aided detection (CADe) of salient features, especially masses and "microcalcifications," quality control of imaging, and epidemiological research including broader aspects of patient data. In doing so, it attempted to create a paradigm for practical, grid-based healthcare-oriented projects, particularly those which rely on imaging, where there are large volumes of data with complex structures. Clinicians rarely analyse single images in isolation but rather in a series of related images and in the context of metadata. Metadata that may be required are clinically relevant factors such as patient age, exogenous hormone exposure, family and clinical history; for the population, natural anatomical and physiological variations; and for the technology, image acquisition parameters, including breast compression and exposure data.

As a research project, MammoGrid encompassed three selected clinical problems:

1. Quality control: The effect on clinical mammography of image variability due to differences in acquisition parameters and processing algorithms;
2. Epidemiological studies: The effects of population variability, regional differences such as diet or body habitus, and the relationship to mammographic density (a potential biomarker of breast cancer), which may be affected by such factors;
3. Support for radiologists, in the form of tele-collaboration, second opinion, training and quality control of images.

The MammoGrid proof-of-concept prototype enables clinicians to store digitized mammograms along with appropriately anonymized patient metadata; the prototype provides controlled access to mammograms both locally and remotely stored. A typical database comprising several thousand mammograms was created for user tests of clinicians' queries. The prototype comprises (a) a high-quality clinician visualization workstation (used for data acquisition and inspection); (b) an interface to a set of medical services (annotation, security, image analysis, data storage and queries) accessed through a so-called *GridBox*; and (c) secure access to a network of other *GridBoxes* connected through grid middleware. The *GridBoxes* may therefore be seen as gateways to the grid (Warren et al., 2007a)

The prototype provides a medical information infrastructure delivered in a service-based grid framework. It encompasses geographical regions with different clinical protocols and diagnostic procedures, as well as lifestyles and dietary patterns. The system allows, among other things, mammogram data mining for knowledge discovery, diverse and complex epidemiological studies, statistical analyses, and CADe; it also permits the deployment of different versions of the image standardization software and other services, for quality control and comparative study. (Warren et al., 2007b)

It was always the intention of MammoGrid to get rapid feedback from a real clinical community about the use of such a simple grid platform to inform the next generation of grid projects in healthcare. In fact, a Spanish company has already entered into negotiations to commercialize the project and to deliver a real, MammoGrid-based radiology service in the region of Extremadura. Thus, many ideas which came up as questions, issues or obstacles in research, must be solved in a real-life system within the next two or three years.

We may now imaginatively consider what may happen in the course of a consultation and diagnosis using the MammoGrid system. A patient is seen and mammograms are taken. The radiologist is sufficiently concerned about the appearance of one of these that he or she wishes to investigate further. In the absence of any other method, he or she may refer the patient for a biopsy, an invasive procedure; however, she also knows that in the majority of cases, the initial diagnosis turns out to have been a false positive, so the patient has been put through a lot of anxiety and physical trauma unnecessarily. Given the degree of uncertainty, a cautious radiologist may seek a second opinion: how can the MammoGrid system support her? He or she may invoke a CADe service; the best among these can identify features which are not visible to the naked eye. Another possibility is to seek out similar images from the grid database of mammograms and examine the history to see what has happened in those other cases. However, since each mammogram is taken under different conditions, according to the judgement of a radiographer ("radiologic technician") it is not possible to compare them as they are. Fortunately, a service exists which standardizes and summarizes the images, provided certain parameters are available—the type of X-ray machine and its settings when the mammograms were taken. Perhaps at this particular moment the radiologist's workstation is already working at full capacity because of other imaging tasks, so it is necessary for the image to be transmitted to a different node for processing. Since our grid is distributed across Europe, it now matters whether the node, which will perform the standardization is in the same country or not. Let us suppose that it is a different country. A conservative outcome is to ensure that, provided the regulatory conditions in the country of origin and in the country where the processing will take place are mutually compatible (i.e. logically consistent, capable of simultaneous satisfaction) that they are both complied with. If one set requires encryption, say, but the other does not, the data must be encrypted. If both sets of regulations allow the image to be transmitted unencrypted but one country requires all associated data transmitted with the image to be pseudonymized, the data must be at least pseudonymized. These are human decisions, but it is clear that they can be automated. It is not entirely clear how the question of responsibility would be answered even if all decisions were taken explicitly by professionals, but it will be further confounded if technology is implicated in some way (e.g., through a decision process which may have been misprogrammed). Indeed, what may go wrong varies widely: confidential data may be inadvertently disclosed, patient identities may be mixed up or the primary clinician may unwittingly fail in his or her duty of care. We lack the legislation to address many of these questions, nor have they been tested in a court of law.

In any case, the story has further ramifications: the whole idea of MammoGrid is to build up a rich enough database of images and case histories to provide a sound basis both for diagnostic comparison and for epidemiology. Once standardized and returned, the image may be stored and made available to others for comparative use, or it may remain outside the system. This choice raises a question of informed consent and technology. Will a service, in the sense we have already used the term, be trusted to determine whether such informed consent as the patient has given covers this question? This is in effect a question of trust in the technology: assuming the question of consent itself can be answered unambiguously by an expert, can an intelligent system be trusted to make the decision on an automated basis.

We now consider the comparison the radiologist wanted to make—the reason for standardizing the image to begin with. The intention is to find images which are sufficiently similar and whose associated history gives an indication of the associated risk. For example, if from among the ten most similar instances, seven turn out to be malignant, there would be good reason to proceed to the more invasive stage of investigation. But how is the database to be queried so as to suggest valid comparisons? Clearly, this goes beyond image similarity. The risks for a childless woman of 65 are very different from a 50-year old mother of three. Image similarity would not be sufficient to warrant a comparison. Thus we must transmit, as part of the database query, data that potentially identify the patient; and the result of the query may provide data which potentially identify patients. On a need-to-know basis, the radiologist has to know details of the cases, but not necessarily the names of the patients, although it would not be difficult to imagine a case where the name reveals something about ethnic background and this turns out to be significant. In a fully deployed system, there may be relevant cases and images from several countries; the system must be capable of "policy bridging," as described above, to ensure that all regulatory conditions are met. Indeed, if the impact of including a case from one particular country would be to render the comparison less useful overall, perhaps the system should be able to reject that particular case—in other words, to apply a criterion which maximizes the information obtained subject to satisfaction of applicable laws and regulations—where the "applicable set" is itself taken to be a variable.

Quality and Quality Control

Acquisition parameters for mammograms include the peak voltage at the X-ray anode and the total energy dosage (measured in kVp for peak kilovolts and mAs for milliampere seconds); the characteristics of the film and of the digitizing scanner (if film is being used, as in MammoGrid) or of the electronic tablet on which the image is captured; and the degree of breast compression. Commonly, these settings are subject to certain protocols but also left to the radiographer's discretion: she will consider the individual patient and set the apparatus accordingly. There are many things that may be amiss in an exposure. Apart from poor physical conditions, such as insufficient compression of the breast when pressure proves painful, less than optimal settings will result in over- or under-exposed X-rays, with poor contrast. The equipment itself requires maintenance and calibration, with images of standard objects ("ghosts") of known structure and opacity used to ensure optimal calibration.

If the aim of a system is to support comparison of mammograms, the least that will be required is a means of standardizing images so that they can be compared as if taken under the same conditions. Indeed, software to do this, based on a detailed mathematical analysis of the entire X-ray process, is available commercially. Using this software in experimental mode, it is possible also to study images for which the settings have not all been recorded (as is sometimes the case) in order to retrospectively suggest the most likely settings used by the radiographer. These experiments allow a body of expertise to be built up which enables radiological services to exercise a degree of quality control over the images taken in regular screening programmes.

For epidemiological use across a number of centres, it is therefore necessary not only to ensure the quality of particular images or of images from each centre individually, but to establish a consistent approach. Cultural differences in what may constitute acceptable practice may exist, so that adherence to an abstract protocol—in the sense of one applicable to all centres equally—will be necessary to ensure consistency. In this context we speak of data having good "provenance," (i.e., precise information about how they were obtained) when and where, using which protocols and respecting which ethical codes, and by whom; this information will extend to the level of qualification of individuals and of certification of the centre, as well as to the equipment used, its calibration and settings.

Quality has an ethical dimension: it is the aspiration and goal of modern "evidence-based practice" in medicine that care is to be based on the "best" information about the patient and the "best" available knowledge. Noting that, even in the simplest cases, information to be used by the clinician may not have originated from a process within his or her control, reliable provenance information should be available with any data. In view of this, it is worth considering the steps taken by the MammoGrid partners in defining minimum standards for collaboration. In order to join the collaboration and add to the pool of patient data, any unit screening for breast cancer and caring for breast cancer patients had to prove that it met the requirements of EUSOMA[3] both in terms of the unit itself (standards of the core team of staff, the equipment, the services offered, and so on) and in terms of its quality assurance processes. Thus any unit wishing to join the programme had to meet the double requirements of adherence to a demanding European standard and to the protocols of the project at the same time. This was the concrete expression of the need for provenance for any data that might be used within the project and was considered to be an adequate guarantee; although it was stated as a "minimum requirement," there is evidently nothing minimal about the demands it placed on anyone wishing to contribute and take advantage of this example healthgrid.

Evidence and Evidence-Based Healthcare

Hitherto, I have given a "naïve" account of one system and its approach to diagnosis. How is such a system to fit into the modern conception of evidence-based medicine (i.e., medicine that is based on scientific results, rather than on the doctor's intuition, personal knowledge and craft skill)? Evidence-based practice rests on three pillars: medical knowledge, as much as possible based on "gold standard" (double-blind, controlled) clinical trials whose results have been peer reviewed and then published; knowledge of the patient, as complete as the record allows; and knowledge of the resources, procedures, and protocols available in the setting where the encounter with the patient is taking place.

There is a very extensive literature on knowledge management and the difficulties and opportunities it presents. Some work currently undertaken in the healthgrid context, such as on ontologies and on knowledge representation, is relevant here. A development which is bringing economics into conflict with the traditional approach to the establishment and dissemination of knowledge is online publication of research results. While in medicine at present this is restricted to electronic publication of papers that have already been peer reviewed and are in the pipeline for printing in a journal, in other fields of science, notably physics, immediate online publication of un-peer reviewed results so that they can be viewed and critically assessed is now common. It has been argued that the open and public scrutiny that ideas receive in this manner is at least as critical as a journal peer review process, while it is evidently quicker. However, there are bound to be some qualms about results that have not *necessarily* been reviewed, and all the more so in fields such as biomedical research.

In another field, the journal *Nature* recently conducted a comparative study of errors in *Wikipedia* and in the *Encyclopaedia Britannica*; the results were equivocal, leading some to argue that an online, user-managed encyclopaedia is less error prone, although there have been many hacking attacks on *Wikipedia*. (Giles, 2005) In the case of medicine, not only malicious postings, but poor research may have serious results. In the case of clinical trials, some have advocated a global databank, so that both successful and, perhaps more importantly, unsuccessful and inconclusive trials are documented. Here it may be said that the traditional approach to knowledge has failed; negative results are often not published and, as certain legal cases have brought to light, even results suggestive of risks are kept under wraps.

Another practice that would benefit from being formally documented is the effective prescription of certain drugs beyond their designed purpose or licence, where nevertheless anecdotal clinical evidence has led practitioners to believe they are effective. This practice is sufficiently widespread to have acquired a name—"off-label prescribing"—and to have been studied in the literature, from the point of view of particular diseases and medications, from the perspective of practice in different countries and in the submissions of pharmaceutical companies.

However, beyond these examples, the MammoGrid application we have described above (and other similar projects) takes us a step further in the direction of "dynamic" construction of knowledge. If images and histories are to be used as part of the diagnostic knowledge in new cases, it is imperative that they are collected with as much care and rigour as the cases in a controlled trial. Therefore, it is essential to know the "provenance" of the data with precise details of how it has been handled (e.g., if standardized and subjected to CADe, which algorithms were used, set to what parameters, by whom, and if capture and interpretation were subject to appropriate practice standards). I have labelled this set of issues "the question of practice-based evidence for evidence-based practice." If this were to be accepted as an appropriate source of diagnostic information, the underlying grid services which maintain it would have to make quality judgements without human intervention.

Integration, Individualized Medicine and Ethico-Legal Consequences

We have suggested that a highly networked, collaborative healthcare subsystem, such as the one envisaged by MammoGrid, would naturally tend to construct its own evidence base. None the less, traditional sources of knowledge would not be

Figure 1. Levels of biosocial organization, knowledge disciplines, pathologies, and informatics(acknowledgement: BIOINFOMED/F. Martin-Sánchez, ©2001 used with permission.)

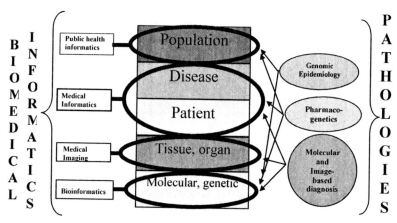

ignored but rather would have to be integrated and managed together with the new evidence accruing from the use of the system itself. It is envisaged that the means of such integration would go beyond the familiar methods of informatics and would itself be informed by an integral view of the human subject and recognition of the inter-relatedness of the different "life science" disciplines, especially in relation to human pathologies.

A major breakthrough in healthcare is anticipated from the association of genetic data with medical knowledge. In the healthgrid research community the Bioinfomed (European Commission, 2001b) study has provided us with a map that has become almost an article of faith (Figure 1).

This view of "life" is in fact shared by many different disciplines, system biology being the most obvious among them. Drug development is increasingly driven by a molecular view of the world, using a variety of models to understand both how drugs act and how their action may be enhanced, inhibited or frustrated. This usually means understanding what proteins are present and, therefore, which genes code for those proteins. In the foreseeable future, we may anticipate certain drugs to be available in subtypes to account for the specific genetic endowment of the patient.

This would suggest that genetic information would have to be accessed routinely in the course of healthcare. Viewing this as part of the information held on a patient raises a number of difficult problems. Among these are the predictive value and the shared nature of genetic information. Knowing a person's genotype could mean knowing what diseases they may or may not be susceptible to. Knowing one person's genetic map also reveals that of his or her siblings' in large measure. This introduces a range of questions, from confidentiality to "duty of care" issues. If physicians will be held liable both for what they do and what they do not do, is it necessary for the underlying knowledge technology to "be aware" and to inform them of the possibilities?

It is generally held that data protection legislation and duty of care may conflict in particular cases and indeed that only case law is likely to clear up this issue, in the sense that case-by-case clarification of what is and is not defensible to do in different circumstances for different patients may require particular judgements.[4] The complexity of interactions between different laws may well be more easily untangled by an automatic system that could at least provide first line advice whether reference to a legal expert is indicated.

Grid and Electronic Health Records

The grid could provide the infrastructure for a complete "electronic health record" with opportunities to link both traditional patient data and genetic information to bring us closer to the ideal of genomic medicine. Among many questions being investigated in current projects is a set concerning development and illness in childhood, especially conditions in which genetic predisposition is at least suspected and in the diagnosis of which imaging is also essential. Physicians want to know how certain genes impact the development of diseases and radiologists want to know what the earliest imaging signs are that are indicative of a disease. For example, the Health-e-Child project (European Commission, 2005a) is investigating paediatric rheumatology, cardiac dysmorphology and childhood brain tumours using this approach. Consider its aims:

1. To gain a comprehensive view of a child's health by vertically integrating biomedical data, information, and knowledge, that spans the entire spectrum from genetic to clinical to epidemiological;

2. To develop a biomedical information platform, supported by sophisticated and robust search, optimization, and matching techniques for heterogeneous information, empowered by the grid;

3. To build enabling tools and services on top of the health-e-child platform, that will lead to innovative and better healthcare solutions in Europe:
   - Integrated disease models exploiting all available information levels;
   - Database-guided biomedical decision support systems provisioning novel clinical practices and personalized healthcare for children;
   - Large-scale, cross-modality, and longitudinal information fusion and data mining for biomedical knowledge discovery.

With major companies looking to translate research results into products, successful outcomes from this and other projects would bring the scenario described above closer to reality.

Next Steps

The SHARE project, a so-called "specific support action" within the European Information Societies Technology programme, will over the two years 2006-2007 be seeking to define a research road map that will allow not only the technology to be developed but the social issues also to be addressed, with the goal of establishing a healthgrid as the infrastructure of choice for European biomedical activity in the next ten years. The SHARE collaboration includes both computer scientists, experts on social requirements and medical law specialists. The project begins with the fundamental assumption that technical and social requirements must be addressed concurrently. It has identified these challenges to the modernization of health systems (European Commission, 2005b):

- Creating and populating, connecting and understanding patient records across organization boundaries and, in due course, across different national health systems;
- Increasing the openness and accessibility of systems (e.g., providing patients with ownership of their healthcare record); while
- Ensuring privacy, confidentiality and ethical compliance in the socio-legal plane, and
- Maintaining data integrity, security and authenticity (e.g., provenance and semantics) in the technical plane;
- Providing appropriate levels of authorization and authentication of users across all the services and the citizen;
- Discovering, grading and certificating trustworthy sources of knowledge and case information to guide future action; finally,
- Winning the trust and commitment of the medical professions at a time of immense change and economic pressure.

At present it seems unlikely that technology will be allowed to determine answers to questions of a legal nature, much less so of an ethical nature. Yet the extent to which we trust financial affairs to the Internet and the extent to which we have allowed privacy to be invaded by online transactions, "cookies" and preference tracking (to say nothing of store loyalty schemes) (Freedman, 2006) suggests that we may be more flexible in our attitudes that our legal attitudes may imply. Indeed, as far as personal data are concerned, the financial analogy has been made before in the concept of a personal data bank. Would patients be less trusting of a "bank" with their health record than they are with their money?

I have argued that "healthgrid," the augmented application of grid computing to health, presents an opportunity to review not only information technology for health—a major enough task—but also our approach to the complex issues of ethical, legal and regulatory compliance as mediated by the technology. The case in favour of the technology, in terms of improved information and knowledge for clinicians, patients, public health officials, administrators and governments, is not difficult to make. The need for ethical and legal safeguards cannot be circumvented, but in itself this may prove an insuperable obstacle for the deployment of the new technology. One way forward is to analyse precisely these "social" requirements and enhance the technology with the means to apply them automatically with minimal human intervention.

Acknowledgment

This work would not have arisen were it not for questions asked by colleagues on the MammoGrid, SHARE, and Health-e-Child projects, in our organization, HealthGrid, and by my co-authors of the "White Paper." In relation to legal, ethical, security and trust issues, I am deeply indebted to Isabelle Andoulsi, Brecht Claerhout, Celine Van Doosselaere, Jean Herveg, James Lawford-Davies, Veli Stroetmann, and Petra Wilson, as well as to my students, Mark Olive and Hanene Rahmouni.

References

Ahmedin, J., Ward, E., & Thun, M. J. (2007). Recent trends in breast cancer incidence rates by age and tumor characteristics among U.S. women *Breast Cancer Research 9*:R28 (doi:10.1186/bcr1672) 9.3 Retrieved from http://breast-cancer-research.com/content/9/3/R28.

Cancer Research UK. (2006) *Cancer Research UK Scientific Yearbook 2005-06.* Retrieved from http://www.cancerresearchuk.org/aboutus/whoweare/our-reportsandaccounts/scientific_yearbook05_06/[5]

European Commission. (2001a). The information societies technology project: *MammoGrid—A European federated mammogram database implemented on a Grid infrastructure*, EC Contract IST-2001-37614.

European Commission. (2001b) The information societies technology study: *BIOINFOMED Study Prospective analysis on the relationships and synergy between MEDical informatics and BIOINFOrmatics*, EC Contract Number IST 2001-35024.[6]

European Commission. (2005a). The information societies technology integrated project. *Health-e-Child—An integrated platform for European paediatrics based on a grid-enabled network of leading clinical centres*, EC Contract Number IST-2005-027749.

European Commission. (2005b) The information societies technology specific support action. *SHARE*, EU Contract Number IST-2005-027694.

Freedman, D. H. (2006). *Why privacy won't matter. Newsweek (International Edition)*, issue of 3rd April. Retrieved from http://www.msnbc.msn.com/id/12017579/site/newsweek/

Giles, J. (2005). Internet encyclopaedias go head to head. *Nature* 438, 900-01; note also response by Britannica at http://corporate.britannica.com/britannica_nature_response.pdf.

Oh, H., Rizo, C., Enkin, M., & Jadad, A. (2005). What Is eHealth (3): A systematic review of published definitions. *J Med Internet Res, 7*(1), e1. Retrieved from http://www.jmir.org/2005/1/e1/[7]

Warren, R., Solomonides, A. E., del Frate, C., Warsi, I., Ding, J., Odeh, M., McClatchey, R., Tromans, C., Brady, M., Highnam, R., Cordell, M., Estrella, F., Bazzocchi, M., & Amendolia, S. R. (2007a) MammoGrid—A prototype distributed mammographic database for Europe. *Clinical Radiology, 62*(11),1044-1051.

Warren, R., Thompson, D., del Frate, C., Cordell, M., Highnam, R., Tromans, C., Warsi, I., Ding, J., Sala, E., Estrella, F., Solomonides, A. E., Odeh, M., McClatchey, R., Bazzocchi, M., Amendolia, S. R., & Brady, M. (2007b). A comparison of some anthropometric parameters between an Italian and a UK population: "proof of principle" of a European project using MammoGrid. *Clinical Radiology, 62*(11), 1052-1060.

Endnotes

[1] This chapter has its origins in a workshop held at the 16th International Congress on Medical Law (Toulouse 2006) where an early draft was presented to highlight and illustrate these anticipated legal and ethical difficulties.

[2] In [6] the MammoGrid research team provide evidence from the project that breast density per se is a risk factor for breast cancer.

[3] EUSOMA is the abbreviated name of the European Society of Mastology, the branch of medicine related to care of the breast. EUSOMA's mission is to define gold standards in the management of breast diseases, favouring a rapid transfer of knowledge from research centres to clinical practice. (www.eusoma.org)

[4] An Industrial Tribunal in the UK in 2007 found in favour of a care worker who had, against his employer's rules, contacted a client's General Practitioner because he believed the client to be suicidal. The Tribunal found that the action was entirely justified in the circumstances, even if it entailed breach of confidentiality.

⁵   See also http://info.cancerresearchuk.org/cancerstats/types/breast/ and links from there for incidence, mortality and survival statistics as well as risk factors and other scientific issues.

⁶   See also the Information Societies Technology Network of Excellence *INFO-BIOMED Structuring European Biomedical Informatics to Support Individualised Healthcare*, EC Contract IST-2004-507585 at http://www.infobiomed.org/

⁷   All web references accessed on 21st July 2007.

Chapter VIII

Clinical Safety and Quality Management in Health IT

Benedict Stanberry, Medical Imaging Group Limited, UK

Abstract

This chapter describes the principle risks that are associated with the supply of healthcare information systems, services, and technologies and the emerging best clinical safety and quality management practices that are being adopted by both users and suppliers in order to mitigate or remove these risks. It states that there are two principle sources of risk: one derived from the potential harm that could be caused to patients and users in a care environment and the other derived from possible failures to achieve the specifications and service levels demanded by a buyer. It argues that for a health IT supplier, implementing industry best practices in an effective way not only provides a high level of protection from both sources of risk but has in any event now become a minimum expectation on the part of users such as the NHS Connecting for Health programme. The chapter concludes that although quality, safety and performance standards in health IT still lag behind other, more established sectors of healthcare innovation—such as pharmaceuticals and medical devices—new standards for clinical safety and quality management are rapidly emerging, introducing a new dimension into informatics standardisation and substantially but necessarily raising the barriers to entry into the health IT market place.

Risks and Liabilities

Sources of Risk in Health IT

There are four basic sources of risk to which a provider of information systems, services, or technologies for use in health or social care can be exposed:

- Hardware defects
- Software defects which affect an automated physical process
- Software defects which affect the advice given to a user
- Organisational and human failures

This classification is complicated by the fact that hardware, software, organisations, and people all interact and it may require a detailed analysis to discover the precise cause or causes of an adverse incident. This is especially the case in health and social care, where a typical care pathway may carry a patient and their information through several different care environments and perhaps through different settings within those environments, where they will come into contact with a diverse range of technologies, equipment, drugs, skills, and expertise. Given the complex interactions that are taking place it is inevitable that sometimes things will go wrong.

Within the immediate care environment, risk management and patient safety are crucial components of the overall quality management system known as "clinical governance." But they are no less important outside of that environment. Every supplier of products and services, which are used in a health or social care setting must recognise that these products and services are being used in a safety-critical environment and must, as is discussed in depth in this chapter, conform to the best quality, safety and risk assurance and management practices that are presently available.

Indeed, when supplying such products and serviced there are two principle sources of risk. One is the external source associated with clinical safety and previously described, which derives from the potential harm that could be caused to patients and users of a product or service in a care environment. The other, however, is an internal and subtly different risk: that of failing to achieve the specifications and service levels defined in a contract to supply these products and services, which will lead to the payment of financial penalties to a client. For a supplier of healthcare IT products, systems and services, implementing industry best practices in an effective way can provide a high level of protection from both sources of risk.

Performance Failures

Significant risks can be associated with delivering health IT products and services to clients in accordance with their contractual requirements in terms of time, cost, quality, and quantity. The most important existing and future users of such products and services—such as the UK's National Programme for Information Technology in the National Health Service (known as NHS *Connecting for Health*)—are likely to buy products and services at fixed competitive prices, transferring financial and delivery risk to the supplier. In such circumstances, the supplier will not be paid until the contracted products and services are delivered and working. The payment of "performance deductions," "delay deductions" and other types of liquidated financial damages by the supplier to a client where specifications, service levels and other delivery milestones have not been achieved will act as a strong incentive for it to tightly manage the risks involved, even where it is possible to win these deductions back through improved performance during the remainder of a contract. For example, within NHS *Connecting for Health* some £241 million was budgeted to be paid to Local Service Providers in 2004-05 but, as a result of delays in delivery of systems and following negotiation on Contract Change Notices (CCNs), £133 million was actually paid (i.e., approximately 55% of the revenue that suppliers had anticipated receiving during that financial year). Consequently, some suppliers received less income from the National Programme than was originally forecast in their accounts, which had to be re-stated (National Audit Office, 2006).

The Director-General of NHS *Connecting for Health,* Richard Granger, has stated:

I use a husky dog-sled racing analogy when I am talking to suppliers.... If one of a pack of huskies is lame, you kill it and feed it to the others. This speeds up the pack in three ways: it is not held back by the lame dog; the other dogs go faster because they are better fed; and the remaining dogs also know what will happen to them if they do not keep up. If a supplier falls behind, we can remove work from them and give it to the supplier who is doing best. It gives the suppliers who fall behind the chance and incentive to catch up, and they can focus more effectively on a diminishing portfolio. We want them to realise how much they stand to lose, much as some of the suppliers involved in the congestion charging ended up hiring specialist subcontractors at their own expense because it still cost them less than the delay-deduction would have done. You need to have a contestable framework and a degree of contestability to make this work. We had to design our procurement process with this in mind. (Toppin & Czerniawska, 2005)

NHS *Connecting for Health* is, moreover, known to use comprehensive due dili-gence, multiple suppliers, parent company guarantees, and "intrusive but supportive" contract management techniques to identify problems and take action to address deficiencies in suppliers' performance. Multiple suppliers have been used to cre-ate competitive tension, with failing suppliers being threatened with termination of contract and replacement by a competitor (a recent example of this policy is the replacement of GE Healthcare—previously known as IDX Systems—with Cerner as the supplier of electronic patient record software in the BT-led London cluster; (e-Health Insider, 2006)). Some adjustment of contractual milestones for the delivery of functionality may be a necessary pragmatic response to difficulties caused by client expectations, which were, with hindsight, overambitious. Nonetheless, there will be little or no margin for error in most contracts of the kind a typical health IT supplier will be entering into for the supply of knowledge-based products and services to NHS *Connecting for Health*.

Figure 1. Adverse incidents by care environment reported as severe or associated with death (statistics from National Patient Safety Agency, 2005)

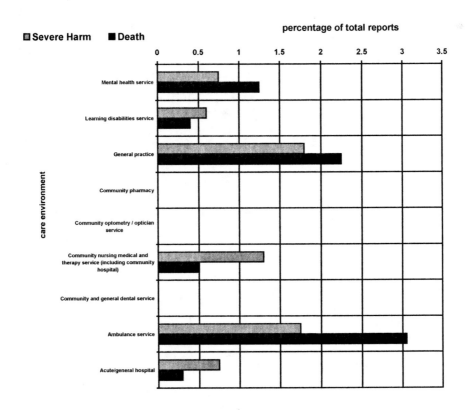

Care Environments

Health IT products and services will typically be used in care environments which are, by their very nature, safety-critical. According to statistics available from the National Patient Safety Agency (NPSA) through their National Reporting and Learning System (NRLS), the majority of occasions where patient safety is compromised in some way (known as "adverse incidents") cause no harm to patients. Adverse incidents leading to severe harm or death account for about one in every 100 incidents. Amongst the 86,142 patients affected by adverse incidents during the period covered by the NPSA's last report, there were 420 deaths and 678 patients who suffered from severe harm. The proportion of incidents in each care environment, which are reported as severe or associated with death is shown in Figure 1. Although these figures are instructive in terms of the comparative "riskinesss" of different care environments, the NPSA has urged that they be used with caution since some environments, such as general practice, may over-report severe harm and death and under-report moderate, low and no harm events. Other settings, such as

Figure 2. Reported adverse incident types in general practice (statistics from National Patient Safety Agency, 2005)

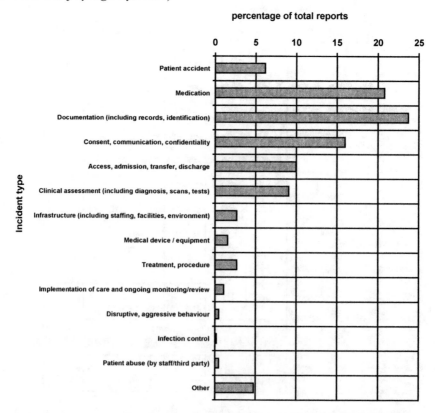

mental health and ambulance services, may have a higher proportion of severe harm and death due to the more serious nature of the pathologies they treat, as compared with, say, community and general dental services.

General Practices

Fewer studies of patient safety incidents have been conducted in primary care than in secondary care. Primary care differs from secondary care in several key respects. It aims to provide longitudinal personalised care that is customised to individual beliefs, needs, values, and preferences across a broad spectrum of concerns relating to health and illness. Given the different population of patients, the different priorities for their care, and the ambiguities of that care in relation to diagnosis and patient choice, delineating "right or wrong" practice is more complex in primary care than in secondary care (Wilson & Sheikh, 2002).

As Figure 2 shows, within general practice the most commonly reported adverse incidents involve improper or insufficient documentation (104 reported incidents,

Figure 3. Reported adverse incident types in ambulance services (statistics from National Patient Safety Agency, 2005)

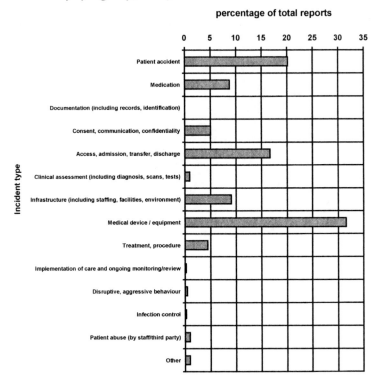

which is 23.7% of the total). This is followed by medication errors (20.8% of the total) and problems around consent, communication, and confidentiality (16.0%). Significant risks also exist around access, admission, transfer and discharge (10.0% of reported incidents) as well as clinical assessment, which includes diagnosis, scans and tests (9.1%). Health IT products and services such as electronic records, clinical information systems and decision-support software are taking a growing role in supporting decision-making in these latter areas, as well as with regards to medication selection, dosage, drug interactions, contra-indications and allergic reactions. These products and services may therefore take a pivotal role in risk reduction but if defective may equally become implicated in an adverse incident.

Ambulance Services

In the period to March 31, 2005, 396 reported incidents took place within ambulance services (see Figure 3). The most frequent incident types are those involving medical

Figure 4. Reported adverse incident types in acute / general hospitals (statistics from National Patient Safety Agency, 2005)

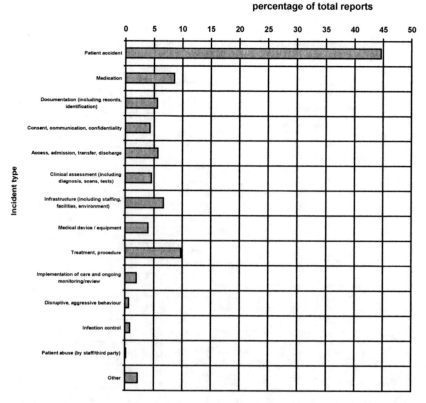

devices and equipment (125 reported incidents, which is 31.6% of the total), patient accidents (20.2% of the total), access, admission, transfer and discharge (16.7%) and medication errors (8.8%).

Acute / General Hospitals

The majority of incidents reported to the NPSA take place in acute / general hospitals and just under half of these incidents are patient accidents such as slips, trips, and falls (30,063 reported incidents, 44.6% of the total). Of the other categories, the most frequent incidents are associated with treatments and procedures (9.8% of the total) and medication (8.6%) - both domains in which clinicians may increasingly rely upon information technologies such as decision-support software, to guide choice.

Other Care Environments

Perhaps the most significant care environment is the one for which the least information regarding adverse incidents is available: the home. We know from the work of organisations such as the Royal Society for the Prevention of Accidents (RoSPA) that more accidents take place in the home than in any other environment, that more than 4,000 deaths are caused by such accidents each year and over 2.7 million people present themselves to Accident and Emergency Departments after an accident in the home (RoSPA, 2007). However, accidents are only one small element of the health and social care needs that arise in the home. At the present time there are no figures available by which to gauge the nature and magnitude of the risks to which a supplier could be exposed by providing health IT products and services - for the monitoring of chronic conditions, for instance - that are directly relied upon by the public in making treatment decisions while at home, about when and how urgently medical intervention should be sought and about where to go for that intervention.

NHS *Direct*—part of the NHS that uses decision-support software to provide 24 hour healthcare advice that is directly relied upon in a home environment - does not participate in the NPSA's National Reporting and Learning System and does not place information about adverse incidents, complaints, or legal claims in the public domain. Hence it is impossible to draw any accurate conclusions about the levels of risk involved in providing such a service.[1] Suffice to say, anecdotal evidence from newspaper articles seems to show that there is the potential for severe harm or death to result from inaccurate medical advice given to and acted upon by people in their homes, but that such serious consequences are very rare. In October 2001, for instance, it was reported that a 60-year old diabetic woman had died after inappropriate advice had been given by an NHS *Direct* nurse. The woman had complained of fluctuating and often very high blood sugar levels, nausea and sweating. The woman's daughter called NHS *Direct* and was advised to give her mother flat lemonade or coke to drink with paracetamol and then to let her sleep. The woman fell into a coma and later died. The Coroner recorded a verdict of death by natural causes to which neglect contributed. NHS *Direct* sacked the nurse adviser concerned and changed its guidelines on diabetes (BBC, 2001).

Sources of Liability

Both performance failures by a health IT supplier as well as adverse incidents in which their products or services are implicated can give rise to legal liability based upon one (or more) of three different potential causes of action:

- Breach of contract
- Product liability
- Negligence

Breach of Contract

If a client (for example, NHS *Connecting for Health*) commissions a supplier to provide health IT products or services, this will certainly create a contract between that client and the supplier, the terms of which will almost always be set out in writing. Subject to any express provisions in the contract setting out the supplier's obligations in more depth, the supplier's contractual liability to their client will be governed by section 13 of the Supply of Goods and Services Act 1982, which implies into the contract a term that the supplier will take "reasonable care." The supplier will be in breach of this term if they fail to take as much care in supplying their products or services as a hypothetical "reasonable supplier" in the same position, professing the same expertise, would have done. It is therefore vital, if the supplier is to fulfil this contractual term that they at the very least conform to the current state of the art in terms of quality and safety management systems and processes. Indeed, any contract with NHS *Connecting for Health* will require the supplier to conform to good industry practice, of which such appropriate quality, safety and risk assurance and management systems are a key feature.

Notwithstanding the provisions of the 1982 Act, present and future health IT users such as the NHS usually describe their quality and safety management expectations in considerably more detail than simply asking a supplier to take "reasonable care." These expectations will almost always be contained in a written contract, which contains detailed specifications and clear provisions for acceptance testing against those specifications, as well as a clear statement of the service levels to be achieved. Failure to achieve these specifications and service levels—or to deliver them within a certain time—would expose the supplier to contractually pre-determined financial penalties, such as service credits or liquidated damages. As we have already discussed, such failures and delays are exposing existing contractors and sub-contractors to NHS *Connecting for Health* to significant financial problems and causing many to have their contracts prematurely terminated. In addition to these detailed specifications, the contracts for the National Programme contain a very broadly defined clause regarding "Expected Standards." By this, NHS *Connecting for Health* imposes a requirement for a contractor to accept and adhere to:

.... using standards, practices, methods and procedures conforming to the law and exercising that degree of skill and care, diligence, prudence and foresight which would reasonably and ordinarily be expected from a skilled and experienced person engaged in a similar type of undertaking and in circumstances where services are being supplied for us in critical clinical environments.

If a supplier has provided similar health IT products and services to a user in the past they may feel confident in giving an absolute warranty that the products and services being supplied in a future contract will perform to that user's exact specifications. However, the supplier may feel that achieving all the functions in a client's specification is not feasible, or not feasible at the price agreed, in which case a qualified warranty - that the supplier will use reasonable care and skill to achieve the specification—may be given instead. Much will depend upon the relative bargaining power of the client in each case, and the specifications and service levels they have demanded.

Under sections 2(2) and (3) of the Unfair Contract Terms Act 1977 it is not possible for a supplier of health IT systems to exclude the term implied by section 13 of the Supply of Good and Services Act 1982 from a contract with a user, unless such an exclusion satisfies a test of reasonableness: that the exclusion is, under the circumstances, a fair and reasonable one.

Such is the nature of the health IT business that there may be some circumstances in which what is being supplied to a user is not classified under English law as goods and services, but as goods alone. This could be the case where a customer purchases an existing product from a supplier which is either sold to them "as is" or with only minor modifications. If this product is sold on physical media, such as software on a CD-ROM, then it is even more likely that it will be classified as being "goods." The reason this classification matters is because under English law the legal classification of software bears very little relation to commercial classifications. While bespoke and custom software are usually classified as "services" (to which section 13 of the Supply of Goods and Services Act 1982 applies), packaged software will normally be classified as "goods," as it is supplied on physical media in multiple copies. "Goods" are not subject to section 13 of the 1982 Act, but to sections 13 and 14 of the Sale of Goods Act 1979, which requires them to be reasonably fit for their common or specific purposes and would not excuse a supplier from liability simply by reason that they took all reasonable precautions to ensure that the goods supplied were reasonably fit for purpose.

Product Liability

The Consumer Protection Act 1987 brings into force, in English law, the EC Directive on Product Liability which renders anyone who produces or supplies a product in the course of business liable to anyone who suffers personal injury or property damage caused by a defect in that product, irrespective of any fault on the producer or supplier's part. A product is "defective" if it does not provide the level of safety (in respect of property as well as the person) that persons generally are entitled to expect.

A "product" is defined in section 1(2) of the 1987 Act as "any goods or electricity" and "goods" are defined in section 45 as including, among other things, "substances." Services do not fall under the Act at all, therefore, and a health IT supplier's products will only fall within the scope of the 1987 Act if they are a "substance," which requires that they are marketed on some form of tangible medium such as paper or a CD-ROM. Since nowadays it is highly unlikely that health IT products will be supplied to customers in this way, it is unlikely that liability will arise under this cause of action, just as it is unlikely that the Sale of Goods Act 1979 will apply, instead of the Supply of Goods and Services Act 1982.

Negligence

For most potential claims against a health IT supplier (other than those arising under contract), the common law of negligence offers the best chances of recovery to a claimant. Moreover, since a claim of negligence does not require a contractual relationship to exist between the potential claimant and the supplier, it is under this cause of action that potential liability to a patient or user of health IT systems is most likely to arise.

Negligence is part of an area of law known as "tort." A tort is a civil wrong that imposes legal liabilities on a person who has acted carelessly or unreasonably omits to do something. The law of negligence is founded upon the legal principle that, under certain circumstances, one person may owe another a "duty of care" and will be liable to compensate the other person if they fail to exercise an appropriate standard of care and the other person is harmed as a result. A claim in negligence does not depend upon the existence of a contract between the two parties. So if a patient or user is harmed as a result of a problem with a supplier's products or services, they will be able to claim against that supplier directly, provided that three essential ingredients are present:

- That the supplier owed the claimant a duty of care.
- That the supplier breached that duty.
- That the claimant was harmed as a direct result of the supplier's breach of duty.

Duty of Care

The landmark case on negligence is *Donoghue* v *Stevenson* (1932) which established that a manufacturer who sold a product in such a way that the purchaser or ultimate consumer could not discover a defect by inspection of the product, is under a legal duty to the ultimate purchaser or consumer to take reasonable care that the article is free from any defect likely to cause injury to health. This duty of care is owed to anyone who it is reasonably foreseeable might be injured by the act or omission of the manufacturer. To this "narrow rule" the judge in this case—Lord Atkin—also added a "wider rule":

You must take reasonable care to avoid acts or omissions which you can reasonably foresee would be likely to injure your neighbour. Who, then, in law is my neighbour? The answer seems to be—persons who are so closely and directly affected by my act that I ought reasonably to have them in contemplation as being so affected when I am directing my mind to the acts or omissions which are called into question.

It should be noted that under this "wider rule," although the supplier will not be potentially liable in negligence to the world at large, they *will* be liable to those persons whom they can reasonably contemplate would be adversely affected by any negligent act or omission on their part. This could include:

- "Client" users (e.g., NHS *Connecting for Health*);
- Other users (e.g., GPs, nurses, pharmacists); and
- Patients and their dependents.

The Standard of Care

To be in breach of their duty of care a health IT supplier must omit to do something, which they could reasonably and prudently be expected to do. Put another way, the law expects a supplier to show the amount of competence—often referred to as the "standard of care"—associated with the proper discharge of the duties of their trade and if they fall short of that and cause harm in consequence, they are not behaving reasonably. The standard of reasonable care is set by law but its application in a particular case is a question of fact that depends upon both the magnitude of the risk, the purpose for which it is being taken and the practicability of the precautions that can be taken against it. Generally speaking, the greater a risk, the less receptive a court of law is likely to be to a defence based simply upon the cost, in terms of money, of the required precautions. Indeed, there may be situations in which an activity must be abandoned altogether if adequate safeguards cannot be provided.

For a health IT supplier the duties of their trade will naturally include a "duty to warn." Where a defect in a product or service becomes known to the supplier they will be under a duty to warn clients and users that could be adversely affected by this defect and to undertake modification or replacement.

Harm

The third essential ingredient necessary for a health IT supplier to be liable in the tort of negligence is that a claimant must have suffered harm. This may take the form of death or physical injury but can also include financial loss. In most situations where outsourced, managed health IT systems and services are being provided to a client it is unlikely that negligence in the provision of that system or service will cause a loss that is not purely financial. However, the safety-critical nature of IT systems and services used in health and social care means that it is certainly foreseeable that careless actions or inactions could cause physical injury or death.

Financial Loss

In the cases of *Junior Books Ltd* v *Veitchi Co Ltd* (1983) and *Caparo Industries plc* v *Dickman* (1990) it has been accepted by the courts that a purely financial loss can be recovered from a defendant where that defendant has undertaken responsibility for achieving a particular result and financial loss was a foreseeable consequence of a failure to meet that responsibility. For a health IT supplier, such a claim in negligence for a purely financial loss is most likely to arise where it is sub-contracted by a software or system provider to supply knowledge-based products and services - such as a structured knowledge base of health treatments, which will be incorporated by the provider into their own products and services. It will therefore be important, in such a case, for a supplier to ensure that they effectively limit their tortious liability using the terms of their written sub-contract with the provider, since where liability in negligence has been effectively limited by the terms of a sub-contract a court is unlikely to be persuaded that it would be fair, just and reasonable to impose a higher liability. This principle also holds true in the case of direct contracts between a supplier and a client user, though it may be more difficult to justify limitations upon liability in such circumstances. As is the case with qualified contractual warranties, much depends upon a supplier's bargaining power relative to that of their client.

Negligent Misstatements

Liability for financial loss, as well as for other types of loss arising from proven negligence on the part of a supplier, might be considered to arise from the fact that the output of a knowledge-based product or service constitutes advice which it is foreseeable—indeed expected—that the user of the product or service will rely upon. Hence incorrect advice has been said, in cases such as *Hedley Byrne & Co Ltd v Heller & Partners* (1964), *JEB Fasteners* v *Marks, Bloom & Co* (1983) and *Re Market Wizard Systems (UK) Ltd* (1998) to be closely analogous to something called a "negligent misstatement" under which anyone in a sufficiently close relationship with a supplier would be able to claim against it for a loss caused by their reliance upon a knowledge-based product or service which produced incorrect advice. Sufficiently close relationships would include:

- Anyone who contracts or sub-contracts the supplier to provide knowledge-based products and services.
- Anyone falling within a class of persons for whose use the products and services were provided, with the intention that they would use and rely upon them.

However, it is very unlikely that a health IT supplier would ever owe a duty of care to patients or the public at large.

"Res Ipsa Loquitur"

In very extreme cases where a electronic record or clinical information system produced incorrect results, the absurdness or obvious inaccuracy of those results might so strongly suggest negligence on the part of its supplier that the legal doctrine of *res ipsa loquitur* (a Latin phrase meaning "the thing speaks for itself") will come into effect. Under this doctrine the burden of proof moves from the claimant to the defendant. Hence it would not be for a claimant to prove negligence on the part of a supplier but for the supplier to disprove it by showing that their quality management system was sufficiently well planned, designed and executed. In a typical case where this doctrine was used, such as *Henderson* v *Henry E Jenkins & Sons* (1970), it was not sufficient that a defendant operated a generic quality management system. The court held that the defendant must have in place a system that was tailored to manage the particular risks and hazards that arose from the products and services they provided, for which the generic system used by the defendant was inadequate.

Standards of Care in Contract and Tort

The standard of care that a health IT supplier must reach in order to fulfil its duty of care under the tort of negligence is, in most practical respects, identical to that demanded under contract: to take reasonable care in the creation, updating, maintenance and presentation of their products, systems and services, as well as in the integration or interfacing of these with other products, systems and services (where it has accepted responsibility for integration).

Damages and Insurance

The most common remedy demanded under any of the causes of action described above is monetary compensation. For insurance purposes the sources of risk specified at the beginning of this chapter essentially fall into two broad liability categories. Hardware and software faults would tend to be covered by third party public and products liability insurance and organisational or human failures will be covered by professional indemnity insurance. It is common practice for an NHS client procuring information technologies or systems to require their supplier to carry both these types of insurance with suitable limits of indemnity. There is usually some scope for negotiation as respects these limits, provided that the supplier takes out suitable policies of insurance, in accordance with good industry practice and the law.

The minimum limit of indemnity demanded by a client will vary greatly from contract to contract and from circumstance to circumstance. It will depend upon both the size of the contract and the magnitude of any potential harm that could result from its breach or from negligence on the part of the supplier. In recent years it has become standard practice for NHS contracts to demand a minimum limit of indemnity of £5,000,000, which is generally considered adequate to cover the highest compensation awards that could be made in respect of death, personal injury, property damage or financial loss.

Standards

Sources of Standards

While the established sectors of healthcare innovation—principally pharmaceuticals and medical devices—are subject to a significant level of regulation and control as regards quality, safety and performance, healthcare information technologies remain largely unburdened by the need for clinical trials and safety studies to have taken place prior to being placed on the market or implemented in clinical settings. Though the regulatory barriers to entry into this, the newest sector of healthcare innovation, are in this sense unsubstantial, the considerations of risk and liability examined in the first part of this chapter require health IT suppliers to have in place formal, auditable systems for quality, safety and risk assurance and management. Such systems should not only assure the supplier's conformance with the standards of care necessary to avoid defects in its products and services causing or contributing to adverse incidents and hence attracting legal liability, but also assure achievement of the specifications, service levels, and delivery milestones demanded by clients.

As has already been considered in the first section of this report, to avoid liability for breach of contract or the tort of negligence, a supplier must achieve the standard of care associated with the proper discharge of the duties of their trade. Both contract and tort law describe this standard as "reasonable care": the standard, which a hypothetical "reasonable supplier" in the same position as the supplier in question, providing the same products and services, would be expected to achieve. Contracts issued by NHS *Connecting for Health* describe the expected standard of care as the use of practices, methods and procedures that conform with the law as well as the exercise of the degree of skill and care, diligence, prudence and foresight which would reasonably and ordinarily be expected from a skilled and experienced person engaged in a similar type of undertaking and in circumstances where services are being supplied for use in critical clinical environments. Such a standard is normally referred to simply as "best practice."

Best practice in the context of healthcare information systems, services and technologies is an evolving concept. Until 2004, NHS *Connecting for Health* had formal systems for quality assurance and management which largely mirrored those used elsewhere in the NHS, but did not have a specific system, as such, for safety and risk assurance and management. Over the last two years, however, there has been significant activity in this area leading to the implementation—supported by the NPSA—of a comprehensive safety and risk management system, which places significant demands on both the programme and its suppliers.

The Department of Health always expects high standards of quality from its service providers. Wave Two of the £1 billion Independent Sector Procurement (ISP) Programme for outsourced diagnostic services (Sims, 2005) for instance, has required bidders to demonstrate ongoing compliance with:

- Good clinical practice
- NHS requirements
- Good industry practice
- NHS Litigation Authority Risk Management Standards
- The Standards for Better Health and National Minimum Standards and Regulations

Not all of these standards will necessarily apply to the supply of health IT products and services. The latter two in particular - the NHS Litigation Authority's Risk Management Standards and the Standards for Better Health / National Minimum Standards and Regulations—have only been demanded in the ISP Programme because the products and services to be provided include significant elements of direct patient care. However, conformance with good clinical practice, NHS requirements and good industry practice is *always* a minimum expectation in an NHS or similar contract.

Good Clinical Practice

Providers of health IT products and services must ensure that those products and services enable healthcare professionals to conform to good clinical practice. Good clinical practice is a relative rather than an absolute concept, varying from specialty to specialty and from situation to situation, but conformance with it will usually enable a healthcare professional to meet both their professional (i.e., ethical) obligations *and* their legal duty of care. A healthcare professional will have fulfilled their legal duty of care and therefore not be guilty of negligence when they have followed good clinical practice, since in doing so they will almost always have acted "in accordance with a practice accepted as proper by a responsible body of medical men skilled in that particular art." (*Bolam* v *Friern Hospital Management Committee* [1957] 1 WLR 582).

While good clinical practice varies with the clinical circumstances, certain fundamental behaviours such as those described in the General Medical Council's guidance for doctors will be expected. These behaviours include:

- Making an adequate assessment of a patient's condition based on their history and symptoms and, if necessary, an appropriate examination.

- Providing or arranging investigations or treatment where necessary.

- Taking suitable and prompt action when necessary.

- Referring a patient to another practitioner when necessary.

- Being competent when making diagnoses and when giving or arranging treatment.

- Keeping clear, accurate, legible and contemporaneous patient records which report the relevant clinical findings, the decisions made, the information given to patients and any drugs or other treatment prescribed.

- Keeping colleagues well informed when sharing the care of patients.

- Prescribing drugs or treatment, including repeat prescriptions, only where there is adequate knowledge of the patient's health and medical needs.

- Reporting adverse drug reactions as required under the relevant reporting scheme and co-operating with requests for information from organizations monitoring the public health (General Medical Council, 2001).

As respects all these required behaviours, health IT products such as electronic records, clinical information systems and decision-support software have the potential not only to enable healthcare professionals to achieve good clinical practice but to substantially mitigate many of the most significant risks that are frequently present within that practice. Typical contracts that a health IT supplier might be awarded over the coming decade could:

- **Enable relevant clinical information to be accessed at the time of consultation:** Lack of knowledge and lack of timely access to information have been described as major root causes of medical errors (Leape et al., 1995). Clinical information systems and electronic records help avoid these errors.

- **Increase access to knowledge:** Such as textbooks and referenced articles, by putting evidence-based clinical information at a healthcare professional's fingertips.

- **Provide clinical decision support:** So that care is driven by high-quality, evidence-based knowledge. This helps improve the quality and safety of decisions, increase the efficiency of care and satisfy the needs of clinical governance.

- **Improve communication between members of the care team:** Inadequate "handovers" remain the commonest factor contributing towards adverse events (Schmidt & Svarstad, 2002). Linked to an evidence-based knowledge database, hazard alerts in electronic patient records will help reduce errors due to poor communication.

- **Provide information and assistance with calculations:** Such as the prescribing of drugs. Constraints can be placed on the dose or route of administration of a potentially dangerous medication.

- **Assist with the monitoring of patients:** By computerising this process (which can become tedious and therefore an inherent source of error) with "smart" monitors and applications that sift through the wealth of data in real time, looking for trends, highlighting abnormalities and alerting clinicians accordingly. This is particularly beneficial in areas such as intensive care and the out-of-hospital management of long-term conditions. Knowledge-based systems, when linked to such monitoring technology, can enable the "ideal" care pathway for a patient to be mapped and navigated.

- **Provide rapid responses to and tracking of adverse incidents:** Only by measuring outcomes across a health community can the quality and safety of treatments be accurately evaluated. Anonymized and aggregated electronic health records can be mined for information about these outcomes.

NHS Requirements

As already noted, NHS *Connecting for Health* presently provides detailed standards guidance to its contracted suppliers, which must be complied with by them as part of the delivery of both national applications and local systems and services. These standards are supported by an assurance process being run through a "National Integration Centre" but are not presently in the public domain.

The Department of Health does not presently provide technical standards to potential (as opposed to actual) suppliers who are not formally contracted through NHS *Connecting for Health*. It does, however, use a process known as "Standards Enforcement in Procurement" (STEP) to assist local sites undergoing IT procurements. STEP is an interactive questionnaire that provides details on those standards with which suppliers of healthcare information systems, services and technologies are expected to conform, together with supporting guidance, under eight broad headings:

- **Frameworks:** Which are essentially a list of standards that can be used in a particular context or within a community. Perhaps the most widely known framework is the e-Government Interoperability Framework (e-GIF), giving a set of standards to be used for communications concerning government systems. This is the only framework currently in use for IT systems in the NHS.

- **Management standards:** Including standards for quality management (BS EN ISO 9001:2000), information security management systems (BS ISO/IEC

17799:2005) and IT service management (BS ISO/IEC 20000:2005). We shall examine these in more detail shortly.

- **Healthcare information standards:** Such as standards for data interchange (HL7, DICOM, IHE and EDIFACT), data standards (the NHS Data Dictionary and CDS Manual), NHS number, clinical terminology (SNOMED CT, Clinical Terms known as "The Read Codes" and the NHS Dictionary of Medicines and Devices), clinical coding standards (ICD-10 and OPCS-4), grouping standards (HRGs), NHS Administrative Codes and the Primary Care Computer Systems Requirements for Accreditation (RFA) which contains detailed specifications for the core functionality of GP systems supported by a testing and accreditation programme.

- **Data integration, information access, and metadata standards:** Including standards for data integration (XML) and access (Web browsers).

- **Security standards:** Including cryptographic services.

- **Communication standards:** For things such as interpersonal mail (including NHSmail and the e-SMTP service), the NHS Data Transfer Service (DTS), directory services, web services (covering SOAP, WSDL and UDDI), internet transfer protocols (covering FTP, HTTP and NNTP) and domain name services (covering DNS).

- **Networking:** Including network connections, LAN interfacing, connections to NHSnet, Wireless LANs, network management systems and structured cabling.

- **Equipment related standards:** Covering safety and standards for human-computer interfaces (e.g., ergonomic standards for computer keyboards).

Under STEP, there are three types of standards. Category 1 standards are mandatory and must be complied with by a potential supplier, unless there are overriding reasons not to. Category 2 standards are desirable and it is seen by NHS clients (such as trusts) as advantageous if systems conform to these standards. Finally, Category 3 standards are advisory only—there can be an advantage for a supplier to conform to them, but this may not be entirely practical in all cases.

Although STEP, by ensuring the interoperability of NHS information systems, is clearly a risk mitigating process, it is the insistence upon standards for the quality management of the processes involved with the production of IT systems (BS EN ISO 9001:2000), the environment in which IT systems are used (BS ISO/IEC 17799:2005) and the services provided with IT systems (BS ISO/IEC 20000:2005) that come closest to describing a complete quality management framework that will substantially mitigate the risks inherent in contracts for the supply of health information services, systems and technologies. As is discussed shortly, however, there are other published and emerging standards that are not only useful but essential in enabling a health IT supplier to properly discharge the duties of their trade.

Good Industry Practice

To the extent that information systems, services and technologies supplied in health-care settings are "safety critical" because their outputs will be directly relied upon by healthcare professionals in reaching clinical decisions, suppliers will be expected to comply with a duty of care covering all aspects of their products' lifecycles. As we examine in more depth below, there are now specific standards for quality, safety and risk assurance and management in healthcare information systems and services, as well as emerging standards of specific application to knowledge-based products and services. These emerging standards recommend that clinicians, managers and patients cannot rely on the peer review process alone and should be offered, and use, knowledge-based products and services which have been treated by additional measures to minimise bias and error.

Quality Management Systems

The "OJEU threshold" is the value above which a contract for the supply of goods or services awarded by a public body must be subject to an open, competitive tendering process under the consolidated Public Sector Directive (2004/18/EC) and the Utilities Directive (2004/17/EC). That threshold is presently £93,898. For procurements above the OJEU threshold a quality management system registered with an accredited body under BS EN ISO 9001:2000 is mandatory under STEP for all the functional units of an NHS supplier that are directly concerned with the supply or integration of an information system or service. Contractors and their material sub-contractors delivering the National Programme are likewise obliged to ensure that all of their services are subject to quality management systems (described in quality manuals and procedures) that conform to internationally recognised standards. They must also submit "quality plans" for approval by the Programme and appoint a quality manager who is approved by the Programme and independent of the supplier's day-to-day operations, prior to commencement. NHS *Connecting for Health* may carry out periodic audits of the supplier's quality management systems.

For procurements outside of NHS *Connecting for Health* and below the OJEU threshold, ISO 9001 registration is desirable but not essential. Although a quality management system does not directly guarantee a fully fit for purpose service or system, the Department of Health considers that companies with a properly imple-mented quality management system in operation are more likely to provide a con-sistent service to their clients. Indeed, the Department also recommends that NHS customers themselves should, at the very least, be familiar with the principles of ISO 9001 and may not experience the full benefits of a supplier's quality management system unless they have comparable procedures in place.

Information Security Management

As a mandatory standard, all information systems and services supplied to the NHS (including NHS *Connecting for Health*) must allow the implementation of the security facilities defined in BS ISO/IEC 17799:2005 (which will shortly be absorbed into the BS ISO/IEC 27001 standard). The standard establishes guidelines and general principles for initiating, implementing, maintaining and improving information security management in an organisation. Where managed IT services are being provided it is considered desirable that the supplier has this certification.

In addition to the BS ISO/IEC 17799:2005 standard, information systems, and services supplied to the NHS must also comply with:

- The BS 7083:1996 guide to the accommodation and operation environment for information technology equipment.
- The recommendations made in the Caldicott Report regarding information security.
- The recommendations and guidance issued by the Department of Health or other relevant NHS bodies.
- All data protection legislation, including relevant Acts and Directive, and any relevant guidance published by the Information Commissioner.

IT Service Management

ISO/IEC 20000:2005 defines the requirements for a service provider to deliver managed services. It is based on BS 15000, which has been superseded. It is commonly used by organisations that are going to tender for their services to provide a consistent approach by all service providers in a supply chain, to benchmark IT service management and demonstrate the ability to meet customer requirements. Certification under ISO/IEC 20000:2005 is presently mandatory for suppliers to NHS *Connecting for Health* but advisory only for procurements taking place outside of the National Programme (though this requirement may change in the future).

The ISO/IEC 20000:2005 requirements are derived from "ITIL"—the IT Infrastructure Library provided by the Office of Government Commerce—which consists of a series of publications giving guidance on the provision of quality IT services together with the accommodation and environmental facilities needed to support IT.

There are obvious benefits to NHS organisations if the suppliers of their managed IT services have this certification. The number of suppliers that have achieved this is, however, currently small. Therefore NHS organisations are advised to consider showing preference to suppliers who have such certification, but not to insist upon it.

Safety and Risk Management Standards in the National Programme for IT in the NHS

Early in the National Programme, a review was undertaken to provide a "first cut" assessment of how patient safety issues were being considered and addressed. That review provided recommendations on a way forward, which would ensure that patient safety improvement opportunities were realised and the introduction of unintended patient safety risks were avoided.

Consequently, NHS *Connecting for Health* undertook a series of actions, including the creation of a "Risk and Safety Board" and the implementation of a safety assurance and management system under which information systems and services supplied through the National Programme must receive a "Clinical Authority to Release' from the Programme's Clinical Safety Committee before they can be deployed.

In March of this year, as the deployments taking place within the Programme became more focused on clinical systems than on administrative systems (as had previously been the case) a second review of patient safety was carried out and a number of further actions were instigated as a result, including:

- The issuing of a Contract Change Notice (CCN) that will make patient safety a formal part of the programme's requirements.

- The recruiting of a new medical director who will have specific responsibility for patient safety assurance and patient safety benefit realisation.

- The extension of the National Programme's safety assurance and management system to cover the *entire* lifecycle of an information system or service, from scoping and specification onwards, and covering all information systems and services supplied to the NHS. This will mean that, in the future, not only will a "clinical authority to release" certificate be required prior to deployment, but a "clinical authority to proceed" certificate will be required at each stage in a system or service's lifecycle.

- A requirement that, henceforth, a risk log must be kept by service providers which will facilitate the management and transfer of patient safety risks during a system or service's lifecycle (National Patient Safety Agency, 2006).

A further change that is likely to take place in NHS *Connecting for Health* is that suppliers that have an internal safety assurance and management system that meets the standards of the National Programme and is appropriately integrated into their workflows and processes will not have to get a new "clinical authority to release" from the Programme's Clinical Safety Committee for minor releases and so-called "bug fixes."

Providing this kind of flexibility to suppliers under NHS *Connecting for Health* will, however, require the National Programme to publish a formal standard for safety and risk assurance and management against which either the Programme or an independent third party can audit a supplier's safety management system. At the present time the Programme uses a safety management system that has been developed in line with the principles of the IEC 61508 standard for the functional safety of safety-related systems. In essence, the safety management system involves three deliverables:

- An **end-to-end hazard assessment**, whereby the products and services being supplied to the National Programme undergo a thorough risk assessment in the clinical context in which they will be used.
- A **safety case**, setting out ways in which identified hazards would be mitigated.
- A **safety closure report**, providing evidence that hazards have been addressed in a satisfactory manner, is produced and submitted to the Clinical Safety Committee.

The IEC 61508 standard is not specific to clinical systems and there is an initiative underway, therefore, to create a medical version of it. Other standards which NHS *Connecting for Health* draws on include ISO 14971:2000 on the application of risk management to medical devices, as well as guidelines published by the NPSA (National Patient Safety Agency, 2003). These latter standards enable the National Programme to ensure the completeness of their safety and risk management system, by including provisions for proactive incident reporting—perhaps via a "helpdesk" and a formal system for sharing and learning lessons on patient safety.

In addition to the safety management requirements described above, suppliers to NHS *Connecting for Health* must manage their risk processes in accordance with the operation of the PRINCE2 methodology and provide monthly risk reports, which include an analysis conducted by the supplier of the key risks in the project and progress made in mitigation of those risks. Suppliers are obliged to undertake regular risk assessments in relation to the supply of information systems and services to the National Programme not less than once every six months.

Emerging Standards for Knowledge-Based Products and Services

Although NHS *Connecting for Health* has established quality, safety and risk assurance and management systems, there are not presently any specific standards for the quality, safety, and risk management of knowledge-based products and services. However, in a recent report to the National Programme by the programme's director of clinical knowledge process and safety, Sir Muir Gray, significant concerns were raised about the poor level of assurance that takes place in the main forms of useable knowledge provided to the NHS (Gray, 2006). The report states that significant improvements need to take place to supplier's existing practices, which are too dependent upon peer review and editing: processes that are argued to have severe limitations.

Specifically, the existing peer-review and editing system is stated by the report to have a number of fundamental flaws:

- **It does not detect poor literature retrieval**—so that, if a research study is based on an inaccurate estimate of the current state of knowledge, its research hypothesis will itself be flawed;

- **It does not detect statistical problems**—significant tests may be inappropriately used for baseline comparisons, methods of randomisation may be poorly described and sub-group findings might be presented without appropriate statistical tests for interaction. Taken together, these failings can lead to exaggerated claims of treatment effects;

- **It does not detect unsystematic systematic reviews**—the word "systematic review," while inferring a high degree of rigour, is misused today. Some reviews that claim to be systematic are not. Indeed, many systematic reviews and meta-analyses have serious or extensive flaws; and

- **It does not detect covert duplicate publication**—which can take place because articles submitted for publication are "masked" by a change of authors or language or by adding extra data. Trials reporting greater treatment effects are significantly more likely to be duplicated.

The general effect of these flaws in the peer review system is to emphasise the beneficial effects of interventions and therefore lead the reader to overestimate the benefits and underestimate the harms of an intervention. These effects are compounded by other factors with the same effect, for example the tendency of authors to submit, and editors to publish, studies with a positive result rather than no result. The combined effect is known as positive publication bias and one estimate is that this bias overestimates the benefits of treatments by up to one-third (Schulz, Chalmers, Haynes, & Altman, 1995).

There is clearly considerable potential for these kinds of flaws to find their way into knowledge-based products and services, such as decision-support software, unless appropriate assurance processes are put in place to protect against this. Indeed, the very fact that busy clinicians and patients do not have the time to find and read journal articles and are becoming increasingly reliant upon synopses and pre-prepared "patient pathways" will mean that a supplier must be sure it is achieving the highest standards as regards:

- **Peer review**—to ensure that research (e.g., randomised controlled trials) is based on a comprehensive synthesis, or systematic review, or previous work in the field;

- **The conduct of research**—to ensure that correct methods were chosen;

- **Complete, honest reporting**—of research outcomes, which means (especially in research supported by the pharmaceutical industry) reporting negative as well as positive findings;

- **Better reporting**—of research outcomes, which can be achieved using guidelines such as CONSORT (Chalmers & Clarke, 1998; Clark, Alderson & Chalmers, 2002; Moher, Schulz, & Altman, 2001)., QUOROM (Moher et al, 2004), STARD (Bossuyt, 2004), STROBE (Von Elm & Egger, 2004) and MOOSE (Stroup, 2000);

- **Selection of better quality articles for clinicians and patients**—by identifying studies of low quality (even though they have been peer reviewed), synthesising the results of high quality studies, writing conclusions in a style that is useful for busy clinicians and patients and keeping the evidence base up-to-date by identifying new studies of high quality for inclusion in the synthesis of research;

- **Systematic reviews**—which should only be treated as such if they fulfil the characteristics of Cochrane Reviews in that they are selected on the basis of explicit quality criteria;

- **Regular updating**—all sources used in knowledge-based products and services should have been updated explicitly and regularly or otherwise treated with caution; and

- **Critical appraisal skills**—a supplier's staff as well as peer reviewers and externally-commissioned authors should be constructively suspicious of everything they read no matter how pre-eminent the author or the venerability of a source. Knowledge sources used for synopses and patient pathways should be appraised not only for their research quality and the quality of reporting but also for their contribution to the solution of the problems of the clinicians and patients who will rely upon them.

These processes are presently being proposed by Sir Muir Gray as best practice for suppliers of knowledge-based products and services to NHS *Connecting for Health* and it is entirely likely that they could, in due course, become contractual requirements with which suppliers to the National Programme will have to demonstrate compliance.

Conclusion

Despite the impression the reader might be left with after reading this chapter, there are relatively few formal regulatory demands presently placed upon the suppliers of health information systems, services and technologies and the barriers to entry into this particular sector of healthcare innovation remain unsubstantial as compared with the pharmaceutical and medical device sectors—where a significant amount of time must be spent carrying out studies which demonstrate clinical efficacy and safety before a marketing authorisation can be issued for a new product.

While there is no compelling evidence to suggest that health IT applications are so scandalously unsafe that they should immediately be subjected to a regime similar to that used for pharmaceuticals and medical devices, the gulf between health IT and its sister sectors is dramatic enough to indicate a market that, while no longer in its infancy, is still not a fully grown adult.

The fact, nonetheless, that a major national health IT programme such as NHS *Connecting for Health* is now putting in place an explicit system of safety and risk management standards demonstrates that medical informatics is no longer the sole preserve of a limited number of trial-blazing sites but is becoming more and more deeply embedded in routine patient care. While this is good news for patients and users, it bodes less well for health IT suppliers that lack the human or financial resources with which to implement the safety and quality management systems that their customers are now entitled to demand.

References

Bossuyt, P. M., Retisma, J. B., Bruns. D. E., Gatsonis, C. A., et al. (2004). Towards complete and accurate reporting of studies of diagnostic accuracy: The START initiative. *Family Practice,* 21, 4-10.

Chalmers, I., & Clarke, M. (1998). Discussion sections in reports of controlled trials published in general medical journals: Islands in search of continents? *JAMA, 280,* 280-2.

Clark, M., Alderson, P., & Chalmers, I. (2002). Discussion sections in reports of controlled trials in general medical journals. *JAMA, 287,* 2799-2801 e-Health Insider. (2006). *NHS officially told of London Cerner switch.* 31 July 2006.

General Medical Council (2001). *Good Medical Practice.* Third Edition, May 2001.

Gray, M. (2006). Best current evidence strategy: Consultation Paper (Version 1.0 –21 March 2006). NHS *Connecting for Health.*

Leape, L. L., Bates, D. W., Cullen, D. J., Cooper, J., Demonaco, H. J., Gallivan, T., Hallisey, R., Ives, J., Laird, N., & Laffel, G. (1995). Systems analysis of adverse drug events. ADE Prevention Study Group. *JAMA, 274*(1), 35-43

Moher, D., Cook, D. J., Eastwood, S., Olkin, I., Rennie, D., & Stroup, D. F. (2004). Improving the quality of reports of meta-analyses of randomised controlled trials: The QUORUM Statement. *Ann. Intern. Med. 141,* 781-8

Moher, D., Schulz, K. F., & Altman, D. G. (2001). The CONSORT statement: Revised recommendations for improving the quality of reports of parallel-group randomised trials. *Lancet, 357,* 1191-4

National Audit Office. (2006). *The National Programme for IT in the NHS.* HC1175. 16 June 2006.

National Patient Safety Agency. (2003). *Seven steps to patient safety.* NPSA: 2003.

National Patient Safety Agency. (2005). *Building a memory: preventing harm, reducing risks and improving patient safety.* July 2005.

National Patient Safety Agency. (2006). *Independent Review of the National Programme for Information Technology's Approach to Patient Safety – Executive Summary and Main Report.* DNV: 26 May 2006.

RoSPA. (2007). *Safety areas.* Retrieved from http://www.rospa.com/safetyareas/index.htm

Schmidt, I. K., & Svarstad, B. L. (2002). Nurse-physician communication and quality of drug use in Swedish nursing homes. *Soc Sci Med, 54,* 1766-77.

Schulz, K. F., Chalmers, I., Haynes, R. J., & Altman, D. G. (1995). Empirical evidence of bias dimensions of methodological quality associated with estimates of treatment effects in controlled trials. *JAMA, 273,* 408-12.

Sims, J. (2005). *Procurement: What are we waiting for?* Healthcare Equipment & Supplies magazine. Retrieved from http://www.hesmagazine.com/story.asp?sectionCode=28&storyCode=2029113

Stroup, D. F., Berlin, J. A., Morton, S. C., Olkin, I., Williamson, G. D., Rennie, D., Moher, D., Bekcer, B. J., Sipa, T. A., & Thacker, S. B. (2000). For the meta-analysis of observational studies in epidemiology (MOOSE) Group. Meta-analysis of observational studies in epidemiology: A proposal for reporting. *JAMA, 283*, 2008-2012.

Toppin, G., & Czerniawska, F. (2005). *The economist guide to business consulting.* London: Profile Books Ltd, 2005 at page 7.

Von Elm, E., & Egger, M. (2004). The scandal of poor epidemiological research. *BMJ, 329*, 868-9.

Wilson, T., & Sheikh, A. (2002). Enhancing public safety in primary care. *BMJ, 324*, 584-7.

Endnotes

[1]   BBC. (2001). Helpline advice "linked to diabetic's death." BBC News. Wednesday, 17 October, 2001. Retrieved from http://news.bbc.co.uk/1/hi/england/1605250.stm

Section V

Privacy and Data Protection Issues Regarding Electronic Healthcare Information

Chapter IX

The Impact of Information Technology in Healthcare Privacy

Maria Yin Ling Fung, University of Auckland, New Zealand

John Paynter, University of Auckland, New Zealand

Abstract

The increased use of the Internet and latest information technologies such as wireless computing is revolutionizing the healthcare industry by improving services and reducing costs. The advances in technology help to empower individuals to understand and take charge of their healthcare needs. Patients can participate in healthcare processes, such as diagnosis and treatment, through secure electronic communication services. Patients can search healthcare information over the Internet and interact with physicians. The same advances in technology have also heightened privacy awareness. Privacy concerns include healthcare Web sites that do not practice the privacy policies they preach, computer break-ins, insider and hacker attacks, temporary and careless employees, virus attacks, human errors, system design faults, and social engineering. This chapter looks at medical privacy issues and how they are handled in the U.S. and New Zealand. A sample of 20 New Zealand health Web sites was investigated.

Introduction

Advances in information technology have increased the efficiency of providing healthcare services to patients. Using Web-based technology, the healthcare team can also include the patient, who must be an informed decision maker and active participant in his or her care. These same advances also improve the features, functions, and capabilities of the electronic medical record systems and potentially increase the number of parties, namely hospitals, insurance companies, marketing agencies, pharmaceutical companies, and employers that may have unauthorized access to private medical information. These systems are justifying themselves in terms of cost and life savings. Accessibility to mobile computing devices in the healthcare industry is also evolving. Wireless computing devices enable physicians, clinicians, and nurses to enter patient data at the point of care (Kimmel & Sensmeier, 2002). Disease management systems provide caregivers with information on efficacy of drugs and treatments at various stages of a medical condition. Using bar-coding technology together with decision support, systems can ensure that patients can receive the correct medication or treatment.

Healthcare organizations must manage a tremendous amount of information, from clinical test results, to financial data, to patient tracking information. While most healthcare organizations have policies and procedures in place to guarantee at least minimum levels of privacy protection, they are not core features of most technology systems in the healthcare industry. This is true despite the fact that unauthorized disclosure of an individual's private medical information can affect one's career, insurance status, and even reputation in the community. Without adequate privacy protection, individuals must take steps to protect themselves from what they consider harmful and intrusive uses of their health information, often at significant costs to their health.

Healthcare privacy is an increasingly complex legal and operational issue facing the healthcare industry. For example, in the areas of mental health, HIV, pharmaceuticals, and genetic information, issues of privacy and the appropriate use of health information have already shown themselves to be particularly sensitive. The public has also become increasingly conscious of privacy issues, such as protection of electronic medical records, commercial uses of health information, and insurer and employer access to patient-identifiable information. The increasing use of the Internet also brings a corresponding need for privacy awareness. The very nature of electronic records makes them more easily transportable and thus accessible.

Healthcare professionals face many challenges as they seek ways to deliver quality healthcare while maximizing efficiency and effectiveness and at the same time ensuring privacy. A substantial barrier to improving the quality of and access to healthcare is the lack of enforceable privacy rules. Individuals share a great deal of sensitive, personal information with their doctors. This information is then shared with others, such as insurance companies, pharmacies, researchers, and employers, for many reasons. Yet unlike other personal information, there is very little legal protection for medical records.

This chapter focuses mainly on the impact that information technology has on health-care privacy and the ways in which privacy can be achieved. We examine this in the context of the situation in the U.S.A. and in New Zealand, which has supposedly the world's strictest privacy legislations in the Privacy Act (1993). Comparisons to other countries are also made where information security technology has been applied in the medical domain.

What is Health Information?

The American Health Information Management Association (AHIMA) (The American Health Information Management Association and the Medical Transcription Industry Alliance, 1998) defines health information as:

- Clinical data captured during the process of diagnosis and treatment.
- Epidemiological databases that aggregate data about a population.
- Demographic data used to identify and communicate with and about an individual.
- Financial data derived from the care process or aggregated for an organization or population.
- Research data gathered as a part of care and used for research or gathered for specific research purposes in clinical trials.
- Clinical data and observations taken by trainees in a teaching hospital.
- Reference data that interacts with the care of the individual or with the health-care delivery systems, like a formula, protocol, care plan, clinical alerts, or reminders.
- Coded data that is translated into a standard nomenclature or classification so that it may be aggregated, analyzed, and compared.

AHIMA further states that healthcare information and data serve important functions, including:

- Evaluation of the adequacy and appropriateness of patient care.
- Use in making decisions regarding healthcare policies, delivery systems, funding, expansion, education, and research.
- Support for insurance and benefit claims.
- Assistance in protecting the legal interests of the patients, healthcare professionals, and healthcare facilities.
- Identification of disease incidence to control outbreaks and improve public health.
- Provision of case studies and epidemiological data for the education of health professionals.
- Provision of data to expand the body of medical knowledge.

What is Healthcare Privacy?

Healthcare is a service industry that relies on information for every aspect of its delivery. Health information is important to the patients, the medical practitioners, the healthcare professionals, and institutions, in addition to society as it directs the health of the population. It must be protected as a valuable asset, and in its primary form as the medical record of a unique individual, it must be safeguarded.

Privacy of health information is a legitimate concern. Such concerns grow as technology is in place to allow confidential medical records and sensitive health information such as: mental illness, HIV, substance abuse, sexually transmitted disease, and genetic information, to be made available to employers, bankers, insurers, credit card companies, and government agencies for making decisions about hiring, firing, loan approval, and for developing consumer marketing.

The application of information technology to healthcare, especially the development of electronic medical records and the linking of clinical databases, has generated growing concerns regarding the privacy and security of health information. The security and integrity of electronic health data must be protected from unauthorized users. However, in the medical field, accessibility for certain authorized functions must overrule any other concerns, that is, when a doctor needs to access the information about a patient in order to provide emergency treatment, it is imperative that the data become available without delay (Ateniese, Curtmola, de Medeiros, & Davis, 2003).

While patients have a strong interest in preserving the privacy of their personal health information, they may also have an interest in medical research and other efforts by healthcare organizations to improve the quality of medical care they receive.

Categories of Healthcare Privacy

In addition to technological revolutions, which are the main cause for privacy concerns, there are three distinct kinds of violations of health information privacy according to the congressional testimony of Janlori Goldman, director of the Health Privacy Project at Georgetown University (Starr, 1999):

- Individual misappropriation of medical records;
- Institutional practices—ambiguous harm to identifiable individuals; and
- Institutional practices—unambiguous harm to identifiable individuals.

Individual Misappropriation of Medical Records

Starr (1999) states that this category involves individuals who misuse medical data, often publicly disclosing sensitive information and typically violating both the policies of the institutions that kept the records and the laws of their state. It is by far the most common type of violation of health information privacy that can be corrected by stronger penalties and more aggressive enforcement of privacy laws and policies. According to *Health Privacy Project: Medical Privacy Stories* (2003), examples include:

- Following the rape accusations against basketball player Kobe Bryant, the alleged victim's medical records were subpoenaed by Bryant's defense lawyers from a Colorado hospital. After a hospital employee released the records to a judge, attorneys for the hospital have asked that judge to throw out the subpoenas and destroy the records already received by him, citing state and federal medical privacy laws. Attorneys for the victim are also attempting to prevent Bryant's defense team from gaining access to her medical records from two other hospitals. However, a number of news stories have published sensitive medical information that reporters allege came from hospital employees (Miller, 2003).

- A hospital clerk at Jackson Memorial Hospital in Miami, Florida stole the social security numbers of 16 patients named Theresa when they registered at the hospital. The hospital clerk then provided the social security numbers and medical record information to a friend, also named Theresa, who opened up over 200 bank and credit card accounts and bought six new cars (Sherman, 2002).

Institutional Practices: Ambiguous Harm to Identifiable Individuals

This category consists of the use of personal health data for marketing and other purposes where the harm to the individual is ambiguous or relatively small. For example, a chemist or pharmacist sells patient prescription records to a direct mail and pharmaceutical company for tracking customers who do not refill prescriptions, and sending patients letters encouraging them to refill and consider alternative treatments. The problem is not so much harmful to the customers, who might have appreciated the reminders; what worries them most is the hands into which such lists might fall. This may also raise the question of the merchandising of health data for purposes unrelated to those for which patients provided the original information.

Institutional Practices: Unambiguous Harm to Identifiable Individuals

This category consists of institutional practices that do cause harm to identifiable individuals. Different from the other two categories, this one raises much more serious privacy issues and needs correction and reform. Starr stresses that the commingling of the insurance and employment functions in the United States has led to serious abuse of confidential medical information; and the development of genetics has made possible a new and insidious form of discrimination. He recommends security measures such as encryption, the use of a universal health identifier, segmentation of medical records, and biometric identifiers for and audit trails of those accessing medical records (Starr, 1999). Examples from *Health Privacy Project: Medical Privacy Stories* (2003) and Starr (1999) include:

- Two hundred and six respondents in a survey reported discrimination as a result of access to genetic information, culminating in loss of employment and insurance coverage or ineligibility for benefits (Science and Engineering Ethics, 1996).

- A survey found that 35% of Fortune 500 Companies look at peoples' medical records before making hiring and promotion decisions (Unpublished study, University of Illinois at Urbana-Champaign, 1996).

- An Atlanta truck driver lost his job in early 1998 after his employer learned from his insurance company that he had sought treatment for a drinking problem (J. Appleby, "File safe? Health Records May Not Be Confidential," *USA Today*, March 23, 2000, p. A1).

Technological Changes

Information technologies, such as the Internet and databases, have advanced substantially in the past few years. With the adoption of these new technologies, the healthcare industry is able to save billions of dollars in administrative and overhead costs. These savings can be used to discover new drugs or expand coverage for the uninsured. Through these new technologies, patient care will also be improved; for example, telemedicine allows medical specialists to "examine" and "treat" patients halfway around the world. Perhaps most importantly, information technologies help to empower individuals to understand and to take charge of their own healthcare needs. Patients become active participants in the healthcare process through secure electronic communication services. Wilson, Leitner, and Moussalli (2004) suggest that by putting the patient at the center of the diagnosis and treatment process, communication is more open, and there is more scope for feedback or complaint. This enhances and supports human rights in the delivery of healthcare.

The Internet and Patients

The use of Internet in the healthcare industry involves confidential health information being developed and implemented electronically. There are already several applications available on the Internet for caregivers and patients to communicate and for the electronic storage of patient data. These applications include: electronic mail, online conversations and discussion lists (online chat and NetMeeting), information retrieval, and bulletin boards. Caregivers and patients use electronic mail and online chat to communicate. Patients can search the Web for information about symptoms, remedies, support groups, and health insurance rates. They can also obtain healthcare services, such as second opinions and medical consultations, and products, such as prescription drugs, online (Choy, Hudson, Pritts, & Goldman, 2002).

Patient databases are stored on the Internet, with some providers storing complete patient records in Internet-accessible sites. Patients can interact with databases to retrieve tailored health information (selection-based on personal profile, disease, or a particular need such as travel or cross-border healthcare) (Wilson et al., 2004). However, the availability of medical information in an electronic form (whether or not available over the Internet) raises privacy issues.

The Internet and Health Professionals

Through the use of the Internet, health professionals will have the most up-to-date information available at the click of a mouse. Hospitals, clinics, laboratories, and medical offices will be digitally linked together, allowing for the quick, efficient transfer and exchange of information. The test results will be digitized, allowing for a speedy transfer from labs to hospitals while gaining back the valuable time lost in physical transport. For example, Telehealth in Canada will make geography disappear on a large scale (Siman, 1999). It is a new initiative that significantly improves health services, particularly to remote and rural areas. It also allows physicians to do a complete physical examination of the patient via a digital link. Diagnosis can be made over long-distance telephone lines, rather than after long-distance travel, thus saving the patient the strain and cost of travel. Physicians and other caregivers may use the Internet to discuss unusual cases and obtain advice from others with expertise in treating a particular disease or condition (Siman, 1999).

The Internet and Health-Related Activities

The Internet can support numerous health-related activities beyond the direct provision of care. By supporting financial and administrative transactions, public health surveillance, professional education, and biomedical research, the Internet can streamline the administrative overhead associated with healthcare, improve the health of the nation's population, and lead to new insight into the nature of disease. In each of these domains, specific applications can be envisioned in which the Internet is used to transfer text, graphics, and video files (and even voice); control remote medical or experimental equipment; search for needed information; and support collaboration, in real time, among members of the health community (*Committee on Enhancing the Internet for Health Applications: Technical requirements and implementation strategies*, 2000). For example, the Internet could do the following (*Committee on Enhancing the Internet for Health Applications: Technical requirements and implementation strategies, 2000*):

- Enable consumers to access their health records, enter data or information on symptoms, and receive computer-generated suggestions for improving health and reducing risk.

- Allow emergency room physicians to identify an unconscious patient and download the patient's medical record from a hospital across town.

- Enable homebound patients to consult with care providers over real-time video connections from home, using medical devices capable of transmitting information over the Internet.

- Support teams of specialists from across the country who wish to plan particularly challenging surgical procedures by manipulating shared three-dimensional images and simulating different operative approaches.

- Allow a health plan to provide instantaneous approval for a referral to a specialist and to schedule an appointment electronically.

- Enable public health officials to detect potential contamination of the public water supply by analyzing data on nonprescription sales of antidiarrheal remedies in local pharmacies.

- Help medical students and practitioners access, from the examining room, clinical information regarding symptoms they have never before encountered.

- Permit biomedical researchers at a local university to create three-dimensional images of a biological structure using an electron microscope 1,000 miles away.

Also called: "Medicine of the Millennium," telemedicine is connecting geographically separate healthcare facilities via telecommunications, video, and information systems. The purpose of telemedicine is for remote clinical diagnosis and treatment, remote continuing, medical education, and access to central data repositories for electronic patient records, test requests, and care outcomes.

However, the increasing use of the Internet brings a corresponding need for privacy awareness. The very nature of electronic records makes them more easily transportable and, thus, accessible. Privacy on the Internet is becoming more and more of a concern as confidential information transmitted via the Internet may be intercepted and read by unauthorized persons. Some commonly used Internet protocols may allow information to be altered or deleted without this being evident to either the sender or receiver. Patients may be totally unaware that their personally identifiable health information is being maintained or transmitted via the Internet, and worse still, they may be subject to discrimination, embarrassment, or other harm if unauthorized individuals access this confidential information. While technology can and should be used to enhance privacy, it can also be used to undermine privacy.

Why are There Healthcare Privacy Concerns?

Undoubtedly, the Internet is a valuable tool for improving healthcare because of its ability to reach millions of Internet users at little or no additional cost and absence of geographic and national boundaries. Unfortunately, the Internet is also an ideal tool for the commission of fraud and other online crime. Examples of such fraud include healthcare scams such as the selling of misbranded and adulterated drugs, and bogus miracle cures.

Many of the bigger healthcare Web sites collect information by inviting users to create a personalized Web page where they can acquire medical information tailored specifically to their age, gender, medical history, diet, weight, and other factors. Some sites offer alerts on special medical conditions, health and fitness quizzes, and even the opportunity to store one's own medical records and prescriptions online in case of emergency (*Medical privacy malpractice: Think before you reveal your medical history*, 2001). Other Web sites collect information using cookies. Cookies are small pieces of data stored by the user's Internet browser on the user's computer hard drive. Cookies will be sent by the user's browser to the Web server when the user revisits the same Web site. Hence the user's information such as number of visits, average time spent, pages viewed, and e-mail address will be collected and used to recognize the user on subsequent visits and provide tailored offerings or content to the user.

The California HealthCare Foundation recently examined the privacy policies and practices of 21 popular health sites including: DrKoop.com, Drugstore.com, and WebMD.com (*Medical privacy malpractice: Think before you reveal your medical history*, 2001). They found that visitors to the sites are not anonymous, and that many leading health Web sites do not practice the privacy policies they preach. In some cases, third-party ad networks run banner ads on the sites that collect information and build detailed profiles of each individual's health conditions.

In New Zealand, no published survey has been previously conducted. In order to examine the privacy policies and practices of the New Zealand health sites, 20 medical related Web sites were chosen from the electronic yellow pages (www. yellowpages.com.nz) and studied for the purpose of this chapter. At this site, the individual listings are arranged such that those that have Web sites appear first. Only unique sites were examined. That is, those with multiple listings or branches were ignored. Those with only a simple banner ad in the electronic yellow pages were also excluded. Of these 20 Web sites, three were medical insurers, or offered a medical insurance policy as one of their services; one was for health professionals to use to support traveling patients; and the rest were medical clinics and hospitals. The result shows that all but one of these Web sites collected personal information, but only one had a privacy statement, and it was very obscure; three used cookies, and none mentioned the purpose for which the information was collected. The New Zealand Information Privacy Principle 3 requires that a well-expressed Web site should have a privacy statement. A privacy statement tells consumers that their privacy right is being considered (Wiles, 1998). The Web sites studied all failed to meet such a requirement. The results of the above studies indicate that healthcare privacy concerns are not just problems in New Zealand, but universal ones.

According to Anderson (1996), many medical records can be easily obtained by private detectives, who typically telephone a general practice, family health services authority, or hospital and pretend to be the secretary of a doctor giving emergency treatment to the person who is the subject of the investigation .

Although privacy is a concern as electronic information is vulnerable to hackers and system errors that can expose patients' most intimate data, the most persistent risk to security and privacy is through the people who have authorized access, much more so than the hackers or inadvertent system errors. As medical information systems are deployed more widely and made more interconnected, security violations are expected to increase in number.

What are the Concerns?

The American Health Information Management Association (1998) estimates that when a patient enters a hospital, roughly 150 people have legitimate access to that person's medical record, including food workers, pharmacists, lab technicians, and nursing staff, each with a specific authority to view components of the record necessary for their job and each with unique ability to act within a system.

The increasing use of the Internet in the healthcare industry has also heightened concerns on privacy. The CERT Coordination Center at Carnegie Mellon University, a national resource for collecting information about Internet security problems and disseminating solutions (*Committee on Enhancing the Internet for Health Applications: Technical requirements and implementation strategies*, 1997), lists seven general areas of vulnerability:

- Compromised system administrator privileges on systems that are unpatched or running old OS versions.
- Compromised user-level accounts that are used to gain further access.
- Packet sniffers and Trojan horse programs.
- Spoofing attacks, in which attackers alter the address from which their messages seem to originate.
- Software piracy.
- Denial of service.
- Network file system and network information system attacks and automated tools to scan for vulnerabilities.

In addition to the above vulnerabilities, other concerns are:

- To whom should organizations be allowed to disclose personal health information with and without patient consent? Under what conditions may such disclosures be made?

- What steps must organizations take to protect personal health information from loss, unauthorized editing, or mischief?
- What types of security technologies and administrative policies will be considered sufficient protection?

Additional Common Threats and Attacks

A threat is any of the capabilities, intentions, and attack methods of adversaries to exploit or cause harm to information or a system. Threats are further defined as being passive (monitoring but no alteration of data) and active (deliberate alteration of information). King, Dalton, and Osmanoglu (2001) define four common threat consequences and the sources of threats in the following sections:

- **Disclosure:** If information or data is revealed to unauthorized persons (breach of confidentiality).
- **Deception:** If corporate information is altered in an unauthorized manner (system or data integrity violation).
- **Disruption:** If corporate resources are rendered unusable or unavailable to authorized users (denial of service).
- **Usurpation:** If the corporate resources are misused by unauthorized persons (violation of authorization).

Temporary or Careless Employees

Electronic health records stored at healthcare organizations are vulnerable to internal or external threats. Although with the protection of firewalls, careless employees, temporary employees, or disgruntled former employees cause far more problems than do hackers. As a company's employees have tremendous access to the company's resources, it is possible that the computer system could be hacked into internally, as well as by third parties. For example, an employee attaches a database of 50,000 names to an e-mail and sends it to a business partner who is working on a marketing campaign at another company. It would be very likely that data could be intercepted or harvested by a third party and used for improper or unauthorized purposes (Silverman, 2002).

Human Errors and Design Faults

A serious threat to the confidentiality of personal health information in hospitals and health authorities is the poor design and lax administration of access controls (Anderson, 1996). In many hospitals, all users may access all records; it is also common for users to share passwords or to leave a terminal permanently logged on for the use of everyone in a ward. This causes a breakdown of clinical and medico-legal accountability and may lead to direct harm. Other design errors include improperly installing and managing equipment or software, accidentally erasing files, updating the wrong file, or neglecting to change a password or backup a hard disk.

Insiders

Another source of threat comes from the trusted personnel (the insiders) who engage in unauthorized activities (copying, stealing, or sabotaging information, and yet their actions may remain undetected) or activities that exceed their authority (abusing their access). The insiders may disable the network operation or otherwise violate safeguards through actions that require no special authorization.

Crackers, Hackers, and Other Intruders

While internal threats consist of authorized system users who abuse their privileges by accessing information for inappropriate reasons or uses, external threats consist of outsiders who are not authorized to use an information system or access its data, but who nevertheless attempt to access or manipulate data or to render the system inoperable. Computer break-ins are proven to have occurred in the healthcare industry. The Health Care Privacy Project, a non-profit corporation in Washington DC, reported that a hacker found a Web page used by the Drexel University College of Medicine in Pennsylvania that linked to a database of 5,500 records of neurosurgical patients (*Health Privacy Project: Medical privacy stories*, 2003). The records included patient addresses, telephone numbers, and detailed information about diseases and treatments. After finding the database through the search engine Google, the hacker was able to access the information by typing in identical usernames and passwords. Drexel University shut down its database upon learning of the vulnerability, and a university spokeswoman stated that officials had been unaware that the database was available online, as it was not a sanctioned university site.

A "2002 Computer Crime and Security" survey conducted by the Computer Security Institute (CSI) with the participation of the San Francisco Federal Bureau of Investigation's (FBI) Computer Intrusion Squad found that the threat from computer crime and other information security breaches continues unabated and that the threat from within the organization is far greater than the threat from outside the organization. Results show that 74% cited their Internet connection as a frequent point of attack than cited their internal systems as a frequent point of attack (33%); 28% suffered unauthorized access or misuse on their Web sites within the last twelve months; 21% said that they did not know if there had been unauthorized access or misuse; 55% reported denial of service; and 12% reported theft of transaction information (*Cyber crime bleeds U.S. corporations, survey shows; Financial losses from attacks climb for third year in a row*, 2002).

Social Engineering

According to King et al. (2001), a social engineering attack involves impersonating an employee with known authority, either in person (disguised) or by using an electronic means of communication (e-mail, fax, or the telephone). For example, an attacker places a phone call to the system administrator claming to be a corporate executive who has lost the modem pool number and forgotten the password. In the hospitals, an outsider places a phone call to an authorized insider, pretending to be a physician in legitimate need of medical information.

Information Warfare

A RAND Corporation study of information warfare scenarios in 1995 suggests that terrorists using hacker technologies could wreak havoc in computer-based systems underlying emergency telephone services, electric power distribution networks, banking and securities systems, train services, pipeline systems, information broadcast channels, and other parts of our information infrastructure (*Committee on Enhancing the Internet for Health Applications: Technical requirements and implementation strategies*, 2000).

Although the above examples do not specifically describe threats to healthcare organizations, they do indicate the growing vulnerability of information systems connected to public infrastructure such as the Internet. As such, the drive for increased use of electronic health information linked together by modern networking technologies could possibly expose sensitive health information to a variety of threats that will need to be appropriately addressed.

Healthcare Privacy Concerns in the United States

According to Ball, Weaver, and Kiel (2004), a national survey of e-health behavior in the U.S. found that 75% of people are concerned about health Web sites sharing information without their permission and that a significant percentage do not and will not engage in certain health-related activities online because of privacy and security concerns. For example, 40% will not give a doctor online access to their medical records; 25% will not buy or refill prescriptions online; and 16% will not register at Web sites. However, nearly 80% said that a privacy policy enabling them to make choices about whether and how their information is shared would make them more willing to use the Internet for their private health information.

A Pew report (2005) documented that 89% of health seekers were concerned about privacy issues, with fully 71% very concerned. When people were made aware of the possibility of the issuance of universal medical ID numbers, a Gallup poll found that 91% opposed the plan; 96% opposed the placement on the Web of information about themselves held by their own doctor (The Gallup Organisation, 2000). On the other hand, the healthcare administrators are aware of security issues and have many safeguards in place. In a recent survey of healthcare information technology executives, participants ranked the protection of health data as their primary concern (Reid, 2004). Hospitals, for example, indicate that current security technologies in use include anti-virus software (100%), firewalls (96%), virtual private networks (83%), data encryption (65%), intrusion detection (60%), vulnerability assessment (57%), public key infractions (20%), and biometrics (10%). Virtually all respondents expected to use all these technologies to some degree during the next two years (The Gallup Organisation, 2000).

Recent evidence indicates that many medical organizations are lagging behind in their implementation of appropriate security systems. A study of 167 U.S. hospitals conducted by research firm HCPro found that 76% had not conducted an information security audit, and only half planned to do so by April 2001 (Johnson, 2001). Of the hospitals that had performed an audit, 51% said that they would need major improvements to, or a complete overhaul of, their security systems, and 49% claimed that they would have to significantly change or replace their security policies. Alarmingly, only 5% said they had an annual budget for HIPAA compliance.

The inadequacy of some medical providers' security systems was recently underscored by the hacking of the University of Washington Medical Center (UWMC) computers (*Thomson Corporation and health data management*, 2005). Security-Focus.com reported that an intruder was able to break into the UWMC computers and view the name, address, and Social Security number and medical procedures of over 4,000 cardiology patients. Theoretically, the UWMC could face potential lawsuits by distressed patients.

Healthcare Privacy Concerns in New Zealand

A survey was conducted in 1998 to study the practice and plans in New Zealand for the collation and retention of health records about identifiable individuals, with particular reference to the implications for privacy arising from the increased use of National Health Index Numbers (NHI) (Stevens, 1998).

What is NHI? The NHI provides a mechanism to uniquely identify healthcare users. It was developed to help protect personally identifying health data held on computer systems and to enable linkage between different information systems whilst still protecting privacy. The NHI database records contain information of each person to whom an NHI number has been allocated, their name, date of birth, date of death, address, gender, ethnicity (up to three entries allowed), residence status, and other names by which they may be known (Stevens, 1998). It, however, does not contain any clinical information, and its availability for research purposes tends to be limited chiefly to a peripheral role in cohort studies and clinical trials (Stevens, 1998).

Alongside the NHI database is the Medical Warnings System (MWS) database, which can only be accessed via the individual's NHI number. The MWS is designed to warn healthcare providers of the presence of any known risk factors that may be important in making clinical decisions about individual patient care.

The MWS database records contain individuals' NHI numbers, donor information (e.g., heart or kidney), contact details for next of kin (name, relationship, and phone number), medical warnings (typically allergies and drug sensitivities, classified as "danger" or "warning" or unverified "report"), medical condition alerts (such as diabetes), and summaries of healthcare events (so far these have been limited to hospital admissions, showing dates of admission and discharge, hospital, and diagnosis or procedure code).

These two databases are maintained by New Zealand Health Care Information Services (NZHIS) formed in 1991, a division of the Ministry of Health. NSHIS is responsible for the collecting, extraction, analysis, and distribution of health information.

In this survey, it is found that a statement on the Ministry Web site states that access to the MWS is "restricted solely for the use of providers in the context of caring for that individual." However, it is estimated that there are some 20,000 people who have direct access to the MWS and a further 70,000 who potentially have access to it, so that in practice, the security of the system probably relies heavily upon the difficulty of getting a hold of the NHI for the individual subject of an unauthorized enquiry (Johnson, 2001).

The survey further reveals that the same Web site document states, in respect of the NHI and MWS systems, "The Privacy Commissioner will be continuously involved in ensuring that the very highest possible standards of integrity and probity are maintained." Yet NZHIS do not appear to have taken any steps either to check with the Privacy Commissioner before making that statement or, having made the statement without the Commissioner's knowledge or agreement, to involve him/her at all in checking arrangements for operation of these databases. At the least, therefore, the statement is misleading in suggesting a form of endorsement by the Privacy Commissioner.

During the survey, more than one doctor contacted admitted that they use a different name for transactions involving their own healthcare, because they do not trust the security of records held by hospitals, laboratories, and other healthcare agencies with which they deal. This implies that the more health records that are to be integrated, the more users that must be concerned about the possibility of security breaches in any one part of the larger system. This also implies that the functions of an information system can be subverted if it does not gain and keep the confidence of both users and subjects.

Who has Access to the Healthcare Information?

There are a variety of organizations and individuals who have an interest in medical data, and they are both within and outside of the healthcare industry. Usually access to the health information requires a patient's agreement by signing a "blanket waiver" or "general consent forms" when the patient obtains medical care. Signing of such a waiver allows healthcare providers to release medical information to employers, insurance companies, medical practitioners, government agencies, court orders or legal proceedings, direct marketers, medical institutions, hospitals, and newsgroups/chat rooms on the Internet.

Employers

Employers have an interest in an employee's fitness to work and fitness to perform particular tasks such as flying airplanes, controlling air traffic, and driving trains, buses, trucks, and cars. Some self-insured businesses establish a fund to cover the insurance claims of employees, which requires employees' medical records to be open for inspection by employers instead of an insurance company.

Insurance Companies

Insurance companies seek to combat rising costs of care by using large amounts of patient data in order to judge the appropriateness of medical procedures. They may also have an interest in healthcare data about a person's injuries and illnesses in relation to medical claims.

In New Zealand, the Accident Rehabilitation and Compensation Insurance Corporation (ACC), whose accident records are used for calculating workplace premium, will be shared with healthcare organizations. For example, to be eligible for weekly compensation, an injured person must be (a) incapacitated through injuries and (b) an earner at the time of the incapacity. ACC obtains medical opinion to clarify incapacity. It also obtains information from Inland Revenue, employers, and accountants to satisfy the second criteria.

Medical Practitioners

The medical practitioners have an explicit statutory obligation to disclose information on patients who have a serious physical condition, notifiable disease, or impairment that the doctor knows is likely to result in significant danger to the public (Clarke, 1990). In some cases it may be important that sensitive health data to be conveyed as part of information provided about a referral, in particular if the patient has been diagnosed as HIV-positive.

Government Agencies

In the U.S., government agencies may request citizens' medical records to verify claims made through Medicare, MediCal, Social Security Disability, and Workers Compensation. In New Zealand, government agencies such as Inland Revenue Department may share the information with healthcare organizations and ACC for tax and benefits purposes.

Medical Institutions and Clinical Researchers

Medical institutions such as hospitals or individual physicians require health information for evaluation of quality of service. This evaluation is required for most hospitals to receive their licenses. Clinical researchers and epidemiologists need health information to answer questions about the effectiveness of specific therapies, patterns of health risks, behavioral risks, environmental hazards, or genetic predisposition for a disease or condition (e.g., birth defects).

Direct Marketers

Drug companies want to know who is taking which drug so that they can conduct post-marketing surveillance to develop marketing strategies. Direct marketers use health-screening tests to collect medical information and build up data banks of businesses for promoting and selling products that are related to the information collected.

Court Orders/Legal Proceedings

In the U.S., medical records may be subpoenaed for court cases for people who are involved in litigation, an administrative hearing, or workers' compensation hearing. In the (less litigatious) New Zealand context, this is more likely to involve the granting of powers of attorney to make decisions on medical matters for patients who are not capable of making such decisions.

Internet Service Providers/Users

The Internet is available for individuals to share information on specific diseases and health conditions. While the Web sites dispense a wide variety of information, there is no guarantee that information disclosed in any of these forums is confidential.

Mechanisms for Addressing Healthcare Privacy

Today, healthcare organizations are confronting the challenge of maintaining easy access to medical/clinical data while increasing data security. Technology is only part of the solution. Many healthcare organizations have deployed, to varying degrees, mechanisms to protect the security and integrity of their medical records, such as the use of strong enterprise-wide authentication, encryption, several levels

Table 1. Functions of technological security tools

Principles	Implementation
Availiability	Ensuring that information is accurate and up to date when needed
Accountability	Ensuring the access to and use of information is based on a legitimate need and right to know
Perimeter indentification	Knowing and controlling the boundaries of trusted access to the information system, both physically and logically
Controlling access	Ensuring the access is only to information essential to the performance of jobs and limiting the access beyond a legitimate need
Comprehensibility and control	Ensuring the record owners, data stewards, and patients understand and have effective control over appropriate aspects of information privacy and access

of role-based access control, auditing trails, computer misuse detection systems, protection of external communications, and disaster protection through system architecture as well as through physically different locations. Among other strategies, databases are also used to address security and access control. One database will have consumer identification (ID) geographic information linked to an ID number. The second database will have actual clinical information indexed by patient ID number but no personal data (Ball et al., 2004). However, there are obstacles to the use of security technologies which are yet to be resolved.

Technological Solution

Technological security tools are essential components of modern distributed healthcare information systems. At the highest level, they serve five key functions, as seen in Table 1 (*Committee on Enhancing the Internet for Health Applications: Technical requirements and implementation strategies*, 1997): availability, accountability, perimeter identification, controlling access, and comprehensibility and control.

However, these types of controls focus more on protecting information *within* healthcare provider institutions and do not address the problems of unrestricted exploitation of information (e.g., for data mining) after it has passed *outside* the provider institution to secondary players or to other stakeholders in the health information services industry (*Committee on Enhancing the Internet for Health Applications: Technical requirements and implementation strategies*, 1997). In New Zealand, the Health Intranet, a communications infrastructure that allows health information to be exchanged between healthcare providers in a secure way, defines six key elements that any security policy must address (New Zealand Health Information Service, 2001): confidentiality, integrity, authenticity, non-repudiation, auditing and accountability.

Table 2. Key elements of a security policy

Principles	Implementation
Confidentiality	Ensuring that the message is not readable by unauthorized parties whilst in transit by applying strong encryption tools, such as Digital Certificates
Integrity	Ensuring that the message is not damaged or altered whilst in transit by using secure private networks and Digital Signatures
Authenticity	Ensuring that the user is a trusted party by using user ID/password and/or Digital Certificates
Auditing	Recording user connectivity and site access for audit purposes
Accountability	Identifying clear responsibilities of organizations and individual users through compliance with Legislation and Security Policies

Security Architecture

The primary goal of a security architecture design in the healthcare industry is the protection of the healthcare provider's assets: hardware, software, network components, and information resources.

Healthcare Finance Administration (HCFA) (*CPRI toolkit: Managing information security in heath care*, 2005) suggests that technical protection measures are traditionally grouped into three high level categories:

- **Confidentiality** measures provide the mechanism to ensure that the privacy of information is maintained. Mechanisms include encryption (e.g., virtual private networks, end-to-end, and link level encryption).

- **Integrity** measures enhance the reliability of information by guarding against unauthorized alteration. Protection measures include: digital signature and strong authentication using certificates provided through the Public Key Infrastructure (PKI) initiative.

- **Availability** measures seek to ensure that information assets are accessible to

Table 3. Security architecture principles and guidelines

Principles	Security Servies	Mechanisms
Confidentiality	Encryption is required over all communications channels (e.g., Internet, ISP-based connections, dial up etc.). Confidential data must be kept encrypted on user laptops and workstations. Such information is to be disclosed only to named individuals on a need-to-know basis	• Firewalls—Used at connection Internet and boundary points. • Physical Control—Central office and Data Center continued physical security; integrated smart card access control. • Encryption—Application-specific, primary DES-based and PKI-based key mgmt; SSL. • Database Security—Proprietary, DBMS-specific; DAC, PKI-enabled, RBAC (role based access control) intergrated; DAC
Integrity	Business unit managed chage control is required. Fiel-level change history must be maintained. Roll-back functionality is required.	Encryption—Application-specific, primarily DES-based and PKI-based key management; SSL (Secure Socket Layer).
Availability	Virus scanning and redundant and high availibility solutions are required. Strong system configuration, change control, and regular backup/restore processes are required.	Virus prevention—Workstation-based and server-based program; signed applications.
Identification and authentication	Strong authentication (encrypted, username and password, token certificate).	Authentication—User ID and password-based with limited smart card pilots; Private key-based with multi-factor identification.

continued on following page

Table 3. continued

Principles	Security Services	Mechanisms
Authorization and access control	Authorization by business unit or function and detailed role-based access control are required.	Access Control - Platform-specific access control lists. RBAC-based, centrally managed access.
Non-repudiation	Strict change controls are required. Field-level file change history must be maintained. Digital signatures for creator and the checker are required.	Electronic Signature - FIPS 140-1 Digital Signature; Escrow for encryption keys (not signing keys)
Auditing and monitoring	System-level for user-access, file changes, failed login attempts, alarms.	• Audit Trail Creation & Analysis—Logs generated on a platform—specific basis. Consistent log content, directive data reduction and analysis. • Intrusion Detection-Automated monitoring of limited entry/exit points; Pro-active with integrated action plan.
Compliance with regulations	Compliance with Legislation.	For example, HIPAA in the U.S., European Union Data Protection Directive or the Health Information Privacy Code 1994 in New Zealand.

internal and external users when needed and guard against "denial of service" attacks. Protection measures include: firewalls and router filters for mitigating availability risks created by denial of service attacks.

While developing guidelines for the clinical security system for BMA (British Medical Association), Ross Anderson (1996) identified a few shortcomings of the NHS (UK National Health Services) wide network, which are useful for any security architectures to be built for the healthcare industry:

- The absence of an agreed common security policy enforced by all the systems that will connect to the network.
- The lack of confidence in the technical security measures such as firewalls.
- Many of the NHS wide network applications are unethical, which make personal health information available to an ever-growing number of administrators and others outside the control of both patient and clinician. Such availability contravenes the ethical principle that personal health information may be shared only with the patient's informed and voluntary consent. For example, the administrative registers will record patients' use of contraceptive and mental health services, while the NHS clearing system will handle contract claims for inpatient hospital treatment and contain a large amount of identifiable clinical information.

- Item of service and other information sent over existing electronic links between general practitioners and family health services authorities. While registration links are fairly innocuous, at least two suppliers are developing software for authorities that enables claims for items of service, prescriptions, and contract data to be pieced together into a "shadow" patient record that is outside clinical control (Advanced information system, Family Health Services computer unit, 1995; Data Logic product information at http://www.datlog.co.uk/).

Table 3 is a typical security architecture, the components of which are formed based on the ten basic security services (physical security; firewalls; intrusion detection; access control; authentication; privacy and integrity (encryption); electronic signature/non-repudiation; virus protection; audit trail creation and analysis; and database security) identified by HCFA and a list of application-specific baseline requirements for the healthcare industry proposed by King et al. (2001). Some of the components and guidelines are also adopted from the Anderson's UK NHS model.

Encryption

There is an increasing number of health practitioners transferring patient health information using electronic mail across wide area networks, for example, using mailbox systems to transfer registration data and item of service claims to family health services authorities, links between general practitioners and hospitals for pathology reports, and the use of Internet electronic mail to communicate with patients that require continuing management. Anderson (1996) suggests that the problem may be tackled using cryptography: encryption and digital signatures can protect personal health information against disclosure and alteration, whether accidental or malicious, while in transit through a network.

Encryption is a tool for preventing the possibility of attack and interception during transmission and storage of data, for assuring confidentiality and integrity of information, and for authenticating the asserted identity of individuals and computer systems by rendering the data meaningless to anyone who does not know the "key." Information that has been cryptographically wrapped cannot be altered without detection. For example, the integrity of a health message is destroyed by removal of personal identifiers or by encryption of crucial pieces of the message. At the destination, the receiver decrypts the message using the same key (symmetrical encryption) or a complementary but different key (asymmetrical encryption) (New Zealand Health Information Service, 2001). Pretty Good Privacy (PGP) and GNU-PGP are commonly used third-party encryption software, which are available free for most common makes of computer.

There are two types of encryption systems: Public-key encryption and private-key encryption. The most commonly used and secure private-key encryption system is the data encryption standard (DES) algorithm developed by IBM in the 1970s, which is gradually replaced by the newer and more efficient algorithm, the advanced encryption standard (AES), which was chosen by the U.S. government after a long, open contest. According to Wayner (2002), the basic design of DES consists of two different and complementary actions: confusion and diffusion. Confusion consists of scrambling up a message or modifying it in some nonlinear way. Diffusion involves taking one part of the message and modifying another part so that each part of the final message depends on many other parts of the message. DES consists of 16 alternating rounds of confusion and diffusion.

Public-key encryption is quite different from the DES. The most popular public-key encryption system is the RSA algorithm, developed in the late 1970s, which uses two keys. If one key encrypts the data, then only the other key can decrypt it. Each person can create a pair of keys and publicize one of the pair, perhaps by listing it in some electronic phone book. The other key is kept secret. If someone wants to send you a message, only the other key can decrypt this message, and only you have a copy of that key. In a very abstract sense, the RSA algorithm works by arranging the set of all possible messages in a long loop in an abstract mathematical space (Wayner, 2002). Public key cryptography is the underlying means for authenticating users, securing information integrity, and protecting privacy. For example, New Zealand North Health is planning to use encryption to encrypt the patients' NHI number and to deposit the information in a database. As such, information about any individual can only be retrieved by means of the encrypted identifier.

In the wide area networks, both secure socket layer (SSL) encryption and IP security (IPSec) should be deployed to allow the continued evaluation of different modes of securing transactions across the Internet. SSL is used to transport the encrypted messages on a communication channel so that no message could be "intercepted" or "faked." It provides authentication through digital certificates and also provides privacy through the use of encryption. (IPSec) protocol, a standards-based method of providing privacy, integrity, and authenticity to information transferred across IP networks, provides IP network-layer encryption.

Virtual Private Network (VPN)

Virtual private networks (VPNs) are standard secure links between companies and their resource users, which allow a company's local networks to be linked together without their traffic being exposed to eavesdropping. It can reduce the exposure to interception of international network traffic. With the increasing use of Internet in the healthcare industry, VPNs play a significant role in securing privacy. VPNs use tunneling and advanced encryption to permit healthcare organizations to establish secure, end-to-end, private network connections over third party networks. Some practical applications that will be used include accessing and updating patient medical records, Tele-consultation for medical and mental health patients, electronic transfer of medical images (x-ray, MRI, mammography, etc.), psychiatric consultations, distance learning, and data vaulting (ScreamingMedia, 1999).

The Hawaii Health Systems Corporation (HHSC) has created a Virtual Private Healthcare Network and Intranet solution that allows for collaboration between its 12 hospitals, 3,200 employees, and 5,000 partners located worldwide. By creating a sophisticated healthcare network that supports high speed, broadband data connectivity, doctors, specialists, and administrators can collaborate throughout the State of Hawaii just as if they were together at the same hospital. This scalable solution also allows existing and future partners, clients, and suppliers to connect to the HHSC network to collaborate and share data. By using a unique subscription profile concept, the network provides impenetrable security and allows for the free and secure flow of mission critical data (ScreamingMedia, 1999).

Firewalls

When private networks carrying confidential data are connected to the Internet, firewalls must be utilized extensively to establish internal security boundaries for protecting the internal private network, computers, data, and other "electronic assets" from tampering or theft by outsiders. Firewalls are a collection of network computing devices such as routers, adaptive hubs, and filters working in tandem and configured to ensure that only expressly permitted packets of data may enter or exit a private network. Firewalls will screen all communication between the internal and external networks according to directives established by the organization. For example, Internet access to an internal patient data system should be entirely prohibited or limited only to those people authenticated by a password or security token (*Committee on Enhancing the Internet for Health Applications: Technical requirements and implementation strategies*, 2000).

Communications security is also important. Some general practices have branch surgeries, and many hospitals have branch clinics, so the possibility of access via a dial up modem from branches is often raised (Anderson, 1996). In such cases, the main additional risk is that an outside hacker might dial up the main system and gain access by guessing a password. In order to avoid that, Anderson (1996) suggests that there should be no direct dial access to the main computer system. Instead, the main system should dial back the branches. Extra effort should also be made to educate users to choose passwords with care, and all incidents should be investigated diligently.

Audit Trails and Intrusion Detection Monitoring

Transaction logs and audit trails are important, as changes to the patient data can be closely monitored and traced. Audit trails record who and when alterations are made to particular files. The use of audit trails is invaluable, as they can be used as evidence in a court of law. The HCFA information systems create audit logs that record, in a centralized repository, logon and logoff; instances where a role is authorized access or denied access; the individual acting in that role; the sensitivity level of the data or other asset accessed; what type of access was performed or attempted (e.g., whether the nature of the requested action was to create, read, update, execute a program, or delete). Anderson (1996) suggests that periodic audits should be carried out, and from time to time these should include penetration tests. For example, a private detective might be paid to obtain the personal health information of a consenting patient. In this way, any channels that have developed to sell information on the black market may be identified and closed off.

Intrusion detection is primarily a reactive function that responds as attacks are identified. HCFA recommends the use of intrusion detection software to monitor network and host-based assets and employ a computer emergency response team to report and respond when incidents occur.

Biometric Systems

New technology called "biometric authentication" is being used to replace passwords and other security measures with digital recognition of fingerprints or other unique attributes. Biometrics uses individual physiological (finger-scan, iris scan, hand-scan, and retina-scan) or behavioral characteristics (voice and signature scans) to determine or verify identity. The most commonly used is the physiological biometrics. Because biometric security is based on a unique feature of an individual's body, for instance, a fingerprint, it is very difficult to copy, steal, or replicate this information (The Independent Research Group, 2002). Iris-scan is very suitable for use by healthcare institutions. Iris-scan can verify or identify a person based on the unique characteristics of the human iris. The strengths of iris-scan include its high resistance to false matching, the stability of the iris over time, and the ability to use this biometric to provide access to healthcare information or entry into physically secure locations, such as a medical record-keeping or information technology department.

A study done in Albuquerque, New Mexico indicates that the most effective technologies currently available for identification verification (i.e., verifying the claimed identity of an individual who has presented a magnetic stripe card, smart card, or PIN) are systems based on retinal, iris, or hand geometry patterns (Stevens, 1998).

On the other hand, single-sign-on technology enables users to log on via user IDs and passwords, biometrics, or other means to gain immediate access to all information systems linked to a network (Clarke, 1990). Single sign-on (SSO) is the capability to authenticate to a given system/application once, and then all participating systems/applications will not require another authentication (King et al., 2001). Both technologies are designed to provide increased security in an unobtrusive manner (Clarke, 1990). St. Vincent Hospital and Health Care Services, Indianapolis had implemented a combined biometric and single-sign-on system in one of its acute care departments using different types of biometric readers to identify physicians and nurses.

Smart Cards

Internet commerce interests are pushing forward aggressively on standards for developing and deploying token-based cryptographic authentication and authorization systems (e.g., the Mastercard-Visa consortium and CyberCash Inc.) (Siman, 1999). Smart Card Token is a smart card about the size of a credit card and has a liquid crystal display on which a number appears that changes every minute or so. Each user card generates a unique sequence of numbers over time and, through a shared secret algorithm for which the user has been assigned access privileges, can generate the corresponding sequence of numbers. The number can be used as a session password. The write-controlled internal memory supports services such as user-specific information storage, authentication, and cryptographic certificate management. Some even have biometric access control features. Employees and appropriate contractors will be issued smart cards or tokens that store a private key and other essential authentication information.

Access Control

A serious threat to the confidentiality of personal health information in hospitals and health authorities is the poor design and lax administration of access controls (Anderson, 1996). Anderson stresses that, in particular, the introduction of networking may turn local vulnerabilities into global ones if the systems with ineffective access controls are connected together in a network, and then instead of the data being available merely to all staff in the hospital, they might become available to everyone on the network.

However, access controls must also be harmonized among networked systems, or moving information from one system to another could result in leaks. The solution for this is to have a common security policy that clearly states who may access what records and under what circumstances. Anderson emphasizes that the following are important to the implementation of effective access controls:

- A senior person such as a hospital manager or partner in general practice must be responsible for security, especially if routine administration is delegated to junior staff. Many security failures result from delegating responsibility to people without the authority to insist on good practice.

- The mechanisms for identifying and authenticating users should be managed carefully. For example, users should be educated to pick passwords that are hard to guess and to change them regularly; and terminals should be logged off automatically after being unused for five minutes.

- Systems should be configured intelligently. Dangerous defaults such as maintenance passwords and anonymous file transfer access supplied by the manufacturer should be removed. User access should be restricted to departments or care teams as appropriate. With hospital systems that hold records on many people, only a few staff should have access to the files of patients not currently receiving treatment.

Password Management

In many hospitals all users may access all records and often share passwords and leave terminals permanently logged on for the use of everyone in a ward. Such behavior causes a breakdown of clinical and medicolegal accountability and may lead to direct harm: one case has been reported in which a psychiatric patient changed prescription information at a terminal that was left logged on (Anderson, 1996).

It is important for administrators to educate all users that passwords issued to an individual should be kept confidential and not be shared with anyone. When a user ID is issued to a temporary user who needs access to a system, it must be deleted from the system when the user has finished his or her work. All passwords should be distinctly different from the user ID, and ideally they should be alphanumeric and at least six characters in length. Also, passwords should be changed regularly, at least every 30 days. Rittinghouse and Ransome (2004) suggest that it is a good security practice for administrators to make a list of frequently used forbidden passwords. Standard passwords that are often used to get access to different systems for maintenance purposes are not recommended.

Database Security

Database authentication and access control will be public key enabled and role-based. This means that a user will employ a multi-factor authentication procedure based on knowledge of his/her private key to obtain access to a database. Once authentication is complete, access, sometimes down to the record level, will be granted or denied based on the user's roles and associated privileges. Database security will be implemented on a discretionary access control (DAC) basis.

Social Engineering and Careless Disclosure Safeguards

The weakest link in security will always be people, and the easiest way to break into a system is to engineer your way into it through the human interface (*CPRI toolkit: Managing information security in heath care*, 2005). The main threat to the confidentiality of clinical records is carelessness in handling telephone/e-mail/fax inquiries, instant messaging and on-site visits, and inadequate disposal of information.

According to King et al. (2001), social engineering safeguards consist of non-technical (procedural) means that include: security training for all corporate users; security awareness training for all system administration personnel with well-documented procedures, handling, and reporting; and security awareness training for personnel responsible for allowing outside visitors into restricted areas (such as assigned escorts).

With regard to careless disclosure, Anderson (1996) developed a set of common sense rules that the best practices have used for years and that are agreed by the UK NHS Executives. Whether records are computerized or not, these rules of best practice can be summed up as clinician-consent-call back-care-commit:

- Only a clinician should release personal health information. It should not be released by a receptionist or secretary.

- The patient's consent must be obtained, except when the patient is known to be receiving treatment from the caller or in the case of emergency or the statutory exemptions. In the latter two cases the patient must be notified as soon as reasonably possible afterward.

- The clinician must call back if the caller is not known personally, and the number must be verified, for example, in the Medical Directory. This procedure must be followed even when an emergency is claimed, as private investigators routinely claim emergencies.

- Care must be taken, especially when the information is or may be highly sensitive, such as HIV status, details of contraception, psychiatric history, or any information about celebrities.

- The clinician must commit a record of the disclosure to a ledger. This should have the patient's name; whether consent was sought at the time (and, if not, the date and means of notification); the number called back and how it was verified; and whether anything highly sensitive was disclosed.

In addition, the guidelines for disclosure by telephone should also apply to faxes. Verifying the identity or, failing that, the location of the caller is just as important as it is when disclosing personal health information over the telephone. It is important, and it is the BMA's established advice that personal health information should be faxed only to a machine that is known to be secure during working hours.

Equipment Theft, Loss, and Damage

Anderson (1996) considers the most serious threat to the continued availability of computerized clinical information in general practice to be theft of the computer that has been experienced by over 10% of general practices surveyed. Data can also be destroyed in other ways such as by fire, flood, equipment failure, and computer viruses. He suggests that physical security measures must be taken; hygiene rules to control the risk of computer virus infestation must be applied together with a tested recovery plan.

Since most organizations do not perform realistic tests of their procedures, with the result that when real disasters strike recovery is usually held up for lack of manuals and suppliers' phone numbers, it is important that a drill based on a realistic scenario, such as the complete destruction of a surgery or hospital computer room by fire must be carried out, and a full system recovery to another machine from back up media held off site must be performed. Another measure is to keep several generations of back ups in cases of equipment failure and virus attacks that it may take time to notice that something has gone wrong. A typical schedule in a well run establishment might involve back ups aged one, two, three, four, eight, and twelve weeks, as well as daily incremental back ups.

Limitations of Security Technologies

Despite an aggressive move toward computerized healthcare records in recent years and ongoing parallel technological improvements, there are still limitations of the security technologies to achieve usable and secure systems (Gillespie, 2001).

Firewalls

Firewalls do not offer perfect protection, as they may be vulnerable to so-called tunneling attacks, in which packets for a forbidden protocol are encapsulated inside packets for an authorized protocol, or to attacks involving internal collusion (Gillespie, 2001). One of the concerns with firewalls is that most firewalls pass traffic that appears to be Web pages and requests more and more, as it is the way to get things to work through the firewall. The solution is to re-implement the whole as Web services (Webmail being a good example). These pressures continually erode the effectiveness of firewalls (Ateniese et al., 2003). For example, the NHS Network in Britain is a private intranet intended for all health service users (family doctors, hospitals, and clinics — a total of 11,000 organizations employing about a million staff in total). Initially, this had a single firewall to the outside world. The designers thought this would be enough, as they expected most traffic to be local (as most of the previous data flows in the health service had been). What they did not anticipate was that as the Internet took off in the mid-1990s, 40% of traffic at every level became international. Doctors and nurses found it very convenient to consult medical reference sites, most of which were in America. Trying to squeeze all this traffic through a single orifice was unrealistic. Also, since almost all attacks on healthcare systems come from people who are already inside the system, it was unclear what this central firewall was ever likely to achieve (Ateniese et al., 2003).

Cryptography

The basis for many of the features desired for security in healthcare information systems depends on deploying cryptographic technologies. However, there are limitations to the use of cryptography. One problem is that security tools based on cryptography are still largely undeployed. One general weakness is poor usage of the system by individuals that includes: easily guessed passwords to the cryptographic system are chosen, or even written down on a sticker and stuck on the notebook, or people use the same password across different systems. The password then becomes as safe as the weakest system that is using it (which will often be something like a Web browser that has been told to remember the password) (Anderson, 2005; Gutmann, 2005). The other problem is that cryptography does not solve the security problem, that is, cryptography transforms the access problem into a key management problem, including authentication, digital signatures, information integrity management, session key exchange, rights management, and so on. It is observed that as the scope of key management services grows, trust in the integrity of key assignments tends to diminish, and the problems of revocation in the case of key compromise become much more difficult (Gillespie, 2001). Although public key infrastructure can help deal with the problem, it has also introduced complexities of its own. This has led to organizations effectively misusing cryptographic keys, as managing them appropriately has become too complex. The simplest example is that everyone in the organization really does get the same key.

Biometrics

The deployment of biometrics is proven to be advantageous to the healthcare providers because it provides added security, convenience, reduction in fraud, and increased accountability. It increases the level of security by providing access to health information to authorized individuals and locking out those with nefarious intent. However, there are drawbacks to the technology. For example, when performing an iris-scan, individuals must remain perfectly still during enrollment and presentation, or the system will not be able to scan the iris, therefore causing false non-matching and failure-to-enroll anomalies to occur. Reid (2004) further identified a few drawbacks to biometrics: hardware costs, user perception, placement, and size. For example, iris-scans require specialized cameras with their own unique light source that can be very expensive. The user perception on having infrared light shined into the eye is quite disconcerting. To get the iris in the proper position can be quite time consuming. Some cameras can use eye recognition techniques to try to auto-pan and focus the camera, but such solutions do increase the cost of the camera and may still require some user coordination. The current size of the camera, which has been reduced to that of a desktop camera on steroids, is still very large. It needs further reduction to be able to work efficiently on a desk.

Hardware and Software Costs

The costs of putting secure technologies in place can be tremendous. Very often the implementation of secured systems requires procurement of new software and hardware as the legacy system becomes obsolete. Unfortunately, there are not many commercial tools readily available in the market to integrate legacy systems into modern distributed computing environments. Furthermore, such integration will involve many database content inconsistencies that need to be overcome, including patient identifier systems, metadata standards, information types, and units of measurement.

Overall the lack of standards for security controls and for vendor products that interoperate between disparate systems will hinder the implementation and enforcement of effective security solutions.

Legislation

The importance of assuring the privacy and confidentiality of health information has always been acknowledged. However, up until recently the legal protection for personal information has been patchy and disorganized (ScreamingMedia, 1999).

U.S. Legislation

The healthcare industry is currently going through an overhaul to meet government-mandated regulations stemming from HIPAA to ensure patient confidentiality, privacy, and efficiency. HIPAA, which was passed in 1996 and effective in 2001, gives consumers the right to their medical records, to limit disclosure, and to add or amend their records. Providers must have complied by April 2003. Entities covered include health insurers, physicians, hospitals, pharmacists, and alternative practitioners such as acupuncturists.

HIPAA requires all healthcare providers, health insurers, and claims clearinghouses to develop and implement administrative, technical, and physical safeguards to ensure the security, integrity, and availability of individually identifiable electronic health data. Failure to comply with HIPAA can result in civil fines of up to $25,000 a year for each violation of a standard. Because HIPAA encompasses dozens of standards, the fines can add up quickly, and wrongful disclosure of health information carries a criminal fine of up to $250,000, 10 years imprisonment, or both (King et al., 2001).

N.Z. Legislation

In New Zealand, the Privacy Act, which came into force on July 1, 1993, provides a measure of legal protection for all personal information, including health information, and applies to the public and private sectors and to information held in both paper and electronic formats.

The Health Information Privacy Code 1994, which is consistent with the provisions of the Privacy Act 1993 (s.46), was issued by the Privacy Commissioner specifically to protect the privacy of personal health information. While the code protects personal health information relating to an identifiable individual, it does not apply to statistical or anonymous information that does not enable the identification of an individual.

The Medicines Act 1981 was issued by the Ministry of Health to penalize any unauthorized sale of prescription medicines, publication of advertisements containing insufficient information about precautions and side effects, and advertising the availability of new medicines before their approval for use in New Zealand. Under Section 20, the maximum penalty for an individual is up to six months imprisonment or a fine not exceeding $20,000. Sections 57 and 18 have a maximum penalty for an individual of three months imprisonment and a fine not exceeding $500.

The Privacy Commission also considered the application of the Privacy Act to the process of caching (Anderson, 2001). Caching occurs when a Web page accessed by users is temporarily stored by the user's computer (client caching) or by the network server that provides the user with Internet access (proxy caching). It also considered that the Privacy Act applied to the use of cookies within New Zealand and offered sufficient protection. It is proposed that using cookies for the purpose of collecting, holding, or giving access to personal information would be an offence unless the Web site indicated such information would be gathered. However, the Privacy Commissioner did not support the creation of such an offense.

European Union Data Protection Directive

International action may further affect the ways in which personal health information is transmitted over the Internet. The EU Data Protection Directive, which went into effect on October 25, 1998, requires EU member states to block outbound transmissions of data to countries that do not have laws providing a level of privacy protection similar to that in the country where the data originated (Siman, 1999). The directive affords the people to whom the data refer a host of rights, including the right to be notified of data collection practices, to access information collected about them, and to correct inaccuracies (Stevens, 1998). In 1998, New Zealand addressed three aspects of the Privacy Act to ensure it is adequate for the purposes of the EU directive. This is important for New Zealand businesses dealing in personal data originating from Europe because the directive limits the exportation of data to third countries (countries outside the EU) that do not have an adequate privacy protection (Wiles, 1998). The three aspects are:

- The channeling of data from Europe through New Zealand to unprotected data havens;
- Limits on who may exercise rights of access and correction under the Privacy Act; and
- The complaints process. "With a long queue of complaints awaiting investigation, the EU may have concerns that our complaints system is not sufficiently resourced to provide timely resolution of complaints."

In view of the above, the Privacy Commissioner addressed that the Privacy Act is built upon a desire that the collection, holding, use, and disclosure of personal information should be carefully considered and that all activities in this area should be as open as possible.

Future Trends

The growth of wireless computing in healthcare will take place for two reasons (The Independent Research Group, 2002):

- For all electronic medical record systems to work, physicians cannot be tied down to wired PC workstations. They will need to use some type of wireless device that allows them access to the relevant hospital databases.
- As the cost of healthcare continues to rise, many individuals are being treated on an outpatient basis. To keep track of an outpatient's vital statistics or signal when the patient needs immediate medical attention, many pervasive devices, such as toilet seats, scales, smart shirts, smart socks, and pacemakers, are being developed that collect relevant patient information. Collected data can then be transmitted via a wireless device using a wireless or mobile network to the patient's physician, who can then decide on possible interventions.

In the recent years, the technological advancements in sophisticated applications and interoperability has increased the popularity of wireless LAN (WLAN) and the use of wireless technology in healthcare. Also with the faster connection speeds of broadband LANs, the healthcare providers have developed a number of applications to improve patient safety and the healthcare delivery process. According to Kourey (2005), the use of personal digital assistants (PDAs) has become increasingly popular. It is because, "PDAs provide access to data and e-mail, store and retrieve personal and professional information and facilitate communication in wireless environments, their use among healthcare professionals has skyrocketed. Industry experts predict the trend to continue. In 2001, 26% of American physicians used handheld devices for tasks related to patient care. While some experts predict this number to reach 50% by 2005." Increasingly, clinicians can check on patient data or order treatments through secure wireless networks from anywhere in the hospital. For example (Hermann & Norine, 2004):

- A nurse is automatically notified on a handheld wireless device that a patient's blood pressure is falling.
- A doctor on rounds receives the results of an important blood test on a wireless PDA instead of having to call the lab for the information.

- A telemetry system records the vitals signs of dozens of patients in critical care and sends them wirelessly to a central control station for continuous, around-the-clock monitoring.

- A surgeon completing a procedure writes after-care orders while still in the operating room and transmits them to the clinical information system, making them instantly part of the patient's electronic record.

Rittinghouse and Ransome (2004) stress that employees who have not been properly educated about wireless security may not realize the dangers a wireless network can pose to an organization, given wireless computing is still a very new technology. They classify WLAN security attacks into two types:

- **Passive attacks:** An unauthorized party simply gains access to an asset and does not modify its content (i.e., eavesdropping). While an attacker is eavesdropping, he or she simply monitors network transmissions, evaluating packets for specific message content. For example, a person is listening to the transmissions between two workstations broadcast on an LAN or that he or she is running into transmissions that take place between a wireless handset and a base station.

- **Active attacks:** An unauthorized party makes deliberate modifications to messages, data streams, or files. It is possible to detect this type of attack, but it is often not preventable. Active attacks usually take one of four forms (or some combination of such):

  1. **Masquerading:** The attacker will successfully impersonate an authorized network user and gain that user's level of privileges.

  2. **Replay:** The attacker monitors transmissions (passive attack) and retransmits messages as if they were sent by a legitimate messages user.

  3. **Message modification:** It occurs when an attacker alters legitimate messages by deleting, adding, changing, or reordering the content of the message.

  4. **Denial-of-service (DoS):** It is a condition that occurs when the attacker prevents normal use of a network.

When patient information is sent wirelessly, additional security measures are advisable, although a well-defined wireless utility basically protects confidentiality and restricts where the signal travels (Hermann & Norine, 2004). Tabar (2000) suggests that the growth of new technology also creates a unique security threat and requires user authentication protocols. For example, PDAs, laptops, and even mobile carts can fall into unauthorized hands; the electronic ID must be stored elsewhere. Vendors are working on solutions such as: hardware ID tokens that are inserted into the mobile devices before use and radio transmitter-tracking devices. Other browser-based only applications on the mobile computing device are also used such that the patient data resides only on the server and cannot be accessed by the mobile computing device once it is outside the WLAN coverage area. Turisco and Case (2001) argue that while vendors are responsible for code sets, encryption, privacy, and audit trails, user organizations need to manage the device with extreme care or cautions. Physical security is of paramount concern in the wireless communications. The device needs to be turned off when not in use and be kept in a safe place. Tabar (2000) concurs that the greatest hurdle in information security still rests with the user, and no technology can make up for slack policies and procedures. "Changing perceptions, culture and behavior will be the biggest challenges," says Monica Summers, IS Director at Beaufort Memorial Hospital, Beaufort, S.C. "It's not just the technology. You could slap down $5 million in technology, and it won't stop people from giving out their password." (Tabar, 2000).

Conclusion

Privacy is not just about security measures, but is at least as much about what information is collected and collated and practically recoverable. Health information has always been regarded as highly sensitive, which must be protected by medical ethics and privacy legislations. The emergence of new technology and new organizational structures in the healthcare industry has opened up the means and the desire to collect and collate such information in ways never previously considered.

The increased use of the Internet and latest information technologies such as wireless computing are revolutionizing the healthcare industry by improving healthcare services, and perhaps most importantly, empowering individuals to understand and take charge of their own healthcare needs. Patients become involved and actively participate in the healthcare processes, such as diagnosis and treatment through secure electronic communication services. Patients can search healthcare information over the Internet and interact with physicians. This enhances and supports human rights in the delivery of healthcare. The same technologies have also heightened privacy awareness. Privacy concerns include: healthcare Web sites that do not practice the privacy policies they preach, computer break-ins, insider and hacker attacks, temporary and careless employees, virus attacks, human errors, system design faults, and social engineering. Other concerns are the collection, collation, and disclosure of health information. Healthcare providers and professionals must take into account the confidentiality and security of the information they collect and retain. They must also ensure that their privacy policies or secure technologies meet the public expectation and abide by the law. Such policies and technologies must also be implemented to ensure the confidentiality, availability, and integrity of the medical records. If this is not done, resources could be wasted in developing secure systems, which never reach fruition, and the new systems will never gain the confidence of the public or of the health professionals who are expected to use them.

Technology is, to a large extent, both the cause of and the solution to concerns about the protection of personal health information. However, there are limitations to the secure technologies that need on-going research and development. Technologies, if coupled with physical security control, employee education, and disaster recovery plans, will be more effective in securing healthcare privacy. Further advances of new information technologies, if designed and monitored carefully, will continue to benefit the healthcare industry. Yet patients must be assured that the use of such technologies does not come at the expense of their privacy.

References

Anderson, R. (1996, January 2). *Clinical system security: Interim guidelines.* Retrieved June 2005, from http://www.ftp.cl.cam.ac.uk/ftp/users/rja14/guidelines.txt

Anderson, R. (2001). *Security engineering: A guide to building dependable distributed systems.* Wiley. Retrieved June 2005, from http://www.ftp.cl.cam.ac.uk/ftp/users/rja14/c18_anderson.pdf

Andreson, R. (n.d.). *Why cryptosystems fail.* Retrieved June 2005, from http://www.cl.cam.ac.uk/users/rja14/

Ateniese, G., Curtmola, R., de Medeiros, B., & Davis, D. (2003, February 21). *Medical information privacy assurance: Cryptographic and system aspects.* Retrieved June 2005, from http://www.cs.jhu.edu/~ateniese/papers/scn.02.pdf

Ball, M., Weaver, C., & Kiel, J. (2004). *Healthcare information management systems: Cases, strategies, and solutions* (3rd ed.). New York: Springer-Verlag.

Carter, M. (2000). Integrated electronic health records and patient privacy: Possible benefits but real dangers. *MJA 2000, 172,* 28-30. Retrieved 2001, from http://www.mja.com.au/public/issues/172_01_030100/carter/carter.html

Choy, A., Hudson, Z., Pritts, J., & Goldman, J., (2002, April). *Exposed online: Why the new federal health privacy regulation doesn't offer much protection to Internet users* (Report of the Pew Internet & American Life Project). Retrieved June 2005, from http://www.pesinternetorg/pdfs/PIP_HPP_HealthPriv_report.pdf

Clarke, R. (1990). Paper presented to the Australian Medical Informatics Association, Pert. Australian National University. Retrieved 2001, from http://www.anu.edu.au/people/Rogger.Clarke/DV/PaperMedical.html

Committee on Enhancing the Internet for Health Applications: Technical requirements and implementation strategies. (1997). For the record: Protecting electronic health information. National Academy Press: Washington. Retrieved 2001, from http://bob.nap.edu/html/for/contents.html

Committee on Enhancing the Internet for Health Applications: Technical requirements and implementation strategies. (2000). Networking health: Prescriptions for the Internet. National Academy Press: Washington. Retrieved 2001, from htttp://www.nap.edu/books/0309068436/html

Constantinides, H., & Swenson, J. (2000). *Credibility and medical Web sites: A literature review.* Retrieved 2001, from http://www.isc.umn.edu/research/papers/medcred.pdf

CPRI toolkit: Managing information security in heath care. (n.d.). Target it architecture Vol. 6. Security architecture version 1. The Centers for Medicare & Medicaid Services (CMS) Information Security (previously Health Care Financing Administration). Retrieved June 2005, from http://www.cms.hhs.gov/it/security/docs/ITAv6.pdf

Cyber crime bleeds U.S. corporations, survey shows; financial losses from attacks climb for third year in a row. (2002, April 7). Retrieved June 2005, from http://www.gocsi.com/press/20020407.jhtml?_requestid=953064

DeadMan's handle and cryptography. (n.d.). Retrieved June 2005, from http://www.deadmanshandle.com/papers/DMHAndCryptology.pdf

E-commerce, privacy laws must mesh. (2001, February/April). *News from the Office of The Privacy Commissioner,* (39). Retrieved 2001, from http://www.privacy.org.nz/privword/pwtop.html

Fox, S. (n.d.). *Vital decisions.* Pew Internet & American Life Project. Retrieved June 2005, from http://www.pewinternet.org

Fox S., & Wilson R. (n.d.). *HIPAA regulations: Final. HIPAA Regs 2003.* Retrieved June 2005, from http://www.hipaadvisory.com/regs/

Gillespie, G. (2001). *CIOs strive to increase security while decreasing the 'obstacles' between users and data.* Retrieved 2001, from http://www.health datamanagement.com/html/current/CurrentIssueStory.cfm?PostID=9059

Gutmann, P. *Lessons learned in implementing and deploying crypto software.* Retrieved June 2005, from http://www.cs.auckland.ac.nz/~pgut001/

Health Insurance Portablity and Accountability Act of 1996. Public Law No. 104-191. Section 1173, USC 101. (1996).

Health privacy (About 1.4 million computer records for in-home supportive service breached). (2004, October 21). *California Healthline.* Retrieved June 2005, from http://www.californiahealthline.org/index.cfm?Action=dspItem&itemID=106520&ClassCD=CL141

Health Privacy Project: Medical privacy stories. (2003). Retrieved June 2005, from http:/www.healthprivacy.org/usr_doc/Storiesupd.pdf

Hermann, J., & Norine P. (2004). *Harnessing the power of wireless technology in healthcare.* Retrieved April 2005, from http://www.johnsoncontrols.com/cg-

iHealthbeat. (2001). Business and Finance: Survey. Retrieved June 2005, from http://www.ihealthbeat.org/members/basecontentwireless/pdfs/healthcare.pdf

Johnson, A. (2001). *The Camelot Avalon: Healthcare procrastinates on HIPAA.* Retrieved 2001, from http://www.camelot.com/newsletter.asp?PageID=326&SpageId=504

Kimmel, K., & Sensmeier, J. (2002). *A technological approach to enhancing patient safety* (White Paper). The Healthcare Information and Management Systems Society (HIMSS) (sponsored by Eclipsys Corporation). Retrieved June 2005, from http://www.eclipsys.com/About/IndustryIssues/HIMSS-TechApproach-to-PatientSafety-6-02-FORMATTED.pdf

King, C., Dalton, C., & Osmanoglu, T. (2001). *Security architecture: Design, deployment & operations.* USA: Osborne/McGraw Hill.

Kourey, T. (n.d.). *Handheld in healthcare part two: Understanding challenges, solutions and future trends.* Retrieved March 2005, from http://www.dell-4healthcare.com/offers/article_229.pdf

Medical Privacy Malpractice: Think before you reveal your medical history. (n.d.). Retrieved 2001, from http://www.perfectlyprivate.com/beware_medical.asp

Miller, M. (2003, September 8). Issues of privacy in Bryant case. *Los Angeles Times.*

Ministry of Health Press Release. (2001). *Conviction for Internet drugs warning to other.* Retrieved 2001, from http://www.http://www.moh.govt.nz/moh.nsf/aa6c02e6249e77359cc256e7f0005521d/5332afe9b6839587cc256ae800647e1b? OpenDocument

More prosecutions tipped for online drugs. (2001, October 19). Retrieved 2001, from http://www.stuff.co.nz/inl/index/0,1008,978172a1896,FF.html

New Zealand Health Information Service. (2001). *Health intranet: Health information standards.* Retrieved 2001, from http://www.nzhis.govt.nz/intranet/standards.html

Null, C. (2003, March 4). Google: Net hacker tool du jour. *Wired News.*

Paynter, J., & Chung, W. (2002, January). Privacy issues on the Internet. In *Proceedings of the Thirty-Fifth Hawaii International Conference on System Sciences (HICSS-35),* Hawaii, USA.

Reid, P. (2004). *Biometrics for network security.* New Jersey: Prentice Hall.

Rogers, R. D. (1998). *Information protection in healthcare: Knowledge at what price? We're drowning in information and starving for knowledge*. Retrieved 2001, from http://www.privacy.org.nz/media/aichelth.html

Rossman, R. (2001). *The Camelot Avalon: Despite HIPAA uncertainty, security must prevail*. Retrieved 2001, from http://www.camelot.com/newsletter.asp?Page ID=416&SpageID=504

Rottinghouse, J., & Ransome J. (2004). *Wireless operational security*. USA: Elsevier Digital Press.

ScreamingMedia, Business Wire. (1999). *SevenMountains Software and SCI Healthcare Group to deliver a secure virtual private networking solution to Hawaii Health Systems Corporation*. Retrieved 2001, from http://www.industry.java.sun.com/javanews/stories/story2/0,1072,18810,00.html

Sherman, D. (2002) *Stealing from the sick*. Retrieved May 21, 2002, from http://www.NBC6.net

Silverman, M. (2002). *Inside the minds: Privacy matters*. Retrieved June 2005, from http://www.duanemorris.com/articles/static/SilvermanBookExcerpt.pdf

Siman, A. J. (1999). *The Canada health infoway — Entering a new era in healthcare*. Retrieved 2001, from http://www.hc-sc.gc.ca/ohih-bsi/available/documents/ecompriv_e.html

Stevens, R. (1998). *Medical record databases. Just what you need?* Retrieved 2001, from http://www.privacy.org.nz/people/mrdrep.html

Starr, P. (1999). *Privacy & access to information: Striking the right balance in healthcare* (Health and the Right to Privacy, Justice Louis Brandeis Lecture). Massachusetts Health Data Consortium, Boston, USA. Retrieved 2001 and June 2005, from http://www.nchica.org/HIPAAResources/Samples1/privacylessons/P-101%20Massachusetts%20Health%20Data%20Consortium.htm

Tabar, P. (2000). Data security: Healthcare faces a tricky conundrum of confidentiality, data integrity and timeliness. *Healthcare Informatics*. Retrieved April 2005, from http://www.healthcare-informatics.com/issues/2000/02_00/cover.htm

The American Health Information Management Association and the Medical Transcription Industry Alliance. (1998). *AHIMA position statement: Privacy official*. Retrieved 2001, from http://www.ahima.org/infocenter/index.html

The Gallup Organisation. (2000). *Public attitudes towards medical privacy*. The Institute for Health Freedom. Retrieved June 2005, from http://www.forhealthfreedom.org/Gallupsurvey/

The Independent Research Group. (2002). SAFLINK Report. Retrieved 2001, from http://www.cohenresearch.com/reports/sflk_11-05-02.pdf

Thomson Corporation and health data management. Survey: Hospitals boosting data security. (n.d.). Retrieved June 2005, from http://www.healthdataman-agement.com/html/

Turisco, F., & Case J. (2001). *Wireless and mobile computing.* Retrieved April 2005, from http://www.chcf.org/documents/ihealth/WirelessAndMobileComputing.pdf

Wayner, P. (2002). *Disappearing cryptography. Information hiding: Steganography & watermarking* (2nd ed.). USA: Elsevier Science.

Wiles, A. (1998). *Integrated care and capitation: New challenges for information protection.* Retrieved 2001, from http://www.privacy.org.nz/shealthf.html

Wilson, P., Leitner, C., & Moussalli, A. (2004). *Mapping the potential of eHealth: Empowering the citizen through eHealth tools and services.* Retrieved June 2005, from http://www.cybertherapy.info/pages/e_health_2004.pdf

Chapter X

Compiling Medical Data into National Medical Databases:
Legitimate Practice or Data Protection Concern?

Boštjan Berčič, Institute for Economics, Law and Informatics, Ljubljana, Slovenia

Carlisle George, Middlesex University, UK

Abstract

In recent years, various national medical databases have been set up in the EU from disparate local databases and file systems. Medical records contain personal data and are as such protected by EU and member states' legislation. Medical data, in addition to being personal data, is also defined in the EU legislation as being especially sensitive and warrants special measures to protect it. It therefore follows that various legal issues and concerns arise in connection with these processes. Such issues relate to the merits of compiling a nationwide database, deciding on who has access to such a database, legitimate uses of medical data held, protection of medical data, and subject access rights amongst others. This chapter examines some of these issues and argues that such databases are inevitable due to technological change; however there are major legal and information security caveats that have to be addressed. Many of these caveats have not yet been resolved satisfactorily, hence making medical databases that already exist problematic.

Introduction

Medical data consists of information used in the provision of healthcare such as observations of patients (e.g., test results), medical histories, symptoms, prescriptions, and treatments. It is essential that such data are properly recorded and accessible in order to support the care of patients. Specifically, medical data can be used for various purposes such as to: create a historical record of a patient, provide a reference for future treatment, provide a communication mechanism among different medical professionals, anticipate future health problems, provide a legal record, and support clinical research (Shortliffe & Barnett, 2001).

The use of information technology in healthcare has created new possibilities including the digitisation of medical data (from passive paper-based patient records). An important consequence of this is the creation of the electronic health record (EHR), which can be defined as:

a longitudinal electronic record of patient health information generated by one or more encounters in any care delivery setting. Included in this information are patient demographics, progress notes, problems, medications, vital signs, past medical history, immunizations, laboratory data and radiology reports. (Healthcare Information and Management Systems Society, 2007)

EHRs are generally stored in a database system and their contents can vary according to the specific national legal framework under which they are regulated. They provide many advantages over traditional paper-based patient records leading to an improved quality of healthcare (by facilitating new methods of delivering healthcare and better data management). Some benefits of EHRs include: non-exclusive, continuous and multiple access to a patient's data; improved accuracy, reliability and integrity of data; standardised data record formats; ease of data access; ease of data integration; and stronger protections for confidentiality and security (Hunter, 2002).

Traditionally, EHRs have been stored in database systems that were locally developed, maintained and stored by organisations (such as hospitals, doctors' surgeries and other healthcare providers) in order to improve their quality of service. The advent of new information and communication technologies, improved networks and the need for new data processing capabilities (e.g., demographic healthcare studies) have resulted in the creation of (or attempt to create) national medical databases. For example in June 2002, the United Kingdom (UK) Government (Department of Health) published a National Strategic Programme for the use of information technology in the National Health Service (NHS). Amongst key elements outlined in the strategy was the delivery of core national services that can be used throughout the NHS such as an electronic health record service (having core data and reference links to local medical databases) accessible nationally for out of hours reference, (Department of Health, 2002).

A national medical database can be described as the aggregation of various disparate local medical registries/databases compiled at the national level. Such databases are characterised by their extensive coverage/storage of medical data, both in terms of their content (they integrate different medical databases) and geographic coverage (they integrate data from an entire country). They can lead to improved healthcare services coordinated (and planned) at a national level. Improvements are due to factors such as: the provision of medical information (e.g., for an emergency) any-time and anywhere, nationally standardised medical records generally leading to an improved quality of medical data, access to a large volume of medical data for clinical research, the ability to undergo epidemiology research, the central control of medical data, the ability to plan services for populations, and better management of scarce national medical resources (see Department of Health, 2003). The nature of national medical databases (compared to local databases), especially the fact that they are accessible nationally raises greater legal concerns regarding the protection (and potential unauthorised disclosure and use) of medical data. This is especially poignant for national medical databases created and maintained by non-governmental organisations (e.g., private medical companies).

In the UK, in order to address predicted future healthcare trends, a national medical database appears to be a necessity. In 2006 a royal society report on digital healthcare (Royal Society, 2006) identified various predicted changes (driven and enabled by technology) in the UK healthcare system in 10-15 years. These predicted changes included: an increase in patient-focused service giving patients more choice in how, where and when treatment is received; a change from hospital care to more primary and community care resulting in advantages such as decrease risk of infections in a large institution; the integration of healthcare with other services (e.g., social care) resulting in a multi-organisational service; and an increase in the number of healthcare service providers, including from the private sector. These changes will require the need for patients' medical data to be accessed anywhere, anytime and 'on-demand'. Further, medical data will need to be shared amongst healthcare workers both within and across (public and private sector) organisations. Such developments will essentially require a national medical database in order to coordinate and integrate medical information from various sources.

This chapter focuses on the phenomenon of national medical databases and some data protection concerns (including related legal issues of privacy and confidentiality) that arise from the creation and the operation of such databases. The chapter first briefly discusses examples of national medical databases in two European Union member states namely the United Kingdom (UK) and Slovenia. It then discusses aspects of the European Union (EU) Data Protection Directive 95/46/EC (the basis of EU Member States' data protection legislation) such as what constitutes personal data, data protection principles, obligations of data controllers, and rights of data subjects. Next, some legal concerns specific to national medical database are discussed with a view to suggesting possible solutions for addressing these concerns. The chapter finally concludes by looking at the balance between the benefits and risks associated with national medical databases.

The Cases of the UK and Slovenia

In the UK, under the 2002 National Strategic Programme for the use of information technology in the National Health Service (NHS), a national medical database is being set up (at the time of writing) that will store the information (medical records) of up to 50 million patients in England. These records will include demographic information (e.g., date of birth, name and address) and medical data (e.g., NHS number, allergies, adverse drug reactions, test results, medication, past or continuing treatment details), (NHS Factsheet, 2005). There is the potential in the future to include other categories of medical data such as genetic data, psychiatric records, and others. Implementation of this system began in 2007 through an "early adopter" programme involving general practitioner practices in four primary care trusts. "Early adopters" are required to create summary care records (SCR), which will form part of the care records service (national medical database) in England. The SCR is formed by the uploading of a patient's current medication, known allergies, and adverse reactions into a database.

There has been much debate over issues such as who will have access to such records, how will the privacy of patients be preserved, and how will the system be protected amongst others. Further there has been speculation about whether the designed system is fully compatible with internationally binding agreements (e.g., Council of Europe recommendation no R(97)5 on the protection of medical data, to which Britain is a signatory or the Declaration of Helsinki on ethical principles for medical research, Anderson, 2007). However, the UK Department of Health has proposed various practices for the implementation and operation of this new national healthcare system. These practices (discussed further on) have been approved by the UK Information Commissioner (who oversees the implementation of the Data Protection Act 1998) as being consistent with the requirements of the (Data Protection) Act (Information Commissioner's Office, 2007).

In Slovenia, around 50 different medical databases are interconnectable on the national level by reference to some unique identifier (mainly national identification number (NINo), but also social security number and healthcare card number) and held by a few governmental agencies (mainly by the national Institute for the Preservation of Health). The collection and processing of these data is regulated by the 2000 Healthcare Databases Act. At present, no single physically integrated (compiled) national medical database exists, but a variety of medical data on individuals is obtainable if data in the various databases (within departments and agencies) are combined/collated. If a physically integrated national medical database existed compiled data may be easily available to non-clinical personnel such as clerks, which raises concern. Most data compiled at the national level (from various databases) are in the identifiable/personal form, with some data anonymised (for example drug users, HIV positives, etc.). Data are collected mainly for research and statistical purposes, which would in theory allow anonymisation, however, some databases are used for other purposes and have to be in identifiable/personal form. A database of contractable diseases, for example (vaccinations, rabies), is used in the prevention of epidemics and pandemics and is usually retained in an identifiable/personal form in other to allow linking (with other databases). Two major data protection concerns are whether it would be better to have all data in an anonymised form (since such data is used mainly for statistics which only cares about aggregates) and how best to prevent misuse of data by unscrupulous employees who can sometimes easily link data from various databases with reference to the same unique identifier.

Personal Data and Data Protection Legislation

Directive 95/46/EC of the European Parliament and of the Council of 24 October 1995 (thereafter referred to as the Directive) sets out the legislative framework (variously implemented in the national legislation of EU member states e.g., the UK Data Protection Act 1998 and Slovenian Personal Data Protection Act 1999) for the protection of individuals with regard to the processing of personal data and on the free movement of such data. Article 2 of the Directive defines "personal data" as "*any information relating to an identified or identifiable natural person ('data subject') where an identifiable person is one who can be identified, directly or indirectly, in particular by reference to an identification number or to one or more factors specific to his physical, physiological, mental, economic, cultural or social identity.*" The means of identifying should not cause excessive costs, effort and should not take much time.

The given definition of personal data is very broad, so that when used, almost any information can qualify as personal data (the criteria are met if it applies to an identifiable individual, for example: the mere fact that an individual is wearing a blue shirt can constitute an item of personal data). On the other hand, this definition is semantically also rather vague. Even if we accept the fact that content-wise every item of information can be considered personal data provided it can be related to an individual, the directive's definition is still rather vague structurally (since it is not always clear what kind of internal structure every data record has to have to be considered personal data). In relational database theory, for example, a record structurally consists of two parts: (1) a unique identifier (primary key) of the record viz. entity under consideration and (2) one or several items of data related to it. The directive's definition does not define personal data in this way, hence it is not always clear, for example, whether a unique identifier of a person (such as national identification number referred to as NINo) already constitutes personal data, whether only items of data related to this unique identifier would be considered personal data (for example the fact that someone lives on Oxford Street) or whether only a record that meets both criteria, inclusion of the unique identifier and data related to it would be considered personal data (for example the NINo of a person plus the fact that this person lives on Oxford Street).

In the UK case of *Durant v Financial Services Authority (2003 EWCA Civ 1746)*, the Court of Appeal issued a landmark ruling narrowing the interpretation of what makes data 'personal' (within the meaning of personal data under the EU directive and UK Data Protection Act 1998). The Court ruled that personal data is information which:

is biographical in a significant sense; has to have the individual as its focus; and has to affect an individual's privacy whether in his personal family life, business or professional activity.

At the time of writing, this case is currently being appealed before the European Court of Human Rights citing a breach of Article Eight of the European Convention of Human Rights (i.e., the right to privacy).

The question of what constitutes personal data is not as trivial as it seems, since the Directive only applies to personal data, which is recorded as part of a filing system (Article 3(1)). Hence another very important question is the question of what constitutes a personal data filing system (which, following the directive's definition, is: "*any structured set of personal data which are accessible according to specific criteria, whether centralized, decentralized or dispersed on a functional or geographical basis.*"), and on this, cascading, another very important question, that of what constitutes processing of personal data (which, following the Directive's definition, is:

any operation or set of operations which is performed upon personal data, whether or not by automatic means, such as collection, recording, organization, storage, adaptation or alteration, retrieval, consultation, use, disclosure by transmission, dissemination or otherwise making available, alignment or combination, blocking, erasure or destruction.

This structurally rather imprecise and all inclusive definition of personal data in the end determines whether the Directive can be applied for a particular case involving collected data. In the context of national medical databases, data stored within them will certainly constitute personal data and as such will fall under the legal framework of member states' data protection legislation (implemented from the Directive), notwithstanding the differences in these implementations.

In any data processing context, there exists a data controller and one or more data processors. The Directive defines a "data controller" as a *"natural or legal person, public authority, agency or any other body which alone or jointly with others determines the purposes and means of the processing of personal data"* and a "data processor" as *"any other body which processes personal data on behalf of the controller."*

Article 6(1) of the Directive states five general principles relating to data quality, namely that data must be:

- Processed fairly and lawfully;
- Collected for specified, explicit and legitimate purposes and only processed for those purposes;
- Adequate, relevant and not excessive;
- Accurate and kept up to date;
- Kept in a form which permits identification of data subjects for no longer than is necessary for the purposes for which the data were collected or for which they are further processed.

Article 25 of the Directive also outlines an important principle related to the transfer of data to third countries—namely that member states shall provide that the transfer to a third country of personal data which are undergoing processing or are intended for processing after transfer, may take place only if the third country in question ensures an adequate level of protection.

Obligations of Data Controllers and Rights of Data Subjects

When is Processing Legitimate?

According to Article 7 of the directive, personal data may be processed only if

- The data subject has unambiguously given his consent; or
- Processing is necessary for the performance of a contract to which the data subject is party; or
- Processing is necessary for compliance with a legal obligation; or
- Processing is necessary in order to protect the vital interests of the data subject; or
- Processing is necessary for the performance of a task carried out in the public interest; or
- Processing is necessary for the purposes of the legitimate interests pursued by the controller (or authorised third parties) subject to the rights of data subjects to (e.g., privacy) under Article1 (1).

The processing of personal data on the local level (e.g., primary care, hospitals etc.) usually falls (has to fall) within one of these categories. In Slovenia, the 2000 Healthcare Databases Act governs compilation of various medical databases on the national level. In the absence of such special law there might be other legal titles by reference to which data compilation could be legal, for example, a contract between an individual and a data controller (e.g., a hospital) which would allow the data controller to process personal data because it is necessary for the performance of a contract. However, a contract between the data subject and the data controller at the local level does not automatically empower local data controllers to transfer data to the national level (e.g., national medical database). Another legal title according to which such transfer would be deemed legal is for example the case of transferring data to a national Centre for Disease Control and Prevention (i.e., performance of a task carried out in the public interest).

In the absence of other legal titles, data could be compiled at the national level on the basis of data subjects' consent. A data controller of a national medical database could, for example, obtain such consents (e.g., in written form) by turning directly to subjects whose data it obtained from a local level or with the collection of data from the data subjects themselves. Different countries regulate this differently. In Slovenia for example, personal data in the public sector may be processed only if the processing of personal data is provided for by statute. If no such statute exists, the public sector is not allowed to extract consent from data subjects to collect categories of data, whose collection was not foreseen by the law. This particular provision seeks to ensure that state administration and organs would not impinge on the privacy of its citizens by *ad hoc* collection of various categories of data and compilation of databases not foreseen by the legislator. However, different statutes may provide that certain personal data may be processed by the administration on the basis of the personal consent of the individual and in such cases, and only in such cases, can the state apparatus set about collecting data by consent. Other countries (such as the UK) do not have such provisions in their data protection legislation since the Directive does not specifically require it.

Medical Data as a Special Category of Data

Medical data (along with data revealing racial or ethnic origin, political opinions, religious or philosophical beliefs, trade-union membership, and the processing of data concerning sex life, but interestingly not financial data) is especially sensitive according to the Directive. It is forbidden to process it, except where (Article 8):

- The data subject has given his explicit consent,
- Processing is necessary for the purposes of carrying out the obligations and specific rights of the controller in the field of employment law,
- Processing is necessary to protect the vital interests of the data subject or of another person where the data subject is physically or legally incapable of giving his consent,
- The processing relates to data, which are manifestly made public by the data subject or is necessary for the establishment, exercise or defence of legal claims.

Information to be Given to Data Subject

The directive demands that when collecting data from a data subject (Article 10), (or obtaining from another source, which is not the data subject Article (11)(1)) the controller must provide the data subject with at least the following information related to the processing of his or her data:

- The identity of the controller,
- The purposes of the processing,

- The categories of data concerned,
- The recipients or categories of recipients,
- The existence of the right of access to and the right to rectify the data concerning him.

If a national medical database is compiled, data would probably not come directly from the data subjects themselves, but rather from the providers of primary health services such as clinics and hospitals (as is the case with "early adopters" in the UK) . Whenever such data is compiled on the national level, but no later than the time when the data are first disclosed to third parties, data subjects would have to be informed about it. The recipients of data would also have to be disclosed, which are not always obvious in advance and transfers to such recipients would always need to occur according to an explicit legal title.

This provision is often violated in practice as various data collectors do not present all of the information necessary to data subjects. Hence, the identities of data controllers are often not disclosed (the data controller's data processor is often enlisted instead, for example, a hospital carrying out clinical research instead of the company on whose behalf the research is carried out); some recipients of the data are not disclosed (in the above case, the ultimate recipient could be the national medical database where the data would eventually resurface); and the purposes of processing are sometimes too vaguely defined (such a broad, all encompassing purpose would for example be processing for the purposes of national healthcare, which is void of specific meaning).

Right of Access

According to the Directive, an individual whose data are being processed has the right (subject to some exceptions) to obtain from the controller (Article 12):

- Confirmation as to whether or not data relating to him are being processed and the recipients or categories of recipients to whom the data are disclosed,
- Communication to him of the data undergoing processing and of any available information as to their source,
- Appropriate rectification, erasure or blocking of data the processing of which does not comply with the provisions of this directive,
- Notification to third parties to whom the data have been disclosed of any rectification, erasure or blocking carried out unless this proves impossible or involves a disproportionate effort.

European member states have codified this article differently in their respective national legislation: some have prescribed a duty to notify data subjects of possible receivers of data relating to them, others go as far as prescribing compulsory recording of each data transfer for specified periods of time. In Slovenia, for example, every transfer of personal data to third parties (e.g., local authorities, police) has to be recorded and retained for some period of time (5 years) in case the subject exercises his right to obtain this information. This recording of transfers puts some burden on the data controller but there are signs that it effectively controls data paths and prevents the leaking of data. Each such transfer must be adducible from one of the titles cited in Article 7 of the Directive and this title must be sought prior to it and recorded alongside the receiver of data. Data controllers are less likely to pass on data if they must record such transfers and search for its justification in advance. In the case of creating a national medical database, local health service providers would have to check whether there is a legal instrument to authorise the transfer of such data to the national level (e.g., a statute mandating such transfer to a national medical database) and in the absence of such a legal instrument would have to deny any transfer request. Once at the national level, each transfer from the compiled national medical database should also be recorded to enable post screening of transactions.

Right to Object

Where processing is necessary for the performance of a task carried out in the public interest or for the purposes of the legitimate interests pursued by the controller (Article 7), a data subject has the right (under Article 15) to object (subject to compelling legitimate ground) to the processing of data related to him unless such processing is provided for by national legislation.

Automated Individual Decisions

Under Article 15 of the Directive, every person shall be granted the right not to be subject to a decision which produces legal effects concerning him or significantly affects him and which is based solely on automated processing of data. If data from a national medical database is used automatically, (e.g., if an insurance company makes an automated decision on an insurance claim, based on information accessed from a national medical database) then the rights of the data subject affected would have been violated.

Exemptions to Certain Obligations and Rights

The Directive (Article 13) provides that member states can restrict the scope of obligations and rights given in Articles 6(1), 10, 11(1), 12 (previously discussed) and 21 (relating to the publicising of processing operations) in order to safeguard: national security, defence, public security, the prevention, detection, investigation, and prosecution of crime, economic and financial interests, and the protection of data subjects or the rights and freedom of others.

Some Legal Issues

Allowability of Linking and the Scope of Utilisation of Nationally Compiled Data

Two important issues can be identified with the compilation of national medical databases. The first is allowability of such compilations *per se* (that is, the linking together of data from previously disparate databases), the other is (provided that the first is positively resolved) the scope of use of such compiled data. The first issue, the mere linking of different databases, is not specifically prohibited by the Directive, but the laws of some EU member states have put an effective ban on the linking itself. For example, in Slovenia it is forbidden to permanently link disparate databases in the public sector (Article 20, Slovenian Personal Data Protection Act 1999). The second issue must be resolved with regard to the Directive, which prohibits data to be used for any other purpose than for the one for which it was collected. This means that there must be a legal basis for the collection, compilation, and use of data on the national level. This special legal basis is usually legislation such as a medical database law.

Even in the absence of a linking prohibition, a national medical database can still only be built if it is governed by special law. If such law does not exist, it means that data can be linked or physically aggregated, but it can only be used in such a way as if the data were not linked.

We consider three possible solutions for these problems.

Tightly Controlled Use of Compiled Records

When national medical databases are compiled, the easiest way to store data is for the data controller to have data (records) kept in an identifiable/personal form. This obviates the need for costly and sometimes difficult anonymisation processes, it allows for the subsequent quality control of data sets, makes possible further research on raw data, and the addition of new data about individuals. However, tight access controls must then be implemented with permissions to access data for various profiles. Since data are being processed in their personal form, all duties with respect to such processing as set forth in the Directive's provision must be carried out (e.g., the notification of data subjects).

Anonymisation (De-Identification) of Compiled Data

One possible solution for databases holding national medical records used for research and statistical purposes is anonymisation (the viz. de-identification) of data. Anonymised data can be used freely. It does not fall under the scope of the Directive, since it is not deemed personal data. Anonymisation refers to the procedure in which unique identifiers of records are deleted, leaving data that are still individual but that cannot be traced back to any specific individual. Any personal data can be turned into non-personal data by removing unique identifiers. This can be achieved by various means, such as by decoupling data from explicit identifiers (e.g. name compared to an implicit e.g. ID number) and full identifiers (i.e. one that defines an individual uniquely) and then destroying any other identifiers (by removing appropriate parts of individual records which together amount to full identifiers in such a way, that no combination of remained data amounts to full identifier).

Where records are merely severed into two parts, one with identifiers and the other with data, which by itself does not refer to identifiable individuals (the so called key-coded data, Lowrance, 1997) this, is not enough for anonymisation. This is according to the EU Directive and member states data protection legislation standards, since all necessary data for full identification sill lie with the data controller in this case.

According to the UK Information Commissioner's Legal Guidance on The UK Data Protection Act 1998:

The Commissioner considers anonymisation of personal data difficult to achieve because the data controller may retain the original data set from which the personal identifiers have been stripped to create the "anonymised" data. The fact that the data controller is in possession of this data set which, if linked to the data which have been stripped of all personal identifiers, will enable a living individual to be identified, means that all the data, including the data stripped of personal identifiers, remain personal data in the hands of the data controller and cannot be said to have been anonymised. The fact that the data controller may have no intention of linking these two data sets is immaterial. (Information Commissioner, 2000)

The UK Information Commissioner's concerns are not without foundation because research has shown that data thought to be anonymised have been re-identified by linking or matching such data to other data. For example, Sweeney (2000) was able to re-identify anonymised data by directly linking/matching two data sources (medical data and voter list) on shared attributes (date of birth, zip code, sex). In her later work, Sweeny (2002) concluded that if release information (i.e., anonymised data) is altered to map onto as many people as possible then any linking will be ambiguous and therefore it is less likely that anonymised data can be re-identified.

Prohibition of Compilation (Linking)

The most radical solution is to ban the linking altogether, effectively outlawing any medical database with substantial data of various categories. What is banned, of course, is linking of personal data, which renders any personal data misuse impossible. It is still possible, however, to link (and use in any way) depersonalized personal data (e.g., for research).

Confidentiality and Protection of Records

Due to the fiduciary (trust) relationship that exists between a medical practitioner and a patient, the medical practitioner and associated employees are under a duty of confidence not to disclose medical data provided by a patient unless authorised to do so. This is duty is usually enshrined in law, such as the UK common law of confidence. The directive further enforces the law of confidence (and privacy legislation) by virtue of the first data principle which states that data must be processed (which includes disclosure) lawfully.

Authorisation to disclose medical data may be given by explicit consent from a patient or may be allowed under special circumstances prescribed by law. With regard to medical data, The directive (Article 8(3)) states that patient consent is not required where processing (e.g., disclosure) of medical data is needed for preventive medicine, making a diagnosis, and caring or treating patients, provided that the data is processed by a healthcare professional subject to professional secrecy rules under his/her national laws.

The confidentiality of medical records is of critical importance for both healthcare workers and data subjects. Disclosure of such data can lead to victimisation, humiliation, social exclusion and prejudicial treatment. Confidentially is particularly relevant to national medical databases because of the fact that medical data can be made available anywhere and anytime.

Various studies have shown that the confidentiality and security of medical data are amongst the biggest concerns that healthcare workers and patients have. For example, a study by Health Which? (2003) concluded that the only barrier to the UK public accepting integrated care records to enable the sharing of medical data (amongst medical personnel and patients) was the perception that electronic systems had security issues. Also Ndeti & George (2005) concluded that the main concerns for UK clinicians and patients regarding IT in primary healthcare were patient confidentiality and the security of electronic records.

The UK provides a good example of how the confidentiality of medical records in a database can be managed. In the NHS, confidentiality issues have been addressed by various measures such as the NHS Code of Practice on Confidentiality (Department of Health, 2003) and the Caldicott Principles (developed by the Caldicott Committee chaired by Dame Fiona Caldicott, see Department of Health, 2006). Both of these measures are consistent with the principles and provisions of the directive. The NHS Code of Practice of Confidentiality (Department of Health, 2003), applies to workers within or under contract to NHS organisations. It uses a confidentiality model with four main requirements namely: (i) protecting patient's information; (ii) informing patients about how their information is used; (iii) providing patients with a choice to decide on disclosure and use of information; and (iv) continually improving the preceding three requirements (protect, inform, choice). The Caldicott Principles were published in 1997 by the Caldicott Committee that was set up to review the transfer of patient-identifiable information between NHS organisations (in England) and non-NHS organisations. The six principles state that (i) the purpose(s) for using confidential information must be justified; (ii) confidential information must only be used when absolutely necessary; (iii) the minimum amount of confidential information required should be used; (iv) access to confidential information should be on a strict and need-to-know basis; (v) everyone must understand his or her responsibilities, and (vi) everyone must understand and comply with the law.

Also in the UK, with reference to the creation of Summary Care Records (SCR) which will eventually form part of the national medical database, the UK Department of Health has proposed specific practices to meet current legal obligations to ensure data protection and confidentiality. All patients are notified before uploading of their SCR and given the option: to decline one; limit the future scope of information in the SCR; or view the contents before uploading. The SCR, however will be uploaded without the explicit consent of the patient (but subject to notification and an opportunity to respond). After uploading, patients can remove any or all information uploaded to the SCR, and any subsequent additions to the SCR must be agreed between the patient and his/her doctor. Patients will also be able to limit the information, which can be made visible without their consent. A wide range of access controls have also been adopted. Only staff with a legitimate relationship with a patient will be able to access that patient's SCR. This includes medical staff acting in an emergency such as staff working in an accident and emergency department.

Securing an Audit Trail

In some countries, an audit trail of all operations with respect to the processing of personal data is required. Such operations include any operation or set of operations defined as processing under the Directive and includes collecting, acquisition, recording, organising, storing, adapting or altering, retrieving, consulting, using, disclosing by transmission, communicating, disseminating, or otherwise making available, aligning or linking, blocking, anonymising, erasing or destroying.

Retrieval, in particular, is included in the set of operations for which an audit trail must exist and this can be problematic as it may present a serious hindrance to system performance to monitor and record all retrievals. The hindrance to system performance can be both in terms of the size of space needed to store audit logs and the number of system cycles dedicated to monitoring. This is especially relevant to national medical databases due to their potentially large size.

The Slovenian Data Protection Act, in particular, requires that subsequent determination must be possible of when and by whom individual personal data were entered into a filing system, used or otherwise processed. The storage term for such logs is for the period covered by statutory protection of the rights of individuals due to the unauthorised supply or processing of personal data. In the Slovenian case, all civil claims for the violation of privacy have a statute of limitation of 5 years. The requirement to store log files of every operation for 5 years, with respect to the processing of personal data is an almost overwhelming duty, one that is usually skirted round by Slovenian companies. An audit trail is also sometimes required for a limited set of operations, such as for the transfer of data to third parties. According to the Slovenian Data Protection Act, data controllers are obliged to ensure that for each supply of personal data to third parties, it is subsequently possible to determine which personal data were supplied, to whom, when and on what basis. This is in respect of the period covered by the statutory protection of the rights of data subjects (i.e., 5 years).

In the UK, an audit is not mandatory for the retrieval of data from a database. However, with regard to the setting up of the new UK national medical database, part of the procedures for protecting medical data include that all access to an SCR will be via a smartcard and PIN, and is logged, providing an audit log. All patients will be able to receive a copy of the audit log giving details of access to their SCR. The NHS also guarantees that information in the SCR will not be shared with any organisation without the explicit consent of the patient. However, previous smartcards have proved cumbersome—especially since many share or borrow smartcards. It remains to be seen whether audits will capture any abuses and curtail them.

Conclusion

The technical feasibility of compiling a national medical database from disparate local medical databases and file systems, together with the potential benefits of using a national medical database, may inevitably result in the widespread compilation of such databases. Arguably a national database can improve the quality and scope of a nation's healthcare services. Some benefits include that it can: facilitate the provision of pervasive healthcare by enabling healthcare professionals to access medical data anytime, anywhere, and "on-demand"; facilitate information sharing across organisational and physical boundaries; provide demographic and epidemiological data for research and clinical purposes; facilitate the standardisation of medical records generally leading to improved data quality and integrity; and help in the management of national medical resources.

While national medical databases arguably facilitate an improvement in the access, availability and use of medical data, the potential concerns relating to data protection issues (including the privacy and confidentiality of medical information) remain. In order to address these concerns, there has been much progress in implementing security and access measures such as hardware and software controls, audit trails, and confidentiality policies amongst others. However, the nature of any networked digital infrastructure makes it prone to security breaches, as evidenced by past well publicised breaches of military and financial systems especially in the United States. Further, security breaches may not always be due to unauthorised access, since for example an unscrupulous employee with access to a national medical database may acquire and use medical data for various illegal purposes (such as to sell to private companies).

Compared to a local database, there is a greater risk of unauthorised access to a national medical database due to the fact that it can generally be accessed nationally at anytime, and by multiple users and organisations. Also there is a greater possibility for errors in medical data due to the volume of data handled. A recent UK survey of over 56 million patient records held by general practitioners(GPs) in England and Wales, found evidence for: duplicate registrations; inaccurate and incomplete data capture; errors in medical records; and incomplete transfer of information between systems (Audit Commission, 2006). It is quite possible that such problems (some due to human error and deliberate deception amongst other reasons) may be magnified in a national medical database. Further, the consequences of any illegal or negligent processing of data in a national medical database may have greater consequences for a data subject. This is because an incorrect or inaccurate medical record from a national database can be accessed by multiple healthcare professionals and providers to make decisions regarding a patient (data subject). Correcting errors and inaccuracies on a medical record that has been widely accessed may not always be easy, since incorrect/inaccurate copies of the medical record may exist (and be in use) in many different national organisations at a given time.

Invariably the decision regarding the creation and use of a national medical database will involve striking the right balance between the concerns about data protection (including privacy and confidentiality) of medical data, and the benefits (to the public) of sharing such data. Public health considerations and social objectives may heavily tip the balance towards data sharing. This will invariably lead to some erosion of individual privacy and confidentiality (protected in part by EU data protection legislation).

The possibility of larger scale compilations of identifiable medical data, such as a regional medical database (for example a European Union medical database) provides even more cause for concern with regard to data protection. This is particularly relevant in light of the EU Commission's stated aim (outlined in September 2006), to establish interoperability between member states' healthcare IT systems, and hence share patients' medical details between member states (EU Commission, 2006). Indeed in 2007 the EU began issuing calls for reseach proposals (via the Competitiveness and Innovation Framework Programme (CIP)) to investigate how best to achieve its interoperability objective. The concept of a regionally or globally accessible medical database is not new and already exists. For example, the US Armed Forces Health Longitudinal Technology Application (AHLTA) electronic health record system, services over 9 million worldwide patients (servicemen, veterans and their families) most with medical records online (Elenfield & Carraher, 2006) .

Given many healthcare research initiatives (e.g., EU Commission, 2006), in-depth studies (e.g., Audit Commission, 2006) together with high level policy decisions, it is inevitable that improvements in technology will continue to drive or enable healthcare change. However, it is important that the consequences of such change are carefully balanced with existing rights especially the rights of individuals in a society. Indeed, the creation of national medical databases in the EU, while beneficial (e.g., for epidemiological and demographic purposes) will continue to raise data protection concerns regarding and security and processing of patient data. Such concerns are well placed especially since (in light of the EU Commission's stated aims regarding interoperability) EU national medical databases may eventually be linked to a regional EU-wide healthcare infrastructure.

References

Anderson. (2007). *Security of medical information systems*. Retrieved from http://www.cl.cam.ac.uk/~rja14/#Med

Audit Commission (2006). *National duplicate registration initiative*. Health National report, August 2006. Retrieved from http://www.audit-commission.

gov.uk/Products/NATIONAL-REPORT/009F4715-3D93-4586-A3A0-7BF69405A449/NationalDuplicateRegistrationInitiative02Aug06REP.pdf

Department of Health. (2006). *The Caldicott Guardian Manual 2006*. Retrieved from http://www.connectingforhealth.nhs.uk/systemsandservices/infogov/policy/resources/new_gudance

Department of Health. (2003). *Confidentiality: NHS Code of Practice*. November 2003. Retrieved from http://www.dh.gov.uk/en/Publicationsandstatistics/Publications/PublicationsPolicyAndGuidance/DH_4069253

Department of Health. (2002). *Delivering 21st century IT Support for the NHS*. National Strategy Programme. Retrieved from http://www.dh.gov.uk/prod_consum_dh/groups/dh_digitalassets/@dh/@en/documents/digitalasset/dh_4071684.pdf

Elenfield, V., & Carraher, J. (2006). *Lessons learned in implementing a global electronic health record*. Hiss Annual Conference, February 14, 2006. Retrieved from http://www.himss.org/content/files/lessonslearned_imp_ehr.pdf

EU Commission. (2006). Connected health: Quality and safety for European citizens. Retrieved from http://ec.europa.eu/information_society/activities/health/docs/policy/connected-health_final-covers18092006.pdf

Healthcare Information and Management Systems Society. (2007). *EHR, Electronic Health Record*. Retrieved from http://www.himss.org/ASP/topics_ehr.asp

Health Which? (2003). *The public view on electronic health records, health which?* And NHS National Programme for Information Technology, 7 October 2003. Retrieved from http://www.dh.gov.uk/prod_consum_dh/groups/dh_digitalassets/@dh/@en/documents/digitalasset/dh_4055046.pdf

Hunter, K. (2002). Electronic health records. In S. Englebardt, & R. Nelson (Eds). *Health care informatics, an interdisciplinary approach* (pp. 209-230). Mosby.

Information Commissioner. (2000). *Data Protection Act 1998, Legal Guidance (p14)*. Retrieved from http://pkl.net/~matt/uni/ct218/other%20useful%20documents%20(not%20examinable)/Legal%20Guidance%20on%20DPA.doc

Information Commissioner's Office. (2007). *The information commissioner's view of NHS electronic care records*. Retrieved from http://www.ico.gov.uk/upload/documents/library/data_protection/introductory/information_commissioners_view_of_nhs_electronic_care_reco%E2%80%A6.pdf

Lowrance, W. (1997). Privacy and health research, A report to the U.S. Secretary of Health and Human Services. Retrieved from http://aspe.os.dhhs.gov/datacncl/phr.htm

Ndeti, M., & George, C. E. (2005). Pursuing electronic health: A UK primary health care perspective. In M. Funabashi & A. Grzech (Eds.), *Challenges of expanding Internet:* E-commerce, e-business, and e-government: Proceedings of the 5th IFIP Conference on *e-Commerce, e-Business, and e-Government (I3e'2005)*, October 28-30 2005, Poznan, Poland, USA: Springer

NHS Factsheet. (2005). *The spine.* Retrieved from http://www.connectingforhealth. nhs.uk/resources/comms_tkjune05/spine_factsheet.pdf

Royal Society. (2006). *Digital healthcare: The impact of information can communication technologies on health and healthcare.* Retrieved from http://www. royalsoc.ac.uk/displaypagedoc.asp?id=23835

Shortliffe, E. H., & Barnett, G. O. M. S. (2001). Medical data: Their acquisition, storage, and use. In E. H. Shortliffe & L. E. Perreault (Eds.), Medical informatics, computer applications in health care and biomedicine (pp. 41-75). Springer.

Sweeney, L. (2002). K-anonymity: A model for protecting privacy. *International Journal of Uncertainty, Fuzziness and Knowledge-based systems, 10*(5), 557-570.

Sweeney, L. (2000). Uniqueness of simple demographics in the U.S. Population. LIDAPWP4, Carnegie Mellon University, laboratory for International Data Privacy, Pittsburgh, PA.

Section VI

Emerging Technologies

Chapter XI

Biometrics, Human Body, and Medicine:
A Controversial History

Emilio Mordini, Centre for Science, Society and Citizenship, Rome, Italy

Abstract

Identity is important when it is weak. This apparent paradox is the core of the current debate on identity. Traditionally, verification of identity has been based upon authentication of attributed and biographical characteristics. After small scale societies and large scale, industrial societies, globalisation represents the third period of personal identification. The human body lies at the heart of all strategies for identity management. The tension between human body and personal identity is critical in the health care sector. The health care sector is second only to the financial sector in term of the number of biometric users. Many hospitals and healthcare organisations are in progress to deploy biometric security architecture. Secure identification is critical in the health care system, both to control logic access to centralized archives of digitized patients' data, and to limit physical access to buildings and hospital wards, and to authenticate medical and social support personnel. There is also an increasing need to identify patients with a high degree of certainty. Finally, there is the risk that biometric authentication devices can significantly reveal any health information. All these issues require a careful ethical and political scrutiny.

Introduction

No longer a science fiction solution, biometric technologies are the most important innovation in the IT industry for the next few years. Early biometric identification technology was considered extremely expensive. However, due to constant developments in computer technology and reduction in prices, along with improvements in accuracy, biometrics have begun to see widespread deployment. For example, a fingerprint scanner that cost $3,000 five years ago, with software included, and $500 two years ago, costs less than $50 today. As a result, biometric systems are being developed in many countries for such purposes as social security entitlement, payments, immigration control, and election management.

Broadly defined, biometrics[1] are just methods of observing and measuring relevant attributes of living individuals or populations to identify active properties or unique characteristics. Biometrics can look for patterns of change by measuring attributes over time or look for consistency by measuring attributes of identity or unique differentiation. When looking for patterns of change, biometrics can be considered a tool for research, diagnosis, or medical monitoring. When looking for consistency, biometrics become a useful vehicle for identifying and verifying identities, because they can differentiate individuals. However this distinction, though basic, should be considered partly theoretical. Most biometrics could be used both to differentiate individuals and to identify medical conditions. It depends on its architecture whether a system, designed for verifying consistency, can be turned into a system that looks for specific pattern of change over time. From a mere technical point of view this is often feasible.

Biometric system for measuring consistency (that is to differentiate individuals) can be used in two ways. The first is identification ("who is this person?") in which a subject's identity is determined by comparing a measured biometric against a database of stored records—a one-to-many comparison. The second is verification, also called authentication ("is this person who he claims to be?"), which involves a one-to-one comparison between a measured biometric and one known to come from a particular person. Also this distinction is partly theoretical because it is largely based on the potential of each technology for building large databases. As a matter of fact all biometrics can be used for verification, but different kinds of biometric vary in the extent to which they can be used for identification. Identification mode is also more challenging, time-consuming, and costly than the verification mode.

Biometric identifications systems consist of a reader or scanning device, a software that converts the scanned information into digital form (template), and, wherever the data is to be analyzed, a database that stores the biometric data for comparison with entered biometric data. The incredible variety of human forms and attributes might seem to reveal a large number of potential attributes for biometric identification. Good biometric identifiers, however, must be:

- **Universal:** The biometric element exists in all persons;
- **Unique:** The biometric element must be distinctive to each person;
- **Permanent:** The property of the biometric element remains permanent over time for each person.

Existing biometrical methods of identification include fingerprints, ultrasound fingerprinting, retinal and iris scans, hand geometry, facial feature recognition, ear shape, body odor, signature dynamics, voice verification, computer keystroke dynamics, skin patterns, and foot dynamics. Future biometrics will include DNA analysis, neural wave analysis, and skin luminescence. Multimodal systems, which match different methods, are the current trend and they are rapidly progressing. Multiple biometrics could consist of different types of biometrics, such as combining facial and iris recognition. Experimental results have demonstrated that the identities established by systems that use more than one biometric could be more reliable, be applicable to large target populations, and improve response time. Also behavioral biometrics—which measure behavioral characteristics such as signature, voice (which also has a physical component), keystroke pattern and gait—is expanding. Since authentication takes place instantaneously and usually only once, identity fraud is still possible. An attacker can bypass the biometrics authentication/identification system and continue undisturbed. A cracked or stolen biometric system presents a difficult problem. Unlike passwords or smart cards, which can be changed or reissued, absent serious medical intervention, a fingerprint or iris is forever. Once an attacker has successfully forged those characteristics, the end user must be excluded from the system entirely, raising the possibility of enormous security risks and/or reimplementation costs. Static physical characteristics can be digitally duplicated, for example, the face could be copied using a photograph, a voice print using a voice recording and the fingerprint using various forging methods. In addition static biometrics could be intolerant of changes in physiology such as daily voice changes or appearance changes. Physiological dynamic indicators could address these issues and enhance the reliability and robustness of biometric authentication systems when used in conjunction with the usual biometric techniques. The nature of these physiological features allows the continuous authentication of a person (in the controlled environment), thus presenting a greater challenge to the potential attacker. Systems for the continuous authentication of a person have been proposed to monitor airplane pilots and other people involved in critical functions (underground controllers, people attending in military restricted areas, etc).

Why Identity Matters

Biometric technology, as any other technology, implies some logic pre-assumptions. In particular, biometrics requires criteria for identifying individuals in different contexts, under different descriptions and at different times. In the course of modern history, personal identities have been based on highly diverse notions such as religion, rank, class, estate, gender, ethnicity, race, nationality, politics, virtue, honor, erudition, rationality, and civility (the list is not, of course, exhaustive). Individuals have been identified by legal names, location, token, pseudonyms, and so. Late modernity is characterized—as Giddens (1991) puts it—by a feeling of "ontological insecurity," that is a very basic sense of insecurity about one's personal identity and one's place in the world. The feeling of "ontological insecurity" corresponds to a weak, uncertain, definition of what makes a given individual that very individual. Individualisation becomes therefore an endless identity making process. It has been said indeed that the problem of the identity is typical of periods of transition and crisis (Hellenism, Late Antiquity, Baroque Period, Belle Époque). The argument would run convincingly but for the fact that any historical period could be described as a period "of crisis." However it is unquestionable that today we see signs of the interest for personal identity wherever we go. Arguments on personal identity have been raised by philosophers, social scientists and psychologists in relation with bioethics (e.g., alzheimer's disease and other dementing disorders; genetic engineering; brain manipulation), immigration and ethnicity (e.g., cultural identities, assimilation, integration), globalisation (e.g., cosmopolitism, global citizenship, re-tribalisation processes), young generations (e.g., crisis of identity, pseudo-identities, false identities), and body politics (e.g., transgenderism, cyber-identities, trans-humanism, cosmetic surgery, body arts).

Philosophers usually distinguish between the general issue of "identity" and the specific question of "personal identity." Logically speaking, the problem of identity is puzzling. As Wittgenstein put this question (*Tractatus Logico-Philosophicus, 5.5303*), to say of anything that is identical with itself is to say nothing at all, and to say that it is identical with anything else is nonsense. Actually, with the word "identity" we mean at least two different concepts, we may indicate an exact similarity between two items (qualitative identity) but we can also indicate that what is named twice should be counted once (numerical identity). When we state something about the identity of "A," we assert that, under that specific circumstance, "A" is identical to any other "A" sharing the same properties (e.g., when we state that the identity of an apple is being an apple, we actually state that an apple is identical with any other apple under this specific circumstance). But when we state that "A" is "A," we mean that there are not two different items but only one (e.g., when we state that this apple is the apple we purchased yesterday, we are actually saying that there is only one apple with two different descriptions).

The problem of "personal identity" is nothing but the way in which the logical issue of identity may concern also persons. "Personal identity" means that each individual is understood as having a coherent personality, which is identical in different spatial and temporal contexts (i.e., each individual is one, although he changes over time). The problem arises when we try to understand whether the subjective experience of personal identity corresponds to any real object or is just a useful figment. What properties identify a person as essentially the person she is? Theories of personal identity try to explain what the identity of a person necessarily consists in, what (if anything) survives through life's normal changes of experience.

The general problem of identity and the specific problem of personal identity do not admit easy solutions. Yet we need some criteria to establish identities, either in the sense of qualitative identities or in the sense of numerical identities. These criteria are our categories. In the space-time frame we live, physical items possess properties that are constant enough to allow us to build classes of beings with some commonalities. When we state something about the identity of anything, we actually include it into a class of items. The core of any identity statement is therefore categorisation[2]. This is evident in the case of qualitative identity but it is also true in the case of numerical identity. In the case of numerical identity, we try to enlist an item into the ultimate class that comprises only that specific item. The problem is that this class, which would by definition consist of only one element, does not exist, is merely fictional. Speaking of physical objects[3] we lack classes that distil the essence of an item, which is constant forever and never changes over time. As a consequence, identity statements are all probabilistic, though at different degrees.

Philosophers would argue that none of these questions is really new, yet what makes them new is their current political relevance. Defining the conditions for individual identification does not reduce to specifying conditions for identities of persons, for personal continuity or survival, or for other highly metaphysical questions. Defining the conditions for individual identification also means specifying the characteristics that distinguish or identify the actual identity of a person. In other words, it means to define the conditions for satisfying identity claims, the elements by which a person is distinguished by other persons, and she is re-identified or dis-identified. We are interested in someone being the same individual for many reasons. First, individuals are responsible for their actions and their commitments. Any kind of transactions and the whole legal and financial domains could not be even thinkable if there was no certainty about personal identity. Second, a descriptive scrutiny of personal identity affects the allocation of duties and rights. In times of social and political change obligations and rights are relocated, and the attribution of obligations and rights require the identification of individuals. Finally, the emergence of globalized orders means that the world we live "in" today is unifying the overall human community. Most criteria to establish personal identities in the past are not, or hardly applicable to the global community. Should we define new criteria? Such questions affect our existence in the concrete sense that they involve our life in a myriad of circumstances, from access to workplace, finances and medical records, till to our digital identities in the online world (Castells, 1997).

From Odysseus to the French Revolution

Traditionally, verification of identity has been based upon authentication of attributed and biographical characteristics. For centuries, in small-scale societies, physical and cultural appearance and location answered the "who is it?" question. We recognize individuals from their physical appearance, their body size and shape, their gait, their gestures and, above all, from their face and voice. Yet physical appearance has never been sufficient. The body gets older, faces change, voice can be altered. Time transforms physical appearance but it also leaves signs that is time "writes" persons by carving wrinkles and scars on the skin, and memories in the mind. Wrinkles, scars, and memories are biographical signs, which allow to recognize individuals beyond the mere appearance[4]. The reader of the Odyssey probably remembers the scene in which the nurse Eurycleia recognises Odysseus. We are in the book XIX of the Odyssey. After the long, enduring ten-year journey, Odysseus, disguised as a vagabond, is back on Ithaca. The queen Penelope welcomes the foreigner without recognizing him as her husband. She tells the vagabond of Odysseus who has been gone for twenty years. Odysseus is deeply touched by her story and has to strive hard with himself to not reveal his identity. After they are finished conversing, Penelope has Eurycleia, an old nurse of Odysseus, to clean the tired and worn feet of the beggar. As Eurycleia washes him, she notices an old scar on this leg and realizes that he is Odysseus. She is about to tell the queen when Ulysses sternly admonishes her to keep his identity for the time being. The next morning, Odysseus starts to keep watch of all the servants, trying to see who is still faithful to him. Eumaeus comes to the palace, driving the hogs for slaughter and demonstrates his goodness. Another servant arrives, Philoetius, the chief cowherd, who shows that he also is faithful to Odysseus. Odysseus then takes Eumaeus and Philoetius aside and identifies himself to them by showing the old scar that was recognized by Eurycleia. The reader should now notice the tension between the two events: in both cases, a body sign is used for identification purposes but in the first case it causes a recognition against the will of the hero, in the second case it certifies the (inconceivable) identity between the late king and the present beggar. In such a tension there is already the core of the present debate, that is the political tension between identification as an instrument for surveillance or empowerment.

With large-scale societies and the increased mobility associated with urbanisation and industrialisation, identity came to be determined by full name and reliance on proxy forms such as a passport, and national identity card. Beginning with the French Revolution in 1789 there has been both conceptually and historically an indivisible unity of citizenship and personal identification. The identity of persons becomes their identity of citizens. Modern societies are presumed to be sovereign social entities with a state at their centre, which organises the rights and duties of each member. The most relevant category of state member is "citizen." A citizen is a "native or naturalized person who owes allegiance to a government and is entitled to protection from it" (Merriam-Webster, 2006). The notion of citizenship embodies modern claims to liberty, equality, rights, autonomy, self-determination, individualism, and human agency. Citizenship may normally be gained by birth within a certain territory (*jus loci*), descent from a parent who is a citizen (*jus sanguinis*), or by naturalisation. There have always been many exclusions and exceptions, but largely, being a citizen is due to one of these reasons. The cornerstone of this system is the birth certificate. In August 4 1794, five years after the French Revolution, France enacted the first law in the West that fixed identity and citizenship to birth certificate. The birth certificate is basically an official document that proves the fact, the place and the date of birth and the parentage. In other words the birth certificate proves those elements that are vital to affirm that an individual is citizen of a nation-state. All other identity elements, which have been important in other historical periods, or which are still important in other cultures (e.g., religion, ethnicity, race, cast, etc), become immaterial. The original birth certificate is usually stored at a government record office, and one of the main tasks of modern states is to register birth certificates and to secure their authenticity.

Globalisation and Personal Identity

After small-scale societies and large scale, nation-state based, societies, globalisation represents the third period of personal identification. Globalisation involves weakening of the traditional concept of citizenship and personal identity based upon the notion of a bounded society, because, in its essence globalisation, is the removal of fix boundaries. Globalisation does not cancel borders, but it changes or redefines their nature. Boundaries could be of geography, culture, technology, politics and economy. Globalisation means a "liquid" world (as in Baumann's definition) of constant transit, an extended "borderland" where meanings, norms, and values are continuously created and negotiated. Globalisation is characterized by the development of technologies (fiber-optic cables, jet planes, audiovisual transmissions, digital TV, computer networks, the Internet, satellites, credit cards, faxes, electronic point-of-sale terminals, mobile phones, electronic stock exchanges, high speed trains, and virtual reality), which dramatically transcend national control and regulation, and thus also the traditional identification scheme. These technologies are organized in networks. An example is the network of hub airports, which structure the global flows of the 500 million or so international travelers each year. The flows consist of not just of the flows of people, but also of images, information, money, technologies, and waste that are moved within and especially across national borders and which individual societies are unable or unwilling to control. Technology networks tend to become organized at the global level and the global flows across societal borders makes it less easy for states to mobilize clearly separate and coherent nations in pursuit of societal goals. Moreover the globalized world is confronted with a huge mass of people with weak or absent identities. Most developing countries have weak and unreliable documents and the poorer in these countries don't have even those unreliable documents. In 2000 the UNICEF has calculated that 50 million babies (41% of births worldwide) were not registered and thus without any identity document. Pakistan, Bangladesh, Nepal have not yet made mandatory child registration at birth (UNICEF, 2006).

The development of automated systems for human identification is thus an outcome of globalisation. The tourist who wants to use the same credit card in any part of the globe, the asylum seeker who wants to access social benefits in the host country, the banker who moves in real time huge amount of money from one stock market to another, they all have the same need. They must prove their identities, they must be certain of others' identities. They can no longer rely on traditional means for proving identities such as birth certificates, passports, or ID cards, because of the very nature of globalisation. By providing global networks with the means to establish trusted electronic identities, identification technologies are both the consequence and the building block of globalisation. There is thus an inextricable link between the raise of technologies for human identification, the crisis of the nation-stat and new forms citizenship.

Personal Identification and the Body

As we have seen, the human body lies at the heart of all strategies for identity management, from Homer to globalisation. It is obvious because for most people a sense of personal identity includes an embodied component: when describing themselves they describe those aspects of their physical bodies, which can be easily codified: height, hair color, sex, eye color. People, and policy makers, naively believe that the body cannot lie about identity[5]. They believe that the perfect identifier is ultimately a body identifier. This is manifestly wrong not only because all body features can be spoofed but, still more seriously, because body properties are just coextensive with personal identity. One's personal identity does not necessarily coincide with one's body identity. Indeed the best way to cheat an automated system for human identification is to substitute personal identities without changing bodies. One does not need twins or clones to reach such a result, it is enough to change one's personality. No matter if they used drugs, brainwashing, blackmailing, or sex, spies have always preferred to change personalities to infiltrate the enemy rather than spoofing bodies.

The gap between personal identity and body identity is well illustrated by the difference between an actual human face and a passport photograph. It is difficult to imagine something more remote from an actual human face than a passport photograph "taken with a neutral expression," which leaves only a frozen expression whose concrete liveliness evaporates. Body requires mind—not in the trivial sense that you need a neurological system to animate the body, but in the profound sense that the very structure of our body is communicational. The human body is language and a fundamental means of communication. Body anatomy and physiology are shaped by human need to communicate. The body recognizes and receives communication directly from other bodies, allowing posture, gesture, and imagery to develop as alternative means of transmitting knowledge and feeling of various states of being. Body language is the essence of suggestive communication and has long been in use in several religious, ceremonial, and healing practices. We do not just need words. We are words made flesh. There is a complex hierarchy of body languages, from genetic formations, which are sometimes intrinsically correlated with an expressive quality, to scars (as we have seen in Odysseus' recognition), to involuntary physiological muscle contractions, till voluntary face expressions. Bodies are biographies and can be read as biographies. Not even a corpse is a real silent body; it still tells his past life to those who have ears to listen. The failure to appreciate the communicational value of the human body and its nature of complex symbolic network risks to be the main source of concern about biometrics. Issues such as gender, ethnicity, and physical disabilities are destined to become critical if those who deal with biometric technology do not realize that the body is not only a passport to be read (to use a fortunate metaphor) but it is rather a book full of allegories.

The relation between biometric technology and the human body does not only concern body symbolic dimension and body language. The human body has often been object of political control. In all societies the correct control of the body is part of the costume of a good citizen (let's think of athletics in ancient Greece, but also of the obsession for fitness in contemporary western societies: in both cases there are deep moral and civil implications in the demand for body control). All these elements are strictly interlaced with biometrics. In January of 2004, the Italian philosopher, Giorgio Agamben cancelled a trip to the United States, protesting the dictates of the U.S.-Visit policy—which requires a particular demographic of persons entering the U.S. to be photographed, fingerprinted, and registered in the U.S. biometric database prior to entry. Then Agamben (2004) wrote a brief essay explaining why he would not enter what he describes in *Means Without Ends* as a state of exception and martial law, a state where he asserts the means does not justify the ends. Agamben stated that biometrics was akin to the tattooing that the Nazis did during World War II. The tattooing of concentration camp victims was rationalized as "the most normal and economic" means of regulating large numbers of people. With this logic of utility applied during a similar state of exception in the United States today, the U.S.-Visit's bio-political tattooing enters a territory, which "could well be the precursor to what we will be asked to accept later as the normal identity registration of a good citizen in the state's gears and mechanisms." Agamben envisages the reduction to bare bodies for the whole humanity. For him a new bio-political relationship between citizens and the state is turning citizens into pure biological life and biometrics herald this new world. The theme of the shift between traditional account of citizenship and body-based citizenship is efficaciously described also by Nikolas Rose: "Citizenship was fundamentally national. Many events and forces are placing such a national form of citizenship in question. The nation can no longer be seen as really or ideally, a cultural or religious unity, with a single bounded national economy, and economic and political migration challenge the capacity of states to delimit citizens in terms of place of birth or lineage or race. [...] we use the term 'biological citizenship' descriptively, to encompass all those citizenship projects that have linked their conceptions of citizens to beliefs about the biological existence of human beings, as individuals, as families and lineages, as communities, as population and races, and as a species" (Rose & Novas, 2003).

Some other scholars (e.g., Aas, 2006; Nyers, 2004) have argued that identity technology is gradually becoming a major source of surveillance. The EURODAC system in Europe is often cited as a supporting argument (van der Ploeg, 1999). EURODAC consists of a Central Unit equipped with a computerized central database for comparing the fingerprints of asylum applicants and a system for electronic data transmission between Member States and the database. EURODAC enables Member States to identify asylum-seekers and persons who have crossed an external frontier of the Community in an irregular manner. By comparing fingerprints Member States can determine whether an asylum-seeker or a foreign national found illegally present within a Member State has previously claimed asylum in another Member State. People enrolled in the system are identified only by their biometrics (fingerprints): no name, no nationality, no profession, no ethnicity, nor any other data are collected but the place and date of the asylum application and a reference number. Eventually their identity will be their biometrics together with their entry in the EURODAC system. It is difficult to avoid thinking that we are actually facing a new outcast. Yet first impressions are often misleading. People in the EURODAC system are identified only by their biometrics chiefly for protecting them from being traced back in case they are political refugees. This leads us to the other side of the coin.

As we pointed out speaking of the myth of Odysseus, body signs and body identification have always had two opposite meanings. Body identification has been undoubtedly an instrument for dehumanizing people. Branding citizens has a long and sad history in Europe (Caplan, 2000). In late ancient regime France, for example, those sentenced to hard labor were marked on the upper arm with "TF" (for travaux forcés), with a life sentence being signified through the letter P (en perpétuité). UK offenders were sometimes branded on the thumb (with a "T" for theft, "F" for felon, or "M" for murder). In Primo Levi's memoir, *The Drowned and the Saved,* he describes the tattoo as a "pure offense," as a hallmark by which "slaves are branded and cattle sent to slaughter" (Levi, 1989, p. 119). Yet few know that in the Nazi regime the larger group of compulsory tattooed people was not made up by prisoners but the Waffen-SS. All members of the Waffen-SS were required to have a tattoo on their left arm verifying their blood group. This included also any of the high-ranking officers. Officially, the purpose of the tattoo was to be able to perform a blood transfusion at the front to save a wounded mans life. Yet the coincidence (the tattoo in gothic lettering was about 7 mm in length and was placed on the underside of the left arm, about 20 cm up from the elbow) is very suggestive: both *untermensche* and *ubermenschen* were hallmarked. Body signs, such tattoos, scars, piercing, are also instruments to establish power relations and to affirm identities. One could not understand the upsurge in hitherto "primitive" body modification practices among modern people if one does not appreciate that body signs provide important "social cues" between people. In traditional societies, ritual body modification practices connect people and their bodies to the reproduction of social positions. The rise of body modifications in contemporary, post industrial, societies (tattoos, piercing, ritual cicatrisation, etc.) undoubtedly serves the function of individuating the self from society (Giddens, 1991), but it is also an attempt to retain some form of power in an increasingly complex world (Shilling, 1998).

This leads us to the other side of the coin, identification technologies are also a critical instrument for protecting and empowering people. In a world system where nearly all States in developing countries are not able to provide their citizens with reliable identity documents, biometrics is likely to be the sole hope for most third world inhabitants to have trustworthy identity documents. This is critical for many reasons, not the least because identity documents are essential to ensure respect for fundamental rights. You are who your papers say you are. Take away those papers and you have no identity. Human rights are unthinkable without "identifiable people." One can be entitled with rights only if he has an identity. No political, civil, and social right can be enforced on anonymous crowds. Even the right to anonymity can be enforced only if one has an identity to hide. In the ancient Greece, slaves were called "faceless" *aprosopon.* The word that in Greek designates the face, *prosopon,* it is also at the origin of the Latin word *persona,* person. The person is thus an individual with a face. Biometrics and other identification technologies can give a face to faceless people, this is to say, out of metaphor, they can turn anonymous, dispersed, people into citizens bestowed with duties and rights. This should never be overlooked in any discussion on ethical issues raised by biometrics.

Biometrics and Medicine

We have till now described some elements of the tension between human body, biometric technology and personal identity. Such a tension is critical in the health care sector. Medical issues in biometrics are usually categorized under two main headings[6]:

1. The potential risk for health arising from the use of biometrics, known as direct medical implication (DMI)
2. The potential ethical risk arising from the violation of medical information, known as indirect medical implication (IMI)

We shall not strictly follow such a classification, which is hardly helpful. Indeed current biometric techniques, although they may imply a certain degree of invasiveness for the subject, do not present any specific health risk. The fear of contamination by contact or of injuries by radiation is totally unjustified and requires educational campaigns rather than ethical awareness. On the contrary the potential for ethical risk due to violation of medical information is complex and requires an in depth discussion and a more articulated classification. Finally, we shall hint at an interesting psychological effect that can also have some ethical implications.

The health care sector is second only to the financial sector in term of the number of biometric users[7]. This is chiefly a consequence of health care system transitions from paper-based to electronic, due to the recent availability of a standard for the exchange of diagnostic images (Dicom) and the significant decrease of data storage costs. Digitisation of patient records improves health care, reduces fraud, reduces medical errors, and saves lives. But digitized information is subject to a new category of risk, as it is illustrated by the recent case occurred in the U.S. Veteran Administration (VA). In May 2006, a UNISYS data analyst working in VA took home electronic data that was stored on a laptop computer and external hard drive. He was not authorized to take this data home. The employee's home was burglarized and the computer equipment was stolen. The electronic data stored on this computer included identifying information for 26.5 million individuals of veterans, including 1.1 million military members on active duty. The data included individual's name, date of birth, and social security number. In some cases, spousal information were included. The stolen equipment has been then recovered and the Federal Bureau of Investigation (FBI) has determined that information stored was not accessed or compromised (U.S. Dept. for Veteran Affairs, 2006). This story—though its (likely) happy end—can be taken as a serious warning about what can happen with digitized medical data when they are not effectively protected. Of course biometrics cannot prevent a lap top to be stolen but they could probably prevent any unauthorized access to stored data even if they have been stolen.

Many hospitals and healthcare organisations are in progress to deploy biometric security architecture. For instance the Copenhagen Hospital Corporation – a public organisation of seven hospitals, with 4500 beds and 20000 employees, which provides 20% of Danish hospital services - has recently entered into an agreement with Danish Biometrics for testing, research and development on biometric recognition based on 4 biometrics: fingerprint (match-on-card), fingerprint (smart card with integrated finger scanner + OTP + PKI), iris scanner, and voice recognition. The objective of the agreement is to result in solutions for secure log-on procedures when doctors and nurses for instance are entering the electronic patient records (EPR) as part of their daily routines. High security needs (tracking) and privacy rules are required as EPR contains information about health, which is regarded as sensitive personal data. At the same time, hospital staff must have quick and effective access to the case record and the patient data, which are needed due to the treatment. Biometrics is an approach to solve both challenges at the same time. An operation, which can be performed within 1-2 seconds with the use of a single finger touch, iris scanning or maybe another biometric option, would provide an advantage for the staff. Simultaneously the process ensures access to the right person as the biometric identifier is unique between individual. In the future a biometric log-on system could be extended to other parts of the health care system (e.g., homecare service, general practitioners, pharmacies, and last not least in relation to each individual patient for the use of a multi-service smart card with the biometric data of each individual stored in the microchip).

Biometrics for Medical Data Protection

Secure identification is critical in the health care system, both to control logic access to centralized archives of digitized patients' data, and to limit physical access to buildings and hospital wards, and to authenticate medical and social support personnel. Secure identification is also requested to control physical and logic access to medical banks (genetic, organ, tissue, cell banks) and to protect communication between healthcare services and global health networks (e.g., for organ exchange, in international drug trials, etc.).

Biometrics to limit physical access to medical facilities and to authenticate medical and social support personnel are likely to have vast applications. Given the sensitive nature of medical data, there are little doubts that there is a just proportionality between use of biometrics and purposes of the scheme. Obviously biometric data of medical and support personnel should be adequately protected and respect for the rights of the data subjects should be ensured. In case biometrics data should be transferred abroad (e.g., international medical research) clear rules should be defined in advance. Some difficulties arise from the inclusion of so called "emergency modes" that will allow the availability of medical data to non-enrolled medical personnel in case of emergency (with associated legal issues).

Secure identification is also vital for controlling logic access to databanks and centralized patients' archives. Unauthorized access to digitized medical data (patients' archives, biological banks, results of clinical trials, etc.) is a serious crime underresearched and under-documented. It is essentially performed for three reasons:

1. To investigate illicitly one or more archives;
2. To manipulate, destroy or to alter data surreptitiously;
3. To steal medical identities.

Illegal search on medical archives and data manipulation are well known information crimes that are performed for specific and limited reasons (e.g., to manipulate results of a clinical trials, to obtain covertly medical information on one or more individuals, etc.). Stealing medical identities is on the contrary quite a new crime. All levels of the medical system may be involved in medical identity theft: doctors, clinics, billing specialists, nurses, and other members of the medical profession. The essence of this crime is the use of a medical identity by a criminal, and the lack of knowledge by the victim. Medical identities are readily found in medical files and insurance records. "Medical identity theft occurs when someone uses a person's name and sometimes other parts of their identity—such as insurance information—without the person's knowledge or consent to obtain medical services or goods, or uses the person's identity information to make false claims for medical services or goods. Medical identity theft frequently results in erroneous entries being put into existing medical records, and can involve the creation of fictitious medical records in the victim's name" (The World Privacy Forum, 2006).

Medical identity theft is usually performed with the aim to fraud health insurances or the public health system. In USA, there is a long and well-substantiated history of criminals using lists of patient names in medical identity theft operations. The USA Federal Trade Commission has recorded that a total of 19.428 individuals have filed complaints specifically concerning medical identity theft at the Federal Trade Commission from January 1, 1992 to April 12, 2006. Medical identity theft is a crime that can cause great harm to its victims. It is also the most difficult to fix after the fact, because victims have limited rights and recourses. Medical identity theft typically leaves a trail of falsified information in medical records that can plague victims' medical and financial lives for years. Medical identity theft may also harm its victims by creating false entries in their health records at hospitals, doctors' offices, pharmacies, and insurance companies. Sometimes the changes are put in files intentionally; sometimes the changes are secondary consequences of the theft. Victims of medical identity theft may receive the wrong medical treatment, find their health insurance exhausted, and could become uninsurable for both life and health insurance coverage. They may fail physical exams for employment due to the presence of diseases in their health record that do not belong to them.

Identity theft is also a menace in Europe, though less frequent and costly. This is because of various reasons. First, the European Data Protection Directive, implemented in 1996, gives people the right to access their information, change inaccuracies, and deny permission for it to be shared. Moreover, it places the cost of mistakes on the companies that collect the data, not on individuals. Then, in Europe companies are not allowed to create or sell databases of people's former addresses and phone numbers. Such databases in the U.S. are often used to contact neighbors or relatives of people who owe debts in an attempt to find out current data on a debtor. Finally most Europeans—with the exception of UK citizens—have national identity cards. It is thus much more difficult to steal identity of European citizens for the simple reason that the key piece of information an identity thief needs is a person's national ID number, and that appears in a lot fewer places than social security numbers do in the U.S.

Biometrics can protect medical archives and, above all, may substitute traditional identifiers, such as Social Security numbers, making more difficult—if not impossible—to steal medical identities. It necessarily means to shift to a biometric scheme for patients' identification. This implies some issues that we are going to discuss in the next chapter.

Biometrics for Patients' Identification

The need to identify patients with a high degree of certainty comes from three basic requirements:

1. Reducing medical errors
2. Reducing risks of fraud
3. Improving capacity to react to medical emergencies

A substantial body of evidence points to medical errors as a relevant cause of death and injury. Studies in different countries estimate that around 10-16% of hospitalized patients experience an adverse event related to clinical care, with a mortality rate in these patients of 5-8%. In the U.S., medical errors cause up to 98,000 deaths and 770,000 adverse effects annually, representing the eighth leading cause of morbidity in the United States, exceeding that of motor vehicles, breast cancer, or AIDS [8]. A recent Eurobarometer survey on the perception of medical errors by Europeans

[9] reveals that almost 4 in 5 EU citizens (78%) classify medical errors as an important problem in their country. Two of the major causes of medical errors are patient misidentification and (wrong) medication administration. Accurate means of identifying patients and staff are therefore a crucial step to reducing medical errors. The combination of various identification technologies might virtually eliminate cases of mistaken identity. For instance, biometrics and RFID (radio frequency identification) are used in combination to identify and track special categories of patients in hospitals, such elderly suffering from dementing disorders, infants, comatose patients, and other categories of patients unable to identify themselves. Pilots are in progress in Italy, Spain, and the Netherlands. There are however a number of ethical problems which are not yet resolved. The most important is likely to be the principle of non-discrimination. For systems to be truly non-discriminatory, it is important that developers and operators consider the needs of those who will experience difficulties—and at the earliest stage of the design cycle. Systems should be designed so that as many people as possible can use them effectively with the minimum of discomfort. Particular attention should be also paid to avoid any discrimination against ageing, given that some biometrics (e.g., fingerprints) can become less readable with age. Problems may arise from patients who cannot provide, permanently or temporarily, the requisite biometric characteristic. In order to reduce risks of discrimination, the biometric system should have been designed so as to minimize the number of failures: false matches, false non-matches, and failures to enroll. The system should have been also tested—preferably by an independent third party—to validate the claims of reliability and security. A second reason for ethical concern regards the concept of "voluntarism" in providing the biometric characteristics. Not only it is highly arguable that hospitalized patients are ever in the real condition to give a free consent, but there is also the issue of patients who suffer from mental disabilities and who are less able to voluntarily consent. It is therefore important to offer patients the choice of biometric and to offer an alternative to disabled who can't use system or who cannot properly process information and voluntarily consent. Respect the patients' privacy is foremost and details of permanent or temporarily disabilities should not be stored without consent. Generally speaking the first requirement should be to avoid identification schemes and to prefer authentication schemes with template-on-card[8].

In Western economies, health care fraud accounts for an estimated 3 to 10% of all health care costs, or 80 to 120 billion dollars of loss per year. Accurate identification and verification of identity is important also to reduce frauds due to medical identity theft (see above) and due to duplication of identities, which is a fraud that involves the collection of more benefits than one is entitled to, by entering the program under two or more identities. Departments in charge of social and health assistance in countries like Spain and the Netherlands are already launching programs for detecting and preventing duplicate benefits. Wide consensus appears to exist concerning the high levels of this type of fraud, and heighten the urgency for establishing new identification practices. The introduction of identity technologies would result in billions of savings on public spending. Unauthorized use of assistance programs (e.g., heroin addicts who participate in methadone maintenance plans) could be tackled by using automatic systems for identification (both to authenticate people and to track medications, for instance by using RFID or other electronic tags). In addition, people are accessing more and more health services over the Web; for this to be secure, establishing people's identity is essential. However, some doubts still remain whether the use of biometrics is proportionate to the purpose of reducing medical frauds and benefit duplication. Proportionality principle requires that the use of biometric is justified in the context of the application, and that no other means of authentication may fulfill equally well the requirements without the need for biometrics. Failure to respect the principle of proportionality exposes users to improper use and increases the potential for function creep[9].

Biometrics have also been used to identify patients in emergencies, where for various reasons, many patients arrive without sufficient documentation to establish their identities. The main emergencies include natural disasters, technological disasters, major transportation accidents, and acts of terrorism including weapons of mass destruction events. Biometric has been recently also used to identify victims, casualties and dispersed persons in natural disasters, such as Tsunami. In emergency, rapid medical diagnosis and treatment is paramount. Casualty location is a continuing problem during natural disasters and other large health emergencies. In emergencies, patients should be properly identified as they arrive for treatment, or before dispensing medicine to them. Incorporating biometrics and biomedical data into a single, portable sensor may provide positive identification of casualties and increase the odds of fast, reliable treatment. The issue of accessibility is however vital. In emergency wards one should always consider the possibility that patients may not be able to be enrolled because of pain, injuries, vast burns, and so on. The risk that any emergence treatment should be delayed because of a failure to enroll a patient in an identification scheme should be excluded a priori. It has also been proposed to provide people with identity and entitlement cards, which could hold—with the consent of the card holder—a limited amount of medical information for use in an emergency (for example, current medication or allergies). This is a huge political, social, and ethical challenge because the application of data protection principles in emergency is complex. First it is not so ethically obvious what sort of emergency medical information would be most useful to display and whether medical information should be coupled with different information such as, for instance, the will to act as an organ donor, as it has been proposed. Second, it is arguable that in emergency it would be ever possible to obtain an informed consent to the processing of biometric data. Third, there are some puzzling issues such as how one can ensure effective fallback procedures if biometric system fails or what legal provisions are necessary for multi-national use of biometric data in international health emergencies like, for instance, natural disasters.

Biometrics and Disclosure of Medical Data

There is currently no evidence that any biometric authentication device can significantly reveal any health information. It is true that injuries or changes in health can prevent recognition, but the technologies have no capability of determining the causes of the recognition failure. There can be medical systems that capture similar images to biometric systems, but they use the information for diagnosis of disease and not identification. Yet it indisputable that most biometric techniques may potentially reveal also medical information. Although most technicians deny this possibility, biometric data can be used to covertly reveal users' state of health because of the very nature of biometrics. Measuring body features to search for consistency over time (as we have initially defined biometrics for identification/verification purposes) is not radically different from measuring to look for patterns of change (as medical biometric do). Biometric images (e.g., face, fingerprint, eye images etc., or voice signals) acquired by the system may show features that can reveal health information. For several reason it can happen that the operator keeps the original images, or is other cases, some information may remain in the template (e.g., if a template stores a compressed version of the image). Certain chromosomal disorders—such as Down's syndrome, Turner's syndrome, and Klinefelter's syndrome—are known to be associated with characteristic fingerprint patterns in a person. Knowing that certain medical disorders are associated with specific biometric patterns, researchers might actively investigate such questions as whether biometric patterns can be linked to behavioral characteristics, or predispositions to medical conditions. Moreover, by comparing selected biometric data captured during initial enrolment and subsequent entries with the current data, biometric technologies may detect several medical conditions. Also future and likely use of genetic test information and DNA profiles in biometrics bears many ethical risks.

Finally a potential weak point of any biometric scheme is represented by liveness checks. Liveness checks are technological countermeasure to spoofing using artefacts. They apply most obviously to biological biometrics such as finger, face, hand and iris, though they might also protect behavioural biometrics in cases where mimicry might be performed by an artificial device (e.g., a signature signing machine). Biometric identification could be fooled by a latex finger, a prosthetic eye, a plaster hand, or a DAT voice recording. Biometric devices must therefore be able to determine whether there is a live characteristic being presented. Liveness checks may detect physical properties of the live biometric (e.g., electrical measurement, thermal measurement, moisture, reflection or absorbance of light or other radiation); the presence of a natural spontaneous signal such as pulse; or the response to an external stimulus (e.g., contraction of the pupil in response to light, muscular contraction in response to electrical signal etc.). By detecting physical reactions, liveness checks may be an important source of medical information (e.g., pupillary responses depend on whether one has been drinking or taking drugs, whether the person is pregnant, and with the variability of age in general; changes in blood flow are typically associated with several medical conditions as well as with emotional responses, etc.). There are also ways in which one might be able to sense the emotional attitudes from some biometrics (e.g., nervousness in a voice pattern and anger from a facial image). There has been some exploratory work in this area and various companies worldwide are currently trying to develop biometric systems provided with behavior-recognition techniques, which are capable to recognize patterns for people with hostile agendas[10]. Also the possibility of continuous authentication of a person (in the controlled environment)—that we mentioned at the beginning of this chapter—can obviously be a source of medical information.

The potential for function creep gives rise to the question of whether there may need to be additional legislative or other measures to address the threats biometrics may pose as a unique identifier in the health sector. This is essentially a question for policy makers and deserves to be discussed at policymaking level.

Technoanimism

One of the most astonishing effects expected from biometric technologies is the creation of a new category of smart objects and environments, with the capacity for recognising human beings. This promises to be relevant to ambient assisted living for elderly and dementing persons, to smart homes and smart workplaces for disable people and other categories of disadvantaged citizens. Yet this is not without any consequence. Human beings show the tendency to regard inanimate objects as living and conscious (animism) and to ascribe them also human characteristics (anthropomorphism). Both tendencies are spontaneous and pervasive in early childhood. Child psychologist Piaget found that the youngest children see virtually all phenomena simultaneously as alive, conscious, and made by humans for human purposes (Piaget, 1962). Tylor (1871) defined animism as a belief that animals, plants and inanimate objects all had souls. For Tylor, animism represented "stone age religion," which still survived among some of the "ruder tribes." In his turn, Piaget believed that animism and anthropomorphism slowly diminish through childhood and, by early adolescence, children's views approximate those of adults. Yet they were probably wrong. In his *Le Dieu Object*, Marc Augé (1988) suggested that all people—also adults, "civilised" people—attribute human shape and qualities (such as agency) to the widest range of objects and phenomena imaginable. In the past few years, several authors, including Guthrie (1993), Bird-David (1999), Ingold (2000), and Harvey (2005) have argued that—rather than a "primitive," "childish" superstition—animism could be understood as alternative responses to universal semiotic anxieties about where or how to draw boundaries between persons and things. These very boundaries are now threatened by info and biometric technologies. Animism is a feeling/belief that things have the ability to recognise humans, observe, gather knowledge, and perform actions in the real world. This is actually what smart technological objects, empowered with biometric sensors, promise to do. In their 1996 book, Reeves and Nass (1996) demonstrated that interactions between humans and ICTs are identical to real social relationships. People automatically extrapolate personalities from little hints. In all human-machine interactions personality can creep in everywhere: the language in error messages, user prompts, methods for navigating options, and fonts chosen. Pesce (2000), one of the early pioneers in Virtual Reality, speaks of "techno-animism" to describe a world pervaded by computational objects. Blogjects (Bleecker, 2005), is a neologism introduced to describe objects that blog, a network of tangible, mobile, chatty objects enabled by the miniaturisation, the ubiquity of consumer electronics and a pervasive Internet. From an ethical point of view, one should carefully consider the implications of "animate" technologies when they are to be used with vulnerable categories of patients, with reduced capacity for informed consent, and potentially compromised mental capacities.

Conclusion

The strange paradox of identity is that it matters when it is weak. It holds true also in the health sector. At all levels of the medical system we see signs of the weakening on traditional schemes for personal identification. Doctors, nurses, and other members of the medical profession are increasingly requested to identify or to authenticate themselves to access electronic databanks and centralized archives. In the era of info technologies medical privacy breaches go well beyond the simple rupture of a medical obligation because their effects involve million patients with enormous consequences. Securing medical personnel identity is not a private business of hospitals and medical agencies but it is a huge policy challenge that involves the whole society. Patients' identity is also an issue. The global health system is increasingly a complex structure, which involves quite a number of international networks, which structure the global flows of people, commodities, medications, body parts (organs, tissues, and cells). Among the most important healthcare issues that directly affect patient safety and quality of care are the ability to correctly identify and track people and materials along the global health networks. In particular, there is an absolute need to identify patients and to confirm the accurate delivery of clinical services for them. Patients' misidentification is not only an important source of medical errors but it also a critical element in the overall architecture of the health system. Biometrics and other identification technology can play a pivotal role in ensuring more reliable identification schemes. Yet one should careful balance benefits with ethical and social risks. Biometrics are techniques that directly affect the human body. Their ethical relevance is not limited to their direct effect on medical systems. Biometrics have important anthropological implications that can be evaluated only long term. Any biometric can act as a powerful unique identifier that can bring together disparate pieces of personal information about an individual. If used in this manner, biometrics enable individuals to be pinpointed and tracked. They also create the potential for personal information from different sources to be linked together to form a detailed personal profile about that individual, unbeknownst to him or her. This represents not only a clear invasion of privacy but it threatens to overturn any current legal, ethical, and social standard.

Policy makers often describe biometrics as a magic bullet, which should allow to identify illegal aliens at borders, terrorists in airports, pedophiles on the Internet, to reduce medical errors and so on. This is not probably the case, but biometrics have however to be taken very seriously by social scientists and philosophers.

Acknowledgment

This work has been funded by a grant from the European Commission—DG Research—Contract—2008217762 HIDE (HOMELAND SECURITY, BIOMETRICS AND PERSONAL IDENTIFICATION ETHICS).

References

Aas, K. F. (2006). The body does not lie: Identity, risk and trust. *Technoculture, Crime, Media, Culture, 2*, 143-158.

Agamben, G. (2004). *No to bio-political tattooing.* From: La Monde, 10 January 2004. Retrieved November 20, 2004, from Www.Infoshop.Org/Inews/Stories. Php?Story=04/01/17/2017978>

Auge, M. (1988). *Le Dieu Objet.* Paris: Flammarion.

Bird-David, N. (1999). Animism. Revisited. Personhood, Environment, And Relational Epistemology. *Current Anthropology, 40*, Supplement, S67-91.

Bleecker, J. (2005). *A manifesto for networked objects—Cohabiting with pigeons, arphids, and aibos in the Internet of things.* Retrieved from Http://Research. Techkwondo.Com/Files/Whythingsmatter.Pdf

Caplan, J. (2000). *Written on the body: The tattoo in European and American History.* Princeton: Princeton Uni Press.

Castells, M. (1997). *The power of identity.* Oxford: Blackwell.

Davies, S. (1994). Touching big brother: How biometric technology will fuse flesh and machine. *Information Technology & People, 7*(4), 7-8.

Eurobarometers. Retrieved July 14, 2006, from Http://Ec.Europa.Eu/Health/Ph_Information/Documents/Eb_64_En.Pdf

Food and Drug Administration Fda. (2006). Retrieved From Www.Fda.Org, Accessed 12/06/06

Giddens, A. (1991). *Modernity and self identity.* Cambridge UK: Polity Press.

Guthrie, S. (1993). *Faces in the clouds: A new theory of religion.* New York: Oxford University Press.

Harvey, G. (2005). *Animism: Respecting the living world.* London: Hurst & Company.

Ingold, T. (2000). *The perception of the environment: Essays in livelihood, dwelling, and skill.* London: Routledge.

Levi, P. (1989). *The drowned and the saved.* New York: Random House.

Merriam-Webster Online Dictionary, Retrieved From Http://Www.M-W.Com/Cgi-Bin/Dictionary?Book=Dictionary&Va=Citizen, Accessed 15/07/2006)

Nyers, P. (2004). What's left of citizenship? *Citizenship Studies, 8*(3), 203-15.

Paiget, J. (1962). *Play, dream, and imitation in childhood.* New York: Norton.

Pesce, M. (2000). *The playful world: How technology is transforming our imagination.* New York: Ballantine Books.

Reeves, B., & Nass, C. (1996). *The media equation.* Cambridge: Cambridge University Press

Rose, N., & Novas, C. (2003). Biological citizenship. In A. Ong & S. Collier (Eds.), *Global anthropology*, Blackwell. Retrieved June 15, 2006, from Http://Www.Lse.Ac.Uk/Collections/Sociology/Pdf/Roseandnovasbiologicalcitizenship2002.Pdf

Shilling, C. (1998). *The body and social theory.* London: Sage.

The World Privacy Forum. (2006). *Medical identity theft: The information crime that can kill you.* Retrieved September 21, 2006, from Http://Www.Worldprivacyforum.Org/Medicalidentitytheft.Html

Tylor, E. B. (1871). *Primitive culture. Researches into the development of mythology, philosophy, religion, language, art, and custom.* London: John Murray.

Unicef. (2006). Retrieved From Http://Www.Unicef.Org/Protection/Files/Birth_Registration.Pdf, Accessed 10/06/2006

U.S. Department For Veteran Affairs. Retrieved On 10/07/2006 From Http://Www.Firstgov.Gov/Veteransinfo.Shtml)

Van Der Ploeg, I. (1999). The illegal body: "Eurodac" and the politics of biometric identification. *Ethics and Information Technology 1*, 295-302.

Endnotes

[1] The word biometrics was coined by Galton (1822-1911), the scientist well known for his theories on improving the human race through eugenics. Galton's application of statistics to the scientific study of evolution is critical and led him to open the Anthropometric Laboratory at the International Health Exhibition in 1884, where he collected biometrics on thousands of people (Bulmer, 2003).

[2] This is a critical point to understand, because most current ethical and political controversies on identity technologies concern the expansion of categorizations associated with people processing. These involve technical measurements and locating the individual relative to others. Such profiled identities (credit risk, IQ, SAT scores, life style categorization for mass marketing, etc) often involve predictions about future behaviour. They may or may not be known to individuals and their existence poses serious ethical and political issues.

[3] Things are quite different with logical objects such mathematical concepts and alike.

[4] In *Poetics* Aristotle writes: "Recognition, as the name indicates, is a change from ignorance to knowledge, producing love or hate between the persons destined by the poet for good or bad fortune[…] the least artistic form [of recognition], which, from poverty of wit, is most commonly employed [is] recognition by signs. Of these some are congenital- such as "the spear which the earth-born race bear on their bodies," or the stars introduced by Carcinus in his Thyestes. Others are acquired after birth; and of these some are bodily marks, as scars; some external tokens, as necklaces, or the little ark in the Tyro by which the discovery is effected. Even these admit of more or less skilful treatment. Thus in the recognition of Odysseus by his scar, the discovery is made in one way by the nurse, in another by the swineherds. The use of tokens for the express purpose of proof- and, indeed, any formal proof with or without tokens- is a less artistic mode of recognition. A better kind is that which comes about by a turn of incident, as in the Bath Scene in the Odyssey. Next, comes the recognitions invented at will by the poet, and on that account wanting in art. For example, Orestes in the Iphigenia reveals the fact that he is Orestes. She, indeed, makes herself known by the letter; but he, by speaking himself, and saying what the poet, not what the plot requires. This, therefore, is nearly allied to the fault above mentioned- for Orestes might as well have brought

tokens with him. Another similar instance is the "voice of the shuttle" in the Tereus of Sophocles. The third kind depends on memory when the sight of some object awakens a feeling: as in the Cyprians of Dicaeogenes, where the hero breaks into tears on seeing the picture; or again in the Lay of Alcinous, where Odysseus, hearing the minstrel play the lyre, recalls the past and weeps; and hence the recognition." (Poetics, Books XI and XVI, translated by S. H. Butcher, HyperText Presentation © 1995 Procyon Publishing, retrieved from http://libertyonline.hypermall.com/Aristotle/Poetics.html)

[5] However in cultures where biological individuals are regarded as hospitable to demonic possession, this is not true. In such cultures, the body per se cannot prove identity. Interestingly, the issue of multiple personalities, which was highly debated in XIX century psychology, is almost ignored in the current debate on personal identity.

[6] For instance compare the report issued by the European JRC, Biometrics at the Frontiers: Assessing the impact on Society, available at www.jrc.cec.eu.int

[7] All pieces of information about the current biometric market cited in the present paper have been retrieved from the *BITE Global Biometric Market and Industry Report*, available at http://www.biteproject.org

[8] All biometric systems operate in essentially the same manner. They capture a biometric sample, perform feature extraction or dataset creation and perform one of two types of searches. They provide either a one-to-one (1:1) or a one-to-many (1:N) search capability. One to many searches (1:N, also known as identification or recognition) are designed to determine identity based solely on biometric information. One to many matching answers the question, "Who am I?" In systems supporting one to many searches a central database must be built containing all biometric templates enrolled in the system. One to one process (1:1, also known as verification, or authentication) check the validity of a claimed identity by comparing a verification template to an enrolment template. One to one authentication answers the question, "Am I whom I claim to be?" Authentication does not require a central database to be built, if the comparison is made against a template stored in a personal device retained by the individual whose identity is to be verified.

[9] "Function creep" (also known as "purpose creep") is the term used to describe the expansion of a process or system, where data collected for one specific purpose is subsequently used for another unintended or unauthorised purpose.

[10] For instance see the COGITO project, http://www.suspectdetection.com/tech.html

Chapter XII

Prospects for Thought Communication:
Brain to Machine and Brain to Brain

Kevin Warwick, University of Reading, UK

Daniela Cerqui, Université de Lausanne, Switzerland

Abstract

In this chapter, we take a look at the realistic future possibility of thought communication—brain to machine and brain to brain. Technical details are presented on experimentation carried out thus far using implant technology and the route ahead involving brain-computer interfaces is described. Some of the social issues raised by such a novel technological development are also developed. Of importance is the fact that, once a new technology is globally accepted, its use tends to be considered as the normal way of being, which may lead to the creation of new disabilities for people unable to use the technology. The two authors agree about the analysis, but, as a result of their two completely different backgrounds, they disagree about how much benefit thought communication can bring to human beings.

Introduction

Talking about informatics applied to medicine will undoubtedly raise a large number of different issues in several different directions, such as medical technology or patients' files. In this chapter, the authors are concerned with the patients themselves, and their physical merger with computers. In particular, technology is now becoming available which is opening up the realistic possibility of thought communication (brain to brain and brain to machine) being achieved in the forthcoming decade, through the use of brain-computer integration. The first trials along these lines are even now occurring in several research labs (Hochberg et al., 2006; Kennedy, Bakay, Moore, Adams, & Goldwaith, 2000; Warwick et al., 2004). New technical methods presently being looked into (e.g., nanotechnology) are only likely to further enhance the results obtained thus far and speed up the rate of progress in this area.

Witnessing the dawning of a completely new and revolutionary technical capability for humans raises a multitude of questions in terms of what it means for all aspects of society and humankind. It is interesting to consider what we can learn by looking back to relevant new directions when they have occurred in the past. In this chapter, the authors make an attempt to indicate the chief areas of interest and have a stab at pointing to pertinent events that relate to the situation as of now, and from which we may take heed.

It is important to realise that it is always extremely difficult, given any new technological discovery or invention, to realistically assess its potential future impact on and in society. At a particular instant, attempting to bring together commercial interests, fashion trends and political alignments is troublesome enough, let alone being faced with the effects of international incidents, extreme weather conditions and natural disasters. Yet all of these can seriously influence not only the immediate reaction to a scientific announcement but also its eventual take up and long-term usage.

The particular new technology considered here is the novel area of direct brain to machine, or brain to brain communication between individuals. This last potentially could change our human concepts of language, individual emotions, and even education. Thus far, a telegraphic form of communication has been successfully achieved between the nervous systems of two humans through neural signalling via implants in the nervous system. The next step, a repeat of the experiment from brain to brain appears to be straightforward enough. But, if successful, which most likely it will be, it will push humanity forward in a way that is perhaps most similar to the era when the first telephone conversations were held.

The following section gives an overview of the state of the art in the field of brain to machine and brain to brain communication. Then, two case studies concerning technological implants—conducted in 1998 and 2002 by one of the authors—are used to discuss some social and ethical issues related to these technological breakthroughs. As the two authors disagree to some extent on how much benefit these technologies are expected to bring, the last part of the text is a dialogue between a position promoting thought communication, and a more reluctant view.

Neural Interfacing

Electronically interfacing the human nervous system has been actively investigated since the 1960s. Recent work in this area has though opened up the possibility of nerve prosthesis technology that will enhance human capabilities rather than simply for restorative purposes, which was the original intent, in an attempt to alleviate the condition of an individual who has suffered trauma due to spinal cord damage or amputation.

One procedure for interfacing with the human nervous system is to directly measure neural activity by implanting electrodes into the brain, see Donoghue (2002) for a review. Such invasive procedures have already given insights into the functionality of the brain. The application of this technology as an aid for patients with locked-in syndrome, (who are alert and cognitively intact but cannot move or speak), has already been shown (Kennedy et al., 2000), allowing them to control a computer cursor merely by thought. The same kind of brain-computer integration was also experienced by Donoghue and his team in June 2006 (Hochberg et al., 2006) to allow a patient suffering quadriplegia to interact with a computer. And in September 2006, an American woman was provided with a bionic arm she can operate by thoughts controlling her own muscles.

Interfacing with the peripheral nervous system has also shown great promise because, in most cases, neurological damage merely interrupts the transfer of electrical signals from sensory receptors to the brain causing impaired sensation and/or from the brain to motor units causing the loss of motor function. By making connections to different nerve fibres, sensation can potentially be restored by bridging the gap or for the closed loop control of externally initiated limb movement (Poboroniuc, Fuhr, Riener, & Donaldson, 2002; Yu, Chen, & Ju, 2001).

However it is when enhancements, rather than therapies, are considered that the situation becomes interesting (Warwick, 2003). In comparison with what some machines can do (especially as far as processing data is concerned), humans are extremely limited, and by linking the human nervous system with a computer, many new possibilities arise. Perhaps the more obvious upgrades are extra mathematical abilities and improved memory, but multi-dimensional thought, wider sensing capabilities and much more powerful communication—through thought signals alone—are all not only apparently achievable but also very good reasons for carrying out the research.

But how far have we come on this path so far?

Microelectrode Array

There are two distinct types of peripheral nerve interface, namely extraneural and intraneural. Extraneural, such as cuff electrodes, wrap tightly around the nerve fibres, and allow a recording of the sum of the signals occurring within the fibres (referred to as the compound action potential) (Loeb & Peck, 1996; Slot, Selmar, Rasmussen, & Sinkjaer, 1997) in a large region of the nerve trunk, or by a form of crudely selective neural stimulation (Naples & Mortimer, 1996; Sweeney & Mortimer, 1990).

A much more useful nerve interface however is one in which highly selective recording and stimulation of distinct neural signals is enabled, and this characteristic is more suited to intraneural electrodes (Kovacs et al., 1994; Lefurge, Goodall, Horch, Stensaas, & Schoenberg, 1991). Certain types of MicroElectrode Arrays (MEAs) (as shown in Figure 1) contain multiple electrodes, which become distributed within the fascicle of the mixed peripheral nerve when inserted into the nerve fibres en block. This provides direct access to nerve fibres from various sense organs or nerve fibres to specific motor units. Such a device allows for a multichannel nerve interface. The 2002 implant experiment, described in the following section, employed just such a MEA, implanted, by neurosurgery, in the median nerve fibres of KW left arm. Again, there was no medical need for this other than in terms of the investigative experimentation that it was wished to carry out.

Figure 1. A 100 electrode, 4X4mm MicroElectrode Array, shown on a UK 1 pence piece for scale

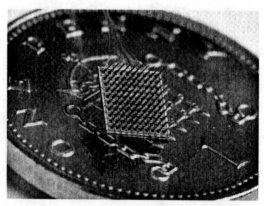

Before progressing, it is worthwhile pointing out that there are other types of Micro-Electrode Arrays that can be used for interfacing between the nervous system and technology. Etched electrode arrays, of which there is quite a variety, actually sit on the outside of the nerve fibres, rather akin to a cuff electrode. The signals obtained are similar to those obtainable via a cuff electrode (i.e., compound signals only can be retrieved) and hence for our purposes this type of array was not selected. To be clear, the type of Microelectrode array employed in the 2002 Experiment consists of an array of spiked electrodes that are inserted (hammered into) into the nerve fibres, rather than being sited adjacent to or in the vicinity of the fibres.

Applications for implanted neural prostheses are increasing, especially now that technology has reached a stage that reliable and efficient microscale interfaces can be brought about. The 2002 Experiment was conducted hand in hand with the Radcliffe Infirmary, Oxford, and the National Spinal Injuries Centre at Stoke Manderville Hospital, Aylesbury, United Kingdom—part of the aim of the experiments being to assess the usefulness of such an implant, in aiding someone with a spinal injury.

The neural interface allowed for a bi-directional information flow. Hence perceivable stimulation current enabled information to be sent onto the nervous system, while control signals could be decoded from neural activity in the region of the electrodes. A radio frequency bi-directional interface (Warwick et al., 2003) was developed (see Figure 2) to interface between the MEA and a remote computing device. In this way, signals could be sent from the nervous system to a computer and also from the computer to be played down onto the nervous system with a signal transmission range of at least 10 metres.

Figure 2. Mobile interface module

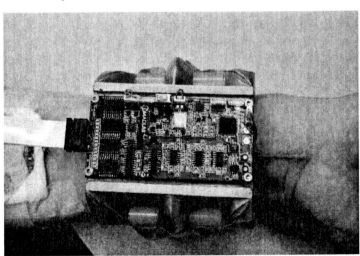

Social and Ethical Issues: Therapy and Enhancement

A wide range of experiments were carried out with the implant in place (Gasson, Hutt, Goodhew, Kyberd, & Warwick, 2005; Warwick et al., 2004). This chapter is focused on those in which neural signals were directly employed to drive a vehicle around, to operate networked technology in order to switch on/off lights and other artefacts and to operate a robot hand across the internet. At the same time, because the implant was bi-directional it was quite possible for the human involved to receive and comprehend incoming ultrasonic signals, to "feel" what the robot hand was feeling and to communicate, in a telegraphic way via the same route.

Concretely, with a finger movement, neural signals on the nervous system were transmitted to a computer and out to a robot hand as shown in Figure 3. Sensors on the hand's fingertips were then employed to pick up signals, which were transmitted back onto the nervous system. Whilst wearing a blindfold, in tests it was not only possible to move the robot hand, with neural signals, but also to discern to a high accuracy, how much force the robot hand was applying to an object being gripped. This experiment was carried out, at one stage, via the internet with KW in Columbia University, New York City, but with the hand in Reading University, in the United Kingdom. What it means is that when the nervous system of a human is linked directly with the internet, this effectively becomes an extension of their nervous system. To all intents and purposes, the body of the individual does not stop as is usual with the human body, but rather extends as far as the internet takes it. In this case, the brain was able to directly control a robot hand on a different continent, across the Atlantic Ocean. It is interesting to point out that such an experiment can be understood in two different ways, opening a philosophical debate how the boundaries of the body are perceived (Cerqui & Warwick, to be published). On the one hand, it could be argued that the body is considered as something of an interference, the main goal

Figure 3. Intelligent anthropomorphic hand prosthesis

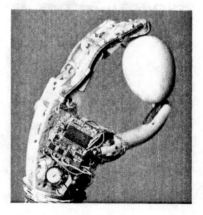

being to connect directly the brain with the environment; on the other hand, it could also be considered that the body is extended by technology.

Moreover, this illustrates how complicated the therapy vs. enhancement topic is. As with many other technologies, this not only has the potential to help relieve suffering from disabilities, but it also opens up the possibility of being used where there is no clear medical benefit, in order to enhance an individual's standard abilities. When a bioethical discussion is held on the possibility of technology being used in this way, the classical reflections are concentrated on fields such as genetics, neuroscience, pharmacology and other areas of biomedicine and do not normally include implant technology and other information technologies merging with the human body. However, the issues and questions raised in the employment of these technologies for this purpose are of far greater significance than those due to such as genetics.

In order to examine the normative challenges posed by this technology in the field of therapy and enhancement, it is firstly important to define these terms, even if, at a later time, it will be necessary to step back from these strict definitions. At least grammatically, the difference between what is a therapy and what constitutes an enhancement appears as a therapy is a treatment for a deficiency or a disorder, which aims to restore health to an unhealthy person. Specifically, it aims to make an individual well, to overcome a deficiency, or to cure a disease. Meanwhile an enhancement is an extension or improvement of some capacity, characteristic, activity, or ability. The goal of enhancement is to make an individual better than well, to optimize capacities, and to take people from standard levels of performance to peak performance. In both of these definitions, when applied to a human, a sense of normality (or norm) is implied, which an individual is either assisted in reaching in the first case or helped to surpass in the latter case.

One usual angle of approach, in the discussions of the committees in charge with ethics or in health policy, is to draw a line between appropriate and inappropriate uses of new technology in respect of a distinction between those targeted at therapeutic goals and those aimed at non-therapeutic enhancement. For instance, there is in the Netherlands an attempt to use the distinction between therapy and enhancement as a guide for care (Davis 1998). Also the report written by the European Group on Ethics in Science and New Technologies (2005) for the European Commission tries to draw a firm line between the two aspects.

Even if considering that the difference between therapy and enhancement is not problematic—but as it will be shown later it is—such a way of thinking does not allow for any decisions in terms of policy about which technologies should be developed and which should not. Indeed, the same technology can perfectly well be used for both goals and a method or technology, which achieves a therapeutic effect in one individual may well also be used to bring about an enhancement in another individual. Manipulating one robotic hand as a prosthesis when you have lost one of your natural hands is clearly in the field of therapy, but directly manipulating one or several hands with a brain signal transmitted across the ocean is an enhancement, as too would be a prosthetic hand that could crush a car. But here both therapy and enhancement use the same technology.

As it happens, controlling objects in a virtual—or in a real—environment by means of electroencephalograph (EEG) signals even when these are collected externally via electrodes should clearly be regarded as an enhancement, quite simply because humans are not born within a virtual environment in which their EEG signals can control artifacts. However, if such an ability is posed as being for training purposes or perhaps even for retraining after an accident then the situation becomes unclear.

The classification between therapy and enhancement is unfortunately even more problematic insofar as the fact that enhancement can mean a variety of things. In January 2003, there was a meeting organized in Brussels by the European Commission on the theme "human augmentation." Related to robotics and information technologies, it was part of the initiative "beyond robotics," launched during the 6th framework by the direction "future and emerging technologies." The goal was to allow researchers involved in the field to meet each other. Amongst others, the two authors of this chapter attended the meeting—the one as a researcher involved in brain–computer interfacing, and the other as an anthropologist interested in the merger between man and machine. It took quite a long time before attendees became aware that there was a huge ambiguity in the discussion. All were talking about "augmentation," but some of them were clearly interested in developing therapies whereas others were talking about enhancing standard abilities. When they realized that were talking of two different things, rather than trying to understand what this difference fundamentally meant, they closed the question by deciding that the only relevant difference is when you are applying the technology: in one case you talk about "patient" and in the other about "volunteer." But that obviously does not solve the problem at all, and this leads to another important issue: the so-considered volunteer of today might perfectly well become a patient tomorrow, because the acceptable norm is continuously shifting according to the most recent technological breakthroughs.

Actually defining a health standard against which either a therapy or enhancement can be measured would appear to be, to all intents and purposes, impossible. The definition of health is dynamic and includes criteria that tend to become more numerous as time passes. First, according to the definition given by the World Health Organization, health is not defined just as an absence of disease. Wellness is also included, which means that the evaluation is necessarily subjective. Even the concept of disease does no longer have any strict definition as, amongst other criteria, Cooper (2002) considers that we can talk about disease if people concerned "could reasonably have hoped to have been otherwise" (2002, p. 276). Again, the definition is subjective, and so it is with the concept of disability (see Harris, 1999), or of quality of life (Beauchamp & Childress, 2001).

In our current society, according to a dynamic conception, being normal means more and more being transformable (Le Blanc, 2002, p. 160). The boundary between what is normal and what is pathological is flexible, and the body has to be plastic (Hottois, 1999, p. 65-66). We are techno-centered (Cerqui, 2002) and we consider that as soon as we can do something, we necessarily ought do it. As a result, the norm is continuously evolving and the definition of what is considered to be normal is an ongoing process. Time is an important element, in that what might well be an enhancement on one day for an individual could easily be a therapy at a later date. Because of changes/improvements in general living conditions, including educational improvements along with the availability of medicines, so the general standard of expectation for humans in a society can be seen to change as effectively the norm is shifted.

Witnessing the dawning of a completely new and revolutionary technical capability for humans raises a multitude of questions in terms of the resultant effects on all aspects of society. It is interesting to consider what we can learn by looking back to relevant new inventions when they have occurred in the past. Whereas techno-logical impact is most of the times unpredictable, at least on a short time scale, all innovations carry many linked in hopes and fears (see Mosco, 2004). For instance, the electric telegraph and the advent of railway trains were already linked to the idea of unifying the world by mastering time and space, as has been the case with the Internet. As Nye argues, "accurate prediction is difficult, even for experts" (2006, p. 36). He refers to research carried out in 1976 focussed on papers that predicted the future, between 1890 and 1940. He showed that only one third were correct, while one third were wrong and one third still unproved. This lack of continuity in development prevents us from predicting with any precision (Gras, 2003).

However, in this field in question we already have the benefit of recent hindsight to some extent, as we can already illustrate how we got used to new devices by looking at the history of Radio Frequency Identification Devices (RFID). In a sense it was the first step on the way to brain to brain and brain to machine communication, when an RFID chip was implanted in a human body with absolutely no medical reason.

RFID Technology

In 1997 Peter Cochrane, then Head of British Telecom Research Labs, wrote "Just a small piece of silicon under the skin is all it would take for us to enjoy the freedom of no cards, passports, or keys. Put your hand out to the car door, computer terminal, the food you wish to purchase, and you would be dealt with efficiently. Think about it: total freedom; no more plastic" (Cochrane, 1997).

In August 1998, one of the authors of this chapter (KW) had an RFID silicon chip surgically implanted. This radio frequency identification device (RFID) was positioned by a doctor in the upper left arm (Scammell, 1999). RFID tags are used for identification purposes, based on the transmission of a signal by radio waves. They are more and more being integrated into different products, however, at this stage, it was the first time a human being was provided with such an implant.

With this in place, on entering the main door of the Cybernetics Department at Reading University, a radio frequency signal across the doorway excited the coil in the transponder, allowing for the transfer of 64 bits of information. This was sufficient for the computer to recognise the entrant and sound out a welcoming "Hello." Elsewhere in the building, on approaching the laboratory, the door opened automatically, again in response to computer recognition of the RFID implant. In fact, the computer kept an accurate record of when the building was entered and when exited, which room was occupied at any time and for how long. A location map held by the computer gave a real-time picture of the situation.

The demonstration was clearly to show just some of the identification possibilities with such an implant. It also realised, only one year on, the first step in Peter Cochrane's 1997 concept. There are currently several commercial applications of this technology. The 1998 Experiment was widely reported in the media—one of the best headlines being in the United Kingdom's tabloid newspaper, The Sun—it read "Hello Mr. Chip." Perhaps unsurprisingly there was, to some extent, also some criticism in the media of the experiment. Some, for example The Register (www.theregister.co.uk), saw it as purely a publicity stunt with no practical value whatsoever. The question was asked succinctly, why would anyone realistically want such an implant and why not use a smart card to open the door, why have an implant like this at all?

A quick search on Google indicates that there are now well over 7,000 such implants in humans—mainly of the "digital angel" type. Some are even used as a fashion item. As an example, a Night club in Barcelona and yet another in Rotterdam (Baja Beach club) allow entry to those with an implant. No credit cards are needed to pay for drinks, it's all done by implant—exactly as Peter Cochrane predicted. But what ethical concerns should have been raised, what commercial practices should have been put in place? In 1998 some people probably didn't understand what it was all about. Others probably didn't care. Whilst some in the media preferred to put their head in the sand and try to conceive that it would have no effect at all.

Rather than simply an implant for identification purposes, other possibilities arise. One example is the use of implants for biometric information. Although this can be, once again, employed for identification—ultimately replacing passports—it also has a medical use, either to indicate to medical personnel what type of mediaction needs to be administered or for transmitting data on a patient's internal functioning to a remote computer, for patient monitoring. Heart rate, temperature, blood pressure can all be (potentially) overseen in this way.

The Benefit of Hindsight

Over 45 years after the invention of the electric telegraph, on March 10th 1876 Alec Bell uttered the words "Mr. Watson—Come here—I want to see you" into a mouthpiece. At the far end of the corridor, via a brass pipe arrangement, Bell's technician Watson heard and understood enough of the words to respond appropriately (Field, 1878; Mackay, 1997). There followed patent arguments, counter claims and denounciations before Bell was widely accepted as the inventor of the telephone. But even he could not have foreseen what worldwide effect it was likely to have. Within a few years the first commercial telephone calls were being made, and by the end of the century, in some circles, the telephone had become an indispensable item. Yet others of Bell's inventions, for example synthesisers and telex machines, took many more years to establish a foothold and when they did they were effectively reinvented (by others) in a slightly different guise.

All of this throws up a multitude of different issues surrounding the introduction of new technology. Society must be ready for it in terms of the infrastructure that exists. Society must also be ready for it in terms of the mental enlightenment of its members—remember that in the case of the telephone it first made an appearance only 5 years after the publication of Charles Darwin's "The Descent of Man," which caused a furore on both sides of the Atlantic. Would things have been the same if the telephone had appeared 10 years earlier? Also, and of extreme importance, other technological developments must be sufficiently established and available to enable any new technology to gain a foothold.

In the earlier part of the 19th Century electricity had become more widely accepted with the invention of the electric motor and generator by Michael Faraday—along with electrolysis and batteries, important ingredients in the foundation of telephones—without the electromagnetic effect there would be no telephones as we know them.

As time passes and people change, so too do the ethical stances taken and views held. What is deemed to be ethically and morally unacceptable at one time becomes perfectly natural only a short time later and what is felt to be normal behavior drowns in the mire of a shift in society and can even become illegal—prime examples in western society would be racial acceptance, drug taking, abortion on demand, and homosexuality. For an extreme example we can look to the state of Virginia where, in 1972, it was still quite possible to be sterilized, whether you were happy with this or not, as the result of a number of factors including a poor score in an intelligence test (Warwick, 2001).

Coming back to the field of information technologies, what is considered as normal is related to what is technically possible. As soon as we are able to do things, we often consider that we ought do them. Therefore, there is a risk that we create new kinds of disabilities for people who, for some reason, are unable to access or to use these new technologies. It is often argued that technology can help in the field of disability. But it can also contribute to create more expectations, and thus more exclusion: rather than being solved, the so-called digital divide might become even more serious with implant technology by creating new haves not in their flesh. Technology is often considered as a tool to help disabled people. This may be true. But we must be aware that technology does also create new disabilities whilst moving the limit of what is considered as acceptable and reducing the margins of what is "normal,"

In the 2002 Experiment, extra sensory input, in the form of signals from ultrasonic sensors, was also investigated as part of the experimentation carried out. In this way the subject was able to obtain an accurate bat-like sense of how far objects were away, even with eyes closed. The results open up the possibility of senses of different types, for example infrared or X-Ray also being fed onto the human nervous system and thus into the human brain. What is clear from the one off trial in 2002 is that it is quite possible for the human brain to cope with new sensations of this type. Nowadays this sixth sense is considered as an extra sense. But what will happen if the technology is generalized? It took six years for RFID to be accepted as a normal device for VIP in the already mentioned nightclubs. How long will it take before we consider that our normal way to interact with our natural and technological environment *must* be operated by six or more senses if we want to be considered normal?

Brain to Brain Communication

The most spectacular part of the tests in the 2002 Experiment was when KW's wife, Irena, also had electrodes positioned directly into her nervous system and motor neural signals were successfully transmitted between the two nervous systems. So when KW moved a finger, a corresponding neural signal appeared on IW's nervous system. In this way a form of telegraphic communication was brought about between the nervous systems of two individuals who were both connected into a network (Gasson et al. 2005). The next step in this research is undoubtedly to bring about the same sort of communication between two individuals whose brains are both networked in the same way.

Therefore, generally speaking, thought communication can alternatively be brain to brain or brain to machine communication. When talking about brain to machine communication, we talk about controlling our environment by exchanging signals and informations directly with it. However, when talking about brain-to-brain communication, we enter something deeper. It is exciting—or frightening, depending on your point of view—to ponder on how far things will go in this direction, for example will it mean an end to language as we know it? Will we have to learn a new language of thought?

It is clear that when we compare the capabilities of machines with those of humans there are obvious differences, this is true both in physical and mental terms. As far as intelligence – defined as an information process, as is more and more done in our society - is concerned, it is apparent that machine intelligence has a variety of advantages over human intelligence. It is these advantages that really express themselves when it comes to linking the human brain directly with a computer network. These advantages then become ways in which a human can be intellectually advanced, also providing motivation and reasoning for making the link in the first place.

Some of the advantages of machine intelligence are the reasons humans make use of computers in the first place. Rapid and highly accurate mathematical abilities, a high speed, almost infinite, Internet knowledge base, and accurate long term memory can all though be added to human brain advantages such as resilience, tolerance to ambiguity and an ability to draw together abstract relationships. However this is just the start.

The human brain exhibits limited sensing abilities, at least in terms of how we presently understand the functioning of a brain. Humans have five senses that we know of, whereas machines offer a view of the world, which includes a much wider range. As discovered in the 2002 Experiment, at least an ultrasonic sense can be endowed on an upgraded human, but other senses will follow. Humans are also limited in that they can only visualise and understand the world around them in terms of a three dimensional perception. Meanwhile computers are quite capable of dealing with hundreds of dimensions and conceptualising relationships between these dimensions.

Perhaps the biggest advantage for machine intelligence is thought communication. The human means of communication, getting an electro-chemical signal from one brain to another, is extremely poor, particularly in terms of speed, power, and precision, involving conversion both to and from mechanical signals, pressure waves in speech communication. When one brain communicates with another there is invariably a high error rate due to the serial form of communication combined with the limited agreement on the meaning of ideas that is the basis of human language. In comparison machines can communicate in parallel, around the world with little/no error.

Overall therefore connecting a human brain, by means of an implant, with a computer network opens up the distinct advantages of machine intelligence to the implanted individual. Clearly even the acquisition of only one or two of these abilities could easily be enough to entice a human to be enhanced thus—indeed how could one refuse?

Of course, depending on which definition of communication one has, such an evolution may be considered as an improvement or as a loss for human beings. The two authors agree on the observation and description we can give of the current trend, but they disagree about how desirable such a situation is for human beings.

As explained, there does not exist a clear cut decision matrix that can be employed mechanistically to select between therapy and enhancement. As an engineer involved in computer-brain invasive integration research, KW thinks that there is a continuum and there is nothing wrong in taking one more step on the path of research. In his view, we should not be frightened while crossing the boundaries of the body: on the contrary, it is exciting and will enable us to achieve more directly our goals. Brain communication will be without interferences. Whatever happens to humans: the human condition might not necessarily be the best condition.

As an anthropologist, DC is more reluctant. In her view, human communication is much more than an electro-signal. What makes us human is our ability to give a meaning to these signals (Cerqui, 2002). Meaning is not necessarily given with the signal itself, and, as several philosophers argue, the context is very important for the understanding (see for instance Fellows, 1995). It is also not sure that thought does not need to be expressed by the way of language in order to exist (Benveniste, 1966). Therefore, thought might not be transmitted without language. Language, as we know it, is an important part of who we are as humans. By removing this basis, we might go into a whole new future, from which we will not return. In a sense it will be an evolutionary milestone, potentially a billion times more disruptive than the introduction of the telephone. We have to wonder if it is what we want. Moreover, we are not purely rational beings, and our body is also responsible for what we are. Connecting brains does not take into account the social part of us.

Had our anthropologist been in Bell's laboratory when he invented the phone, she would for sure have asked him why he did not go into Watson's office to talk to him face to face instead of inventing this mediation! KW's point is that DC is now dependent on her mobile phone, despite the fundamental criticisms she would have developed if she had attended the birth of this device. Which means in KW's view that DC will get used to thought communication, whatever it might mean in terms of loosing some of our human attributes. And DC has to grant that it is perfectly right.

Moreover, the body enhanced by external technology is by definition in some way already extended, and thus its boundary is no longer so clear. However, DC feels concerned about the absence of a clear boundary between inside and outside, and also between what is acceptable and what is not—with the continuous shift in what is considered as normal—because it means that otherwise there is no stop in the process. If it happens, DC will get used to it, as (almost) all of us, but it does not necessarily mean that it will be better for human beings. It just shows that they are flexible. But to what extent? Meanwhile KW is excited by the fact that there is no stop to the process—he simply wishes that the evolutionary train would move a little faster.

Concluding Reflections

The situation with implants is presently not overly clear when, rather than simply repairing ineffective body parts, technology is employed to enhance the normal functioning of the human brain, according to certain values that are very important in our so-called information society: such as the quicker one can access information, the better (Cerqui, 2005).

Whilst external add-ons, as in the case of a military night sight for example, provide a short-term edge, the more permanent implant option has a more direct effect, clearly altering an individual's capabilities, self-opinion, and awareness, especially with regard to themselves—they are clearly a different person. By linking the mental functioning of a human and a machine network, a hybrid identity is created. When the human nervous system is connected directly with technology, this not only affects the nature of an individual's (if they can still be so called) identity, raising questions as to a new meaning for "I," but also it raises serious questions as to that individual's autonomy. Who are you if your brain/nervous system is part human part machine? What about your identity, as an individual, but also as a human being? This process might clearly lead us to our extinction, as a species. A human wearing a night-vision helmet essentially remains a human, whereas a human whose nervous system is directly linked with a computer network puts forward their individuality and identity for questioning.

When an individual's consciousness is based not on a stand alone human brain but rather on a combined human/machine form, this necessarily will affect their choices, their morals, their character and even their concept of ethics (Warwick, 2003). Such individuals may well regard humans with contempt, considering them, for what they are, as intellectually inferior.

In the not too distant future, it appears extremely likely that humans will face the distinct possibility of being able to directly upgrade their mental capabilities by means of implant technology. Extra senses and multi-dimensional thought present themselves as intriguing options. However, it is when we consider the prospects for thought communication that the situation takes on a completely different turn.

Such an ability does not merely give one individual a slight edge or an improved means of interacting, it completely changes who they are as an individual. Obvious questions immediately arise—will one person or a machine be able to read exactly what another person is thinking? The answer is most likely not in the short term. However, with any new technology such as this, it is impossible, with the best will in the world, to know exactly how it can perform until we go there and try.

Hindsight is a wonderful thing. We can all be geniuses and look back at an event and say this or that should have happened. But here we are faced with a dilemma. What do we do about it? Most importantly, what do you do about it? Because it can be suspected that if you, and others, sit back and let it happen or even worse, put your head in the sand, then it will be others, perhaps the Microsoft equivalent in the implant world, who will direct the way things go? If, in the future, you wish to communicate with others by thought alone, you may even need a Windows interface!

References

Beauchamp, T., & Childress, J. (2001). *Principles of biomedical ethics*. Oxford: Oxford University Press.

Benveniste, E. (1966). *Problèmes de linguistique générale. Tome 1*. Paris: Gallimard.

Cerqui, D. (2005). La société de l'information, de la médiation à l'immédiat. In G. Berthoud, A. Kündig, & B. Sitter-Liver (Eds), *Société de l'information: récits et réalités* (pp. 311-321). Fribourg : Academic Press.

Cerqui, D. (2002). The future of humankind in the era of human and computer hybridisation. An anthropological analysis. *Ethics and Information Technology, 4*(2), 1-8.

Cerqui, D., & Warwick, K. (to be published). Une anthropologue chez les cybernéticiens: esquisse de dialogue entre imaginaires concurrents. In C. Fintz (Ed.), *Et si le corps mutant nous était conté... Les imaginaires du corps enchanté, du corps en chantier*, Paris: L'Harmattan.

Cochrane, P. (1997). *Tips for the time travellers*. Orion Business Books.

Cooper R. (2002). Disease. *Studies in History and Philosophy of Biology and Biomedicine, 33*, 263-282.

Davis, K. (1998). The rhetoric of cosmetic surgery: Luxury or welfare? In E. Parens (Ed.), *Enhancing human traits: Ethical and social implications* (pp. 124-134). Washington: Georgetown University Press.

Donoghue, J. P. (2002). Connecting cortex to machines: recent advances in brain interfaces. *Nature Neuroscience, 5* Supplement, November 2002, 1085-88.

European Group on Ethics in Science and New Technologies (EGE). (2005). *Ethical aspects of ICT implants in the human body*. Report to the European Commission. Luxembourg: Office for Official Publications of the European Communities.

Fellows, R. (1995). Welcome to Wales: Searle and the computational theory of mind. In R. Fellows (Ed.), *Philosophy and technology* (pp. 85-97). Cambridge: Cambridge University Press.

Field, K. (1878). *The history of Bell's telephone*. London.

Gasson, M., Hutt, B., Goodhew, I., Kyberd, P., & Warwick, K. (2005). Invasive neural prosthesis for neural signal detection and nerve stimulation. *Proceedings of the International Journal of Adaptive Control and Signal Processing, 19*(5), 365-375.

Gras, A. (2003). *Fragilité de la puissance. Se libérer de l'emprise technologique.* Paris: Fayard.

Harris, J. (1999). Is gene therapy a form of engenics? In E. Kuhse & P. Singer (Eds), *Biethetics. An anthology* (pp. 165-170). Oxford: Blackwell.

Hochberg, L., Serruya, M., Friehs, G., Mukand, J., Saleh, M., Caplan, A., Branner, A., Chen, D., Penn, R., & Donoghue, J. (2006). Neuronal ensemble control of prosthetic devices by a human with tetraplegia. *Nature, 442*(13 July), 164-171.

Hottois, G. (1999). *Essais de philosophie bioéthique et biopolitique*, Paris: Vrin.

Kennedy, P., Bakay, R., Moore, M., Adams, K., & Goldwaith, J. (2000). Direct control of a computer from the human central nervous system. *IEEE Transactions on Rehabilitation Engineering, 8*, 198-202.

Kovacs, G. T., Storment, C. W., Halks Miller, M., Belczynski, C. R., Della Santina, C. C., Lewis, E. R., & Maluf, N. I. (1994). Silicon-substrate microelecrode arrays for parallel recording of neural activity in peripheral and cranial nerves. *IEEE Transactions on Biomedical Engineering, 41*, 567-577.

Le Blanc, G. (2002). L'invention de la normalité. *Esprit, 284*, 145-164.

Lefurge, T., Goodall, E., Horch, K. W., Stensaas, L., & Schoenberg, A. A. (1991). Chronically implanted intrafascicular recording electrodes. *Ann BiomedicalEngineering, 19*, 197-207.

Loeb, G. E., & Peck, R. A. (1996). Cuff electrodes for cronic stimulation and recording of peripheral nerve activity. *Journal of Neurosci Methods, 64*, 95-103.

Mackay, J. (1997). *Sounds out of silence.* Mainstream.

Mosco, V. (2004). *The digital sublime. Myth. Power and cyberspace.* Cambridge: MIT Press.

Naples, G., & Mortimer, J. (1996). A spiral nerve cuff electrode for peripheral nerve stimulation. *IEEE Trans. Biomed. Eng., 35*, 905-916.

Nye, D. (2006). *Technology matters. Questions to live with.* London: MIT Press.

Poboroniuc, M. S., Fuhr, T., Riener, R., & donaldson, n. (2002). closed-loop control for fes-supported Standing Up and Sitting Down. *Proceedings of the 7th Conference of the IFESS* (pp. 307-309). Ljubljana, Slovenia.

Scammell, A. (1999). *I in the Sky:Visions of the Information Future.* Aslib.

Slot, P. J., Selmar, P., Rasmussen, A., & Sinkjaer, T. (1997). Effect of long-term implanted nerve cuff electrodes on the electrophysiological properties of the human sensory nerves. *Artif-Organs, 21*, 207-209.

Sweeney, J., & Mortimer, J. (1990). A nerve cuff technique for selective excitation of peripheral nerve trunk regions. *IEEE Trans. Biomed. Eng., 37,* 706-715.

Warwick, K. (2003). Cyborg morals, Cyborg values, Cyborg ethics. *Ethics and Information Technology, 5*(3), 131-137.

Warwick, K. (2001). *QI: The quest for intelligence.* Piatkus.

Warwick, K., & Cerqui, D. (submitted). Brain-computer integration: Therapy versus enhancement. *American Journal of Bioethics.*

Warwick, K., Gasson, M., Hutt, B., Goodhew, I., Kyberd, P., Andrews, B., Teddy, P., & Shad, A. (2003). The application of implant technology for cybernetic-systems. *Archives of Neurology, 60*(10), 1369-1373.

Warwick, K., Gasson, M., Hutt, B., Goodhew, I., Kyberd, P., Schulzrinne, H., & Wu, X. (2004). Thought communication and control: A first step using radio-telegraphy. *IEE Proceedings on Communications, 151*(3), 185-189.

Yu, N. Y., Chen, J. J., & Ju, M. S. (2001). Closed-loop control of quadriceps/hamstring activation for FES-induced standing-up movement of paraplegics. *Journal of Musculoskeletal Research, 5*(3), 173-184.

About the Contributors

Penny Duquenoy has a first degree in philosophy from the School of Cognitive and Computing Science at Sussex University, UK, and a PhD in Internet ethics. She is a senior lecturer at Middlesex University, London. Dr. Duquenoy has been an active researcher in the field of computer ethics for a number of years, with more than 30 publications on the ethical implications of ICT. Key areas of research are the ethical implications of intelligent technologies in everyday life (described as "ambient intelligence" in European Union research) and medical informatics. She has acted as an expert ethics evaluator for the European Commission (information society and media directorate-general) and has given invited presentations on ethics and ambient technologies at EU level and internationally. She is chair of IFIP Working Group 9.2 (computers and social accountability), member of IFIP Special Interest Group 9.2.2 "Taskforce on Ethics," and manager of the British Computer Society Ethics Forum.

Carlisle George is a lawyer and computer scientist. He holds a master's degree (LLM) in information technology & communications law from the London School of Economics, and a doctorate (PhD) in computer science from the University of London (Goldsmiths). He has also been called to the Bar of England and Wales at Lincoln's Inn (London) and the Bar of the Eastern Caribbean Supreme Court. He is a senior lecturer in the School of Computing Science (Middlesex University, London, UK) and Convenor of the ALERT (aspects of law and ethics related to technology) research group at Middlesex. George is the author of many academic publications and a member of various professional bodies including the Honourable Society of Lincoln's Inn, The Society of Legal Scholars, The Society for Computers and Law, The Eastern Caribbean Bar Association, the Higher Education Academy, and the International Federation for Information processing (IFIP) Working Group 9.2.

Kai K. Kimppa holds a master's degree in philosophy and a doctorate in information technology from the University of Turku. He is a lecturer at the University of Turku, Finland and has been active in research in the field of computer ethics for seven years, with more than 20 publications on the ethical implications of ICT. Key areas of his research include justification of IPRs, ethics of medical informatics and ethics of online computer games. He has given presentations in both academic and business conferences, as well as at EU level. He is secretary of IFIP Working Group 9.2 (computers and social accountability) as well as IFIP Special Interest Group 9.2.2 "Taskforce on Ethics," and a member of the Finnish Information Processing Association Ethics Group, which he also represents as a National Representative in the IFIP SIG 9.2.2.

* * *

Boštjan Berčič is a legal consultant, an economist, and a computer scientist. He has undergraduate degrees in both law and economics. He holds a master's degree in macroeconomics (University of Ljubljana), and a doctorate (PhD) in computer science (University of Ljubljana). He heads the Institute for Economics, Law, and Informatics (Slovenia) which provides consultancy services on matters of economic and information society legislation. His main research interests lie in the interdisciplinary area between economics, law, and informatics. He is the author of several articles, including SCI indexed scientific papers.

Andy Bissett is a senior lecturer in the Faculty of Arts, Computing, Engineering, and Science at Sheffield Hallam University, England. He holds a BSc in electronics from the University of Kent, England, and an MSc in computer studies from Sheffield City Polytechnic. Bissett has worked as an electronic engineer and as a software engineer in a variety of industries. His main area of research is that of the social impact of IT. He is also pursuing doctoral level research into educational matters.

Daniela Cerqui is a sociocultural anthropologist interested in the relationship between technology and society (and, more fundamentally, humankind). She teaches at the Institute of Sociology and Anthropology of the University of Lausanne (Switzerland) where she is involved in teaching and research on the new information technologies, and on the 'information society' they are supposed to create. She recently spent two years conducting research in the Department of Cybernetics of the University of Reading.

Göran Collste, professor of applied ethics, Linköping University, Sweden. Collste's research deals with problems in ethics and applied ethics and his publications include books and articles on the principle of human dignity, work ethics, global justice and ethical issues related to information and communication technologies (ICT-ethics) (i.e., *Ethics and Information Technology* (New Delhi, 1998) and *Is Human Life Special? Religious and Philosophical Perspectives on the Principle of Human Dignity* (Bern, 2002). He is coordinator of the EU-supported Erasmus Mundus Master Programme in Applied Ethics and member of the board of the Swedish Research Council, Section for Humanities and Social Sciences.

Kay Fielden is an associate professor in computing in the School of Computing and Information Technology, Unitec Institute of Technology, Auckland, New Zealand. She is also the research leader for the school, mentors staff research, supervises postgraduate students and teaches postgraduate research methods. Her own research interests are grounded in qualitative research and systems thinking and are most commonly conducted in the context of social informatics.

Hannah H. Gröndahl's research focuses on legal and ethical issues raised by IT and computing, particularly human-computer interaction. She holds a Bachelor's degree from Princeton University and a Master's degree in applied ethics, technology specialisation, from Linköpings universitet in Sweden, where she was a Fulbright Scholar at CTE Centre for Applied Ethics. Gröndahl has also studied IT law at the London School of Economics and has experience working in the legal field. She currently divides her time between Stockholm and London.

Karin Hedström is senior lecturer of informatics at Örebro University, Örebro, Sweden. She holds a PhD in information systems from Linköping University, Sweden. Her research interests concern the ethics of information- and communication technologies (ICT), with a focus on how different interests and values influence the design of ICTs. She is interested in the social and ethical effects of developing and using ICTs. She is especially interested in the development of use of IT in health care. She has published several journal—and conference—articles on the issue of values of IT in health care. She is a member of the research network VITS.

Janne Lahtiranta holds a MSc. in information systems from University of Turku in Finland. From 1999 to 2003, he worked in the field of communication standards and clinical instrumentation for the healthcare market. In 2003, he returned to the academia in order to write his DoctorateThesis on new and emerging technologies used in the field of health and medical informatics. Since 2005, Lahtiranta has worked as a research associate in the University of Turku and as a part-time project manager in the Turku Science Park where his responsibilities include supervising national and international R&D projects in his area of expertise.

Emilio Mordini is a practicing psychoanalyst. Since March 2002 he has been serving as managing director of the Centre for Science, Society and Citizenship (CSSC), an independent research centre whose mission is to attempt to clarify the human (social, cultural and ethical) factors which shape technological innovation. Mordini is an M.D. from the University La Sapienza of Rome and D.Phil. from the Pontifical University S.Thoma. He was non tenure track Professor of Bioethics in the Medical School of the University of Rome "La Sapienza" (1994-2005), member (1994-2000) and secretary (2000-2003) of the Bioethical Commission of the CNR--Italian National Research Council. Mordini is past treasurer (1992-96) and past secretary (1996-98) of the European Association of Centres of Medical Ethics (EACME). He has also served as a member of the board of directors (1996-2000) of the International Association of Bioethics (IAB). Since 1992, he has been main contractor and coordinator of 15 EU funded projects in the field of bioethics and ethics of new and emerging technologies. Mordini has been coordinator of BITE (biometric identification technology ethics), the first international action supported by the EC on ethical implications of biometrics, and he has been the initiator of two transatlantic meetings between the EC and the US DHS on Ethics and Policy of Biometrics. Emilio Mordini has been editor of six books, has published 84 articles or chapters of books in reviewed publications, 160 articles in non-reviewed journals, newsmagazine and newspapers.

Den Pain has recently retired from academic endeavours and enjoys spending his time split between Auckland in NZ and Sheffield in the UK. He met the other authors through his work at Massey University in Auckland and at Sheffield Hallam University.
He worked as a senior lecturer at Massey in information systems researching health informatics and online assessment of students. Previously at Sheffield Hallam in the School of Computing and Management Sciences he taught information systems and was involved with a long-term research project into human-centred office systems.

Rania Shibl is currently working at the University of the Sunshine Coast in Maroochydore as an associate lecturer in Information Systems. Before coming to Australia, Shibl worked at Massey University as an assistant lecturer. Shibl is undertaking a PhD in information systems from The University of the Sunshine Coast. Her PhD topic is in the area of health information systems, focusing on the use of clinical decision support systems and its factors that influence their acceptance. She has a Bachelors of Science (information systems) from the University of Maryland and a Postgraduate Diploma (information systems) from Massey University.

Tony Solomonides is a reader in the School of Computer Science and leads the Biomedical and Healthcare Computing Group. He trained as a mathematician at the University of London and taught and researched in mathematics before entering computing. He formally retrained through the master's in Foundations of Advanced Information Technology (FAIT) at Imperial College and has since worked in logic, logic programming and databases, knowledge-based systems, including foundational work with Francis McCabe on logic & objects. He has applied ideas of logic programming to metadata in the description of component objects and to the extraction of semantics from pathology reports. He has adapted meta-database concepts to epidemiology and sentinel systems, worked on requirements analysis and optimization of the MammoGrid image database, requirements analysis again in Health-e-Child, contributing finally to aspects of ontology integration for the same project. He has since played a leading part in the SHARE and EU PGDcode projects.

As a member of the Centre for Complex Cooperative Systems he worked originally in the application of CRISTAL to medicine, first in the description of a conceptual EU-wide health information system and then in the epidemiology of antibiotic-resistant bacteria. He was then a key contributor to the MammoGrid project, especially in the coordination and integration of diverse contributions from the various research groups. He has co-authored several papers and presented this work and its more recent extensions at numerous conferences and by invitation at events in the US, Russia, and throughout Europe.

He was co-editor of the *HealthGrid White Paper* with Kevin Dean (CISCO) and Vincent Breton (CNRS) and gave a tutorial on healthgrid computing for biomedical research and healthcare at MedInfo 2007. He has published in various software engineering journals, in *Clinical Radiology* and *Methods of Information in Medicine*, and been a regular contributor to and proceedings editor of the HealthGrid conferences.

He is director of Postgraduate Research in the Bristol Institute of Technology at the University of the West of England, where he also chairs the school's Research Ethics Committee. He leads two master's programmes in health informatics and in grid computing.

Benedict Stanberry, having originally intended to pursue a career in medicine, instead chose to read law and received both bachelors and masters degrees in the subject before being appointed as a research fellow and lecturer at Cardiff University. From 1996-2001, he was director of the Centre for Law Ethics and Risk in Telemedicine--a research and consulting unit that spun out of the University as healthcare consulting firm Avienda Limited in March 2001. As a director with Avienda, Ben was a specialist in commercial law with a particular interest in the regulation of both NHS and private sector healthcare providers. He acted as general counsel or legal adviser to a number of NHS bodies and local authorities, to numerous businesses involved in the provision of outsourced or managed healthcare services and to businesses, such as IT consultancies, that support the delivery of modern healthcare. Formerly based in Cardiff, Ben was named Western Mail Welsh Lawyer of the Year (Not in Private Practice) 2004 in recognition of his extensive advisory work with NHS Wales. Now living in London, Ben is an associate member of the Royal Society of Medicine and a full member of the Institute of Directors.

Kevin Warwick is professor of cybernetics at the University of Reading, England, where he carries out research in artificial intelligence, control, robotics, and cyborgs. Warwick is perhaps best known for his self experimentation with biomedical implants, being the first human being to have had a chip linking his nervous system with the internet. He has published over 500 articles including over 100 papers in academic journals and a number of popular science books (e.g., *March of the Machines*). He appears in Google Directory as one of the top four people in the world in the field of artificial intelligence.

Diane Whitehouse is a partner in The Castlegate Consultancy, a UK-based public services and eHealth policy and analysis partnership. Diane works actively in the research, policy, and deployment fields of eHealth, and has clients in a number of national health authorities and ministries. Until February 2007, Whitehouse was a scientific officer in the "ICT for Health" Unit of the European Commission's General Directorate on Information Society and Media. She is a social scientist whose work has focused on the social, organisational, and ethical aspects of ICT, and has 25 years' work experience in European policy including eHealth, academic research/teaching, social action research, human and civic rights, and ICT use by persons with disabilities and by older adults. She has co-written and co-edited a wide range of books and articles. She has worked closely over the years in developing a number of published ideas with both Penny Duquenoy and Kai Kimppa. In August 2007, Diane's services to the international association, the International Federation for Information Processing, were recognised with a silver core award.

Index

A

access control 207, 212
action research project 71, 74
active attacks 221
advanced encryption standard (AES) 209
agentization 113, 115, 120, 129, 132
american health information management
      association (AHIMA) 188
american medical association (AMA)
      7, 46, 110
anthropomorphism 113, 115, 118, 119,
      120, 131, 132, 267
artificial agency 92, 97, 108
artificial intelligence (AI) 85

B

biometrics v, 211, 217, 225, 249, 250,
      259, 260, 261, 263, 265, 266,
      268, 269, 272
black box 91
brain-computer integration 274, 275
brain to brain communication 274
british medical association (BMA) 5

C

CADe 143, 144, 145, 149
caldicott principles 242
careless disclosure safeguards 214
clinical decision support systems (CDSS)
      49, 52
computer security institute (CSI) 198
consumer protection act 1987 112, 166
cryptography 216
cyberdoctors 3

D

data controller 234, 235, 237, 238,
      239, 240
data encryption standard (DES) 209
data integrity 152, 197, 226
data protection act 9, 232, 233, 239,
      240, 243, 246
denial-of-service (DoS) 221
discretionary access control (DAC) 214
distancing 120, 123, 124, 127, 133, 137
duty of care 8, 11, 23, 103, 104, 106,
      145, 150, 166, 167, 168, 169,
      170, 172, 176

E

e-medicine 32, 41
e-science 141
electroencephalograph (EEG) 280
electronic communication services 192
EURODAC 258
european union (EU) data protection directive 231
extra sensory input 284

F

federation of state medical boards
(FGSMB) 6

G

general medical council (GMC) 5
globalisation 255
grid computing 141, 152

H

Health-e-Child 151, 153
healthcare finance administration (HCFA)
206
healthcare industry 187
healthcare privacy 189
HealthGrid 153
health information 187
hippocratic oath 10, 12, 14, 27, 87, 115

I

independent practitioner associations
(IPAs) 52
information warfare 199
integrated care records 242
intentional system 89, 90, 91
internet pharmacies 2, 3, 25, 27
intrusion detection monitoring 211
IPsecurity (IPSec) 209

K

key-coded data 240

M

machine intelligence 285

MammoGrid 142–149, 153, 154
masquerading 221
medical decision support systems (MDSS)
84, 85
message modification 221
microelectrode arrays (MEAs) 276
ministry of health 201, 218, 225

N

national health service (NHS connecting
for health) 158, 230, 231
national identification number (NINo) 232
national medical database 230, 231,
232, 235, 237, 238, 239, 242,
243, 244, 245
national patient safety agency (NPSA) 160
negligent misstatement 8, 10, 101, 102,
103, 107, 112, 169
nerve interface 276
neural interfacing 275

O

online consultations 2, 5, 7, 8, 9, 11, 1
2, 19, 20, 23, 24, 25

P

passive attacks 221
patient autonomy 32, 34, 37, 38, 40,
41, 42
Patient databases 192
patient portal 32, 40
personal digital assistants (PDAs) 220
personal health information 130, 189,
196, 197, 198, 207, 208, 211,
212, 214, 215, 218, 219, 223
principle of autonomy 29, 37
principle of responsibility
29, 34, 36, 37, 40
privacy act 1993 218
professional malpractice 8
provenance 147, 149, 152

Q

quality management system
60, 157, 170, 176, 177

R

radio frequency identification (RFID)
    264, 282
remote prescribing 5, 6
RFID tags 282
royal society for the prevention of acci-
    dents (RoSPA) 163

S

sale of goods act 1979 166
SAVA 66, 71–80
secure socket layer (SSL) 209
SHARE 151, 153
slovenian personal data protection act 1999
    232, 239
smart cards 212
social engineering 214
social services act 67, 71
standard of care 7, 94, 95, 102, 105,
    106, 108, 167, 168, 170, 171
summary care records (SCR) 242
supply of good and services act 1982 165
systems integrator 56, 58

T

technoanimism 267
telemedicine 192
the royal pharmaceutical society of great
    britain (RPSGB) 15
thought communication 273, 274, 275,
    284, 286, 287

U

UK medical act 1983 5
unfair contract terms act 1977 165

V

virtual private networks (VPNs) 209

W

wireless LAN (WLAN) 220
world health organization (WHO) 26, 280

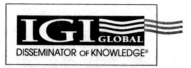
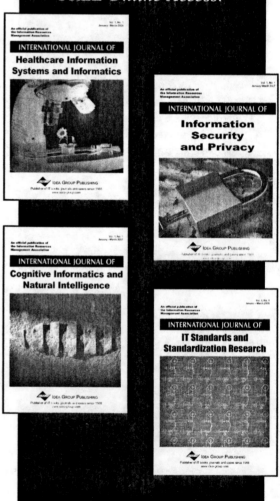